Vocational Rehabilitation
What works, for whom, and when?

Gordon Waddell, CBE, DSc, MD, FRCS, Hon FFOM, FBCA
Centre for Psychosocial and Disability Research, University of Cardiff, UK

A Kim Burton, PhD, DO, Eur.Erg, Hon FFOM
Centre for Health and Social Care Research, University of Huddersfield, UK

Nicholas AS Kendall, PhD, DipClinPsych, MNZCCP
Occupational and Aviation Medicine, University of Otago, NZ

The authors were commissioned by the Vocational Rehabilitation Task Group (a group of stakeholders representing the UK Government, employers, unions and insurers) in association with the Industrial Injuries Advisory Council (IIAC), to conduct this independent review of the scientific evidence. The authors are solely responsible for the scientific content and the views expressed, which do not represent the official views of the Task Group, IIAC, the Department for Work and Pensions (DWP), HM Government or The Stationery Office.

CONTENTS

Acknowledgements

We thank individual members of the Vocational Rehabilitation Task Group and the Industrial Injuries Advisory Council, and the following colleagues for their helpful ideas and comments, and for directing us to useful material during the course of the project:

Mansel Aylward, John Ballard, Antony Billinghurst, Dame Carol Black, Mark Gabbay, Bob Grove, Bill Gunnyeon, Max Henderson, Sayeed Khan, Alistair Leckie, Bob Lewin, John McCracken, Ewan MacDonald, Sir Anthony Newman Taylor, Keith Palmer, Marianne Shelton, Nichole Taske, Andy Vickers, Nerys Williams, Mary Wyatt.

None of them bear any responsibility for the final report, the views expressed, or any errors that remain.

Thanks also to Debbie McStrafick for archiving the data and providing administrative support.

Executive summary

The aim of this review was to provide an evidence base for policy development on vocational rehabilitation:

- To assess the evidence on the effectiveness and cost-effectiveness of vocational rehabilitation interventions.

- To develop practical suggestions on what vocational rehabilitation interventions are likely to work, for whom, and when.

Vocational rehabilitation was defined as *whatever helps someone with a health problem to stay at, return to and remain in work:* it is an idea and an approach as much as an intervention or a service.

The focus was on adults of working age, the common health problems that account for two-thirds of long-term sickness (mild/moderate musculoskeletal, mental health and cardio-respiratory conditions), and work outcomes (staying at, returning to and remaining in work). Data from some 450 scientific reviews and reports, mainly published between 2000 and December 2007, were included in evidence tables. Using a best evidence synthesis, evidence statements were developed in each area, with evidence linking and rating of the strength of the scientific evidence.

Findings

Generic findings:

This review has demonstrated that there is a strong scientific evidence base for many aspects of vocational rehabilitation. There is a good business case for vocational rehabilitation, and more evidence on cost-benefits than for many health and social policy areas.

Common health problems should get high priority, because they account for about two-thirds of long-term sickness absence and incapacity benefits, and much of this should be preventable. Vocational rehabilitation principles and interventions are fundamentally the same for work-related and other comparable health conditions, irrespective of whether they are classified as injury or disease. Return-to-work should be one of the key outcome measures.

Healthcare has a key role, but vocational rehabilitation is not a matter of healthcare alone – the evidence shows that treatment by itself has little impact on work outcomes. Employers also have a key role - there is strong evidence that proactive company approaches to sickness, together with the temporary provision of modified work and accommodations, are effective and cost-effective. (Though there is less evidence on vocational rehabilitation interventions in small and medium enterprises). Overall, the evidence in this review shows that effective vocational rehabilitation depends on work-focused healthcare *and* accommodating workplaces. *Both* are necessary: they are inter-dependent and must be coordinated.

The concept of early intervention is central to vocational rehabilitation, because the longer anyone is off work, the greater the obstacles to return to work and the more difficult vocational rehabilitation becomes. It is simpler, more effective and cost-effective to prevent people with common health problems going on to long-term sickness absence. A 'stepped-care approach' starts with simple, low-intensity, low-cost interventions which will be adequate for most sick or injured workers, and provides progressively more intensive and structured interventions for those who need additional help to return to work. This approach allocates finite resources most appropriately and efficiently to meet individual needs.

Effective vocational rehabilitation depends on communication and coordination between the key players – particularly the individual, healthcare, and the workplace.

Condition specific findings:

There is strong evidence on effective vocational rehabilitation interventions for musculoskeletal conditions. For many years the strongest evidence was on low back pain, but more recent evidence shows that the same principles apply to most people with most common musculoskeletal disorders.

Various medical and psychological treatments for anxiety and depression can improve symptoms and quality of life, but there is limited evidence that they improve work outcomes. There is a lack of scientific clarity about 'stress', and little or no evidence on effective interventions for work outcomes. There is an urgent need to improve vocational rehabilitation interventions for mental health problems. Promising approaches include healthcare which incorporates a focus on return to work, workplaces that are accommodating and non-discriminating, and early intervention to support workers to stay in work and so prevent long-term sickness.

Current cardiac rehabilitation programmes focus almost exclusively on clinical and disease outcomes, with little evidence on what helps work outcomes: a change of focus is required. Workers with occupational asthma who are unable to return to their previous jobs need better support and if necessary retraining.

Practical suggestions

Given that vocational rehabilitation is about *helping people with health problems stay at, return to and remain in work*, the policy question is how to make sure that everyone of working age receives the help they require. Logically, this should start from the needs of people with health problems (at various stages); build on the evidence about effective interventions; and finally consider potential resources and the practicalities of how these interventions might be delivered. From a policy perspective, there are three broad types of clients, who are differentiated mainly by duration out of work, and who have correspondingly different needs:

In the first six weeks or so, most people with common health problems can be helped to return to work by following a few basic principles of healthcare and workplace management. This can be done with existing or minimal additional resources, and is low cost or cost-neutral. Policy should be directed to persuading and supporting health professionals and employers to embrace and implement these principles.

There is strong evidence on effective vocational rehabilitation interventions for the minority (possibly 5-10%) of workers with common health problems who need additional help to return to work after about six weeks, but there is a need to develop system(s) to deliver these interventions on a national scale. These systems should include *both* healthcare and workplace elements that take a proactive approach focused on return to work. To operationalise this requires a universal Gateway that a) identifies people after about 6 weeks' sickness absence, b) directs them to appropriate help, and c) ensures the content and standards of the interventions provided. Pilot studies of service delivery model(s) will be required to improve the evidence base on their effectiveness and cost-benefits in the UK context. This will involve investment but the potential benefits far outweigh the expenditure and the enormous costs of doing nothing.

For people who are out of work more than about 6 months and on benefits, *Pathways to work* is the most effective example to date. There is good evidence that *Pathways* increases the return to work rate of new claimants by 7-9%, with a positive cost-benefit ratio. Continued research and development is required to optimise *Pathways* for claimants with mental health problems and for long-term benefit recipients.

Vocational rehabilitation needs to be underpinned by education to inform the public, health professionals and employers about the value of work for health and recovery, and their part in the return to work process.

Conclusion

There is broad consensus among all the key stakeholders on the need to improve vocational rehabilitation in the UK. This review has demonstrated that there is now a strong scientific evidence base for many aspects of vocational rehabilitation, and a good business case for action. It has identified *what works, for whom, and when* and indicated areas where further research and development is required. Vocational rehabilitation should be a fundamental element of Government strategy to improve the health of working age people.

KEYWORDS: absence, common health problems, case management, disability management, evidence synthesis, healthcare, occupational rehabilitation, policy, return to work, review, sick leave, sickness absence, vocational rehabilitation, work, worker, workplace.

Key messages

1. Vocational rehabilitation is *whatever helps someone with a health problem to stay at, return to and remain in work*. It is an idea and an approach as much as an intervention or a service.

2. This review has demonstrated that there is now a strong scientific evidence base for many aspects of vocational rehabilitation.

3. There is a good business case for vocational rehabilitation, and more evidence on cost-benefits than for many health and social policy areas.

4. Common health problems should get high priority, because they account for about two-thirds of long-term sickness absence and incapacity benefits and much of this should be preventable. Return-to-work should be one of the key outcome measures.

5. Vocational rehabilitation depends on work-focused healthcare *and* accommodating workplaces. To make a real and lasting difference, both need to be addressed and coordinated.

6. Most people with common health problems can be helped to return to work by following a few basic principles of healthcare and workplace management. This can be done with existing or minimal additional resources, and is low cost or cost-neutral. Policy should be directed to persuading and supporting health professionals and employers to implement these principles.

7. There is strong evidence on effective vocational rehabilitation interventions for the minority of workers who need additional help to return to work, but there is a need to develop ways of delivering these on a national scale. There should be pilot studies to improve the evidence base on the effectiveness and cost-benefits of service delivery model(s) in the UK context. This will require investment, but the benefits should far outweigh the expenditure and the enormous costs of doing nothing.

8. There is an urgent need to improve vocational rehabilitation interventions for mental health problems, which are now the largest and fastest growing cause of long-term incapacity. Promising approaches include healthcare which incorporates a focus on return to work, workplaces that are accommodating and non-discriminating, and early intervention to support workers to stay in work and so prevent long-term incapacity.

9. *Pathways to work* increases the return to work rate of new benefit claimants by 7-9%, with a positive cost-benefit ratio. Continued work is required to optimise *Pathways* for claimants with mental health problems and long-term benefit recipients.

10. Vocational rehabilitation should be underpinned by education to inform the public, health professionals, and employers about the value of work for health and recovery.

Introduction

There is consensus among all the key stakeholders – unions, employers, insurers, healthcare professionals - on the need to improve vocational rehabilitation in the UK[1]. This is a fundamental part of the strategy to improve the health of adults of working age (Black 2008; HM Government 2005; HSC 2000). At an individual level, the goals are better health and work outcomes for people who suffer injury, illness or disability (Waddell & Burton 2006). At a policy level, the goals are a) to reduce the number of people who move onto and remain on disability and incapacity benefits when they still have (some) capacity for (some) work[2], and b) to increase employment rates[3].

An increasing number of large UK employers[4] now offer 'vocational rehabilitation', most commonly in the form of access to medical or surgical treatment, occupational health or case management, or flexible working (CBI/AXA 2007). However, there are questions about the nature and effectiveness of the services provided. There are similar questions about whether healthcare is as good as it could be at getting people back to work (Norwich Union Healthcare 2006).

The aim of this review is to provide an evidence base for policy development on vocational rehabilitation:

1.   To assess the evidence on the effectiveness and cost-benefits of vocational rehabilitation interventions.

2.   To develop practical suggestions on what vocational rehabilitation interventions are likely to work, for whom, and when.

---

1   Building capacity for work: a UK framework for vocational rehabilitation (DWP 2004); Vocational Rehabilitation Conference, London 16 June 2007; Vocational Rehabilitation Task Group.

2   It has been estimated that up to 1 million of the 2.7 million recipients of Incapacity Benefit still retain (some) capacity for (some) work (Waddell & Aylward 2005). 34% of people on disability and incapacity benefits say they would like to work (UK Labour Force Survey Summer 2002).

3   Targets include 80% employment for adults of working age (DWP Green Paper *A new deal for welfare: empowering people to work*, January 2006), and increased employment rates for people with disabilities (UK Government's Public Sector Agreement target 2003). For further discussion of these targets, see (DWP 2007; Freud 2007).

4   The term 'employers' is variously used as a shorthand to cover companies, senior management, line managers, human resources and other players in the workplace.

What is Vocational Rehabilitation?

The core objective of rehabilitation is restoration of function (Nocon & Baldwin 1998; WHO 2001). *Vocational* rehabilitation (also called *occupational* rehabilitation or *work* rehabilitation[5]) is directed to employment outcomes.

This review is about 'common health problems' and injuries - the mild/moderate musculoskeletal, mental health and cardio-respiratory conditions that account for about two-thirds of sickness absence, long-term incapacity and ill-health retirement (Waddell & Aylward 2005; Waddell & Burton 2004). Many of these conditions are common in people of working age. They are characterised more by responses to symptoms than by objective impairment. That is not to deny the reality of the symptoms or their impact, but these are essentially whole people whose health conditions *should* be manageable. Long-term incapacity is not inevitable. People with common health problems are therefore prime targets for vocational rehabilitation. People with severe medical conditions (e.g. neurological disease or blindness) may also need rehabilitation, but they have different and specialised rehabilitation needs (BSRM 2000), so were excluded from this review.

In simple language, vocational rehabilitation is *whatever helps someone with a health problem to stay at, return to and remain in work*. It was decided to start from this broad description (DWP 2004; HSA 2008; Irving et al. 2004; TUC 2000), rather than a more technical definition, in order to cover routine healthcare and workplace management in addition to more structured vocational rehabilitation interventions. It is acknowledged that there are other forms of productive activity (Contaldo 2007; Kendall et al. 2006; Saeki et al. 2006), but the remit of this review is *vocational* rehabilitation. Indeed, work[6] is arguably the most important social and economic goal and outcome measure[7] (Waddell & Aylward 2005).

There are many definitions of vocational rehabilitation, some of which reflect a particular perspective, context or legislative framework (Table 1). Analysis of these definitions reveals some key ideas about vocational rehabilitation (see Table 1 Annex for content analysis, evidence linking and references):

---

5   These terms appear to be synonymous in current use.

6   Strictly speaking, this review is about employment rather than work (Waddell & Burton 2006):- *Employment* is typically a contractual relationship between the individual worker and an employer over time for remuneration, as a socially acceptable means of earning a living. *Work* is not only 'a job' or paid employment, but includes unpaid or voluntary work, education and training, family responsibilities and caring.

7   Incapacity for work has a significant detrimental impact on the individual, his or her family, employers, the economy and society. Job retention, return to work and reintegration are therefore the most relevant and important (albeit not the only) goals and outcome measures of vocational rehabilitation (Waddell & Aylward 2005).

- Rehabilitation has traditionally focused on severe medical conditions, but is equally important for people with common health problems.

- Rehabilitation for people with severe and permanent impairments is about overcoming, adapting, or compensating for the impairment. Vocational rehabilitation for common health problems is more about identifying and addressing health-related, personal/psychological and social/occupational obstacles[8] to (return to) work.

- Vocational rehabilitation should be an integral part of all good clinical and workplace management and is not necessarily a separate, second-stage intervention.

- Vocational rehabilitation is not a matter for healthcare alone. It commonly requires a combination of healthcare and workplace interventions, to address the health problem *and* work issues.

- Vocational rehabilitation is goal directed, with the core objective of restoring capacity for work and translating that into participation.

- Vocational rehabilitation is a *process* of active change, facilitating the journey from sickness to work. It is often a *function* of healthcare and the workplace: it is not necessarily a separate programme or service.

- Vocational rehabilitation should be individualised to meet the needs of the person and their health problem.

- Vocational rehabilitation is an active process that depends on the participation, motivation and effort of the individual, *supported by* the workplace and healthcare.

- Vocational rehabilitation requires 'all players onside' – the individual, the workplace and health professional(s) - working together to a common goal.

To operationalise this review, it was important to draw a boundary between vocational rehabilitation interventions and 'treatment' interventions[9]:

Treatment is directed to, and has the primary goal of, treating pathology and/or relieving symptoms. This may be sufficient to enable the person to continue or return to work, but that is an indirect or secondary outcome.

---

8   These factors are variously described as obstacles or barriers: the clinical literature more often describes them as 'obstacles', the disability rights and social policy literatures as 'barriers'. A barrier can be seen as something constructed to prevent access, whereas an obstacle is something that happens to be in the way. Barriers need to be dismantled whilst obstacles can more readily be overcome. The question then is: overcome or dismantled by whom? Return to work and vocational rehabilitation interventions are able to overcome obstacles; dismantling barriers may depend more on systems and society – which may be why different groups tend to use the different terms.

9   In this context, *treatment* refers to specific healthcare interventions, e.g. medication; healthcare *management* is much broader and is part of vocational rehabilitation.

Vocational rehabilitation is directed to, and has the primary goal of, improving capability for work and translating that into actually working. This may secondarily, in the longer term, lead to improved symptoms.

There is a wide spectrum of vocational rehabilitation approaches that vary by type and intensity. Most people with common health problems do not need specialised, multidisciplinary rehabilitation services. Most require a much simpler level of *help to stay at, return to, and remain in work*, which can be delivered in primary healthcare and the workplace by following a few basic principles. At this level, vocational rehabilitation is an idea and an approach more than 'an intervention' or 'a service'. In fact, the very term 'vocational rehabilitation' is unnecessary here: 'facilitating return-to-work' might focus thinking better. However, a small but significant number of people with common health problems do need additional help from more structured vocational rehabilitation interventions. Those who move on to social security benefits and are no longer employed have more complex needs. This review covers all of these stages.

Historically and in most of the literature, vocational rehabilitation has been about *return to work*. More recently, there has been increasing interest in helping people to *stay at work*, recognising that it is better and easier to prevent unnecessary sickness absence and its deleterious effects rather than deal with them after they occur (ACOEM 2006; Varekamp et al. 2006). There is also growing recognition that return to work[10] is not a discrete, all-or-nothing event, but rather a *process* in which the individual prepares for, moves closer to, and engages in work (Wasiak et al. 2007; Young et al. 2005a). Furthermore, people with persistent or recurrent health problems are liable to further sickness absence, so what matters is *sustained* return to work (Bültmann et al. 2007; Franche et al. 2005b; Lotters et al. 2005). Vocational rehabilitation should take account of these various work outcomes.

---

10   Particularly after a prolonged period out of work.

The review

Appendix 1 gives a detailed description of the review methodology.

Throughout the review, broad and inclusive search strategies were used to retrieve as much material as possible, pertinent to the basic question: 'what helps people with common health problems return to work?' The focus was on *what* works, rather than *how* it works. Health promotion, primary prevention, 'presenteeism', disability evaluation, sick certification and disability discrimination were excluded as outside the definition of vocational rehabilitation[11].

In view of the range and amount of evidence, and the time and resources available, the only practical approach was to use existing scientific literature reviews and reports, mainly published from 2000 through December 2007. Data from some 450 included articles were extracted and incorporated into Evidence Tables, from which Evidence Statements were developed in each area, and explicitly linked to the evidence. Where appropriate, the text of the evidence statements was used to expand on the nature or limitations of the underlying evidence, and to offer any caveats or cautions.

Rigorous methods were used to assess the strength of the scientific evidence on effectiveness (Box 1 – adapted from Waddell & Burton 2006).

Box 1: Ratings for the strength of the scientific evidence on effectiveness		
	Evidence Grade	**Definition**
***	**Strong**	Generally consistent findings provided by (systematic) review(s) of multiple high quality studies.
**	**Moderate**	Generally consistent findings provided by review(s) of fewer and/or methodologically weaker studies.
*	**Weak**	Limited evidence – provided by a single high quality study Conflicting evidence – inconsistent findings provided by (review(s) of) multiple studies.
0	-	No high quality **scientific** evidence

---

11   See Appendix 1 for a more detailed discussion of the exclusions.

In a review of this nature, some important issues are inappropriate for scientific experiment or a 'scientific' answer. For these issues, it may be possible to construct a reasoned statement based on various other criteria (Box 2). In appropriate cases this structured approach, which extends beyond consensus, can produce statements that are just as valid as those based on scientific evidence.

Box 2: Criteria used for non-scientific evidence	
#	Background scientific evidence (e.g. epidemiology, indirect or related evidence)
	Logical reasoning
	Worthwhile use of resources
	Direct and indirect evidence on likely benefits

Scientific evidence on cost-effectiveness was incorporated when available. Further evidence was gathered from the policy and business literature on cost-benefit analyses and the business case for vocational rehabilitation.

Evidence findings

Appendix 2 and Table 2 provide the rationale and the evidence that it is reasonable to develop one evidence base for work-related and non work-related conditions. This shows that vocational rehabilitation for work-related and compensable conditions should follow the same principles and use the same interventions as for other comparable health conditions. Importantly, no contradictory evidence was found, though there is a need to pay particular attention to the psychosocial context. In view of the age and working life expectancy of many injured workers, and the good medical prognosis of many of these conditions, vocational rehabilitation is likely to be a worthwhile use of resources.

The evidence on vocational rehabilitation is presented separately for musculoskeletal (Table 3), mental health (Table 4) and cardio-respiratory (Table 5) conditions. This is followed by evidence on 'delivery' (primary healthcare, workplace interventions, specialist rehabilitation services, social security interventions) (Table 6), and on timing and coordination (Table 7). Each section starts with background information, provides Evidence Statements, gives boxed Example(s) to help illustrate what is possible, and concludes with some narrative Interpretation.

Gaps in the evidence and priority areas for further research and development are identified throughout the review. Appendix 3 provides additional suggestions for further research.

MUSCULOSKELETAL DISORDERS

Table 3 lays out the evidence on musculoskeletal disorders.

Most adults of working age (60-80%) experience musculoskeletal symptoms at some time, they are often recurrent and may persist, and they have a variable relationship with work (Hestbaek et al. 2003; Walker-Bone & Cooper 2005). Only for a minority of episodes do people seek healthcare, and about 10% describe it as a 'limiting long-term illness'. Nevertheless, even a small proportion of such a common problem represents a sizable number: musculoskeletal disorders are the most common cause of short- and long-term sickness absence in manual workers (CIPD 2007), and account for around 20% of UK Incapacity Benefits (DWP administrative statistics).

Throughout much of the musculoskeletal literature, there is a broad distinction between specific musculoskeletal diagnoses (e.g. carpal tunnel syndrome or intervertebral disc prolapse) and 'non-specific' disorders (characterised by an absence of identifiable relevant pathology). The terms 'disorder' and 'injury' are not clearly distinguished and are often used interchangeably, though 'injury' is more often used when there is any question of work-relatedness (See Appendix 2).

Reflecting the high prevalence of musculoskeletal disorders and their historical impact on compensation systems, there is a large and varied literature on their vocational rehabilitation (Table 3). The literature on low back pain is most extensive, but recent interest has expanded this to include substantial evidence on other musculoskeletal disorders. Some clinical literature includes return to work, often as a secondary outcome, while the occupational health and rehabilitation literatures commonly have it as the main outcome. Stay at work outcomes are less commonly reported.

Since many musculoskeletal disorders are perceived as work-related, it may be felt that return to work with symptoms is precluded. However, work-relatedness is a complex issue. Undoubtedly musculoskeletal symptoms may be work-relevant (symptom fluctuation in response to work) but that does not mean work was necessarily the primary cause (Burton et al. 2008). Causation is usually multifactorial: work is only one and often not the main cause (Carter & Birrell 2000). Avoidance of work until symptoms have completely resolved is unrealistic and unhelpful in most cases: because work has clear benefits for physical health, workers should be allowed and helped to return as soon as possible.

Evidence Statements

References in this section are to Table 3.

MSD-1   #   There are good epidemiological and clinical reasons and widespread acceptance throughout the literature that early return to work and stay at work approaches are appropriate and beneficial for most people with most musculoskeletal disorders.

(ARMA 2004; ARMA 2007; Bevan et al. 2007; EASHAW 2007; EFILWC 2007; Gobelet et al. 2007b; HSE 2002; Talmage & Melhorn 2005; Waddell & Burton 2004)

MSD-2   ***   A common set of approaches for helping people return to work are effective across the range of musculoskeletal disorders/injuries (accepting that some specific diagnoses require condition-specific treatment).

(Burton et al. 2008; de Buck et al. 2002; Hanson et al. 2006; MacEachen et al. 2006; Seferiadis et al. 2004; Waddell & Burton 2004; Williams et al. 2007; Zampolini et al. 2007)

MSD-3   ***   There is strong evidence that occupational outcomes for most people with most musculoskeletal disorders are improved by (increasing) activity, including early return to (some) work.

(Burton et al. 2008; COST B13 Working Group 2004; EASHAW 2007; Gross et al. 2006; Hagberg 2005; Kool et al. 2004; Kupper et al. 2004; Nash et al. 2004; Staal et al. 2005; Talmage & Melhorn 2005)

MSD-4   ***   Early intervention through delivery of appropriate treatment, positive advice/reassurance about activity and work, and/or workplace accommodation is sufficient for many people with musculoskeletal disorders; those who do not respond in a timely manner may require more structured vocational rehabilitation interventions.

> (Brox et al. 2007; Burton et al. 2008; EASHAW 2007; Guzmán et al. 2001; Heymans et al. 2004; Hlobil et al. 2005; Kool et al. 2004; Loisel et al. 2003; Poiraudeau et al. 2007; Schonstein et al. 2003; Zampolini et al. 2007)

MSD-5   **   Treatments to address any specific pathology and to reduce symptoms are integral to vocational rehabilitation, but treatment *per se* has little impact on occupational outcomes[12].

> (Breen et al. 2007; Burton et al. 2008; Crawford & Laiou 2007; Faber et al. 2006; Gobelet et al. 2007b; Talmage & Melhorn 2005; Waddell & Burton 2004)

MSD-6   **   There is moderate evidence (and wide consensus) that vocational rehabilitation entails a number of elements, which must take account of the individual, their health condition and their work; involvement of the workplace is crucial.

> (Cole et al. 2006; de Buck et al. 2002; Franche et al. 2005b; Karjalainen et al. 2000; Loisel et al. 2003; Ostelo et al. 2005; Waddell & Burton 2004; Williams et al. 2007; Williams & Westmorland 2002)

MSD-7   ***   There is strong evidence that temporarily modified work (transitional work arrangements) can facilitate early return to work.

> (Burton et al. 2008; Carter & Birrell 2000; Hanson et al. 2006; Loisel et al. 2003; Shaw et al. 2007; Waddell & Burton 2004; Weir & Nielson 2001; Williams et al. 2004; Williams et al. 2007)

MSD-8   ***   There is strong evidence that structured multidisciplinary rehabilitation programmes, including cognitive behavioural principles[13] to tackle psychosocial issues, are effective for helping people with persistent musculoskeletal disorders return to work.

> (COST B13 Working Group 2004; Hoffman et al. 2007; MacEachen et al. 2006; Mahalik et al. 2006; Schonstein et al. 2003; Seferiadis et al. 2004)

---

12 Most workers with common health problems do return to work quickly, with or without healthcare. This probably depends mainly on their individual motivation, rather than a direct effect of healthcare.

13 Cognitive behavioural *principles* are incorporated into clinical management and rehabilitation, and delivered by various health professionals. This should be distinguished from cognitive behavioural *therapy* (CBT) which is a *treatment* for mental health problems, delivered by mental health professionals.

MSD-9   ***   There is strong evidence that commitment and coordinated action from all the players is crucial for successful vocational rehabilitation: especially important is communication between healthcare professionals, employers and workers, which should be initiated at an early stage of absence.

(Bongers et al. 2006; Cole et al. 2006; Feldman 2004; Franche et al. 2005b; Hanson et al. 2006; Kunkel & Miller 2002; Loisel et al. 2003; MacEachen et al. 2006; Shaw et al. 2007; Waddell & Burton 2004; Williams et al. 2007; Williams & Westmorland 2002)

MSD-10   *   There is general consensus and limited evidence that successful return to work requires the provision of consistent information and advice (including the correction of unhelpful beliefs and myths) for all the players.

(Crawford & Laiou 2005; de Buck et al. 2002; Feldman 2004; Pengel et al. 2002; Rainville et al. 2005; Shaw et al. 2002; van Geen et al. 2007; Varekamp et al. 2006)

MSD-11   *   There is limited evidence that (some aspects of) vocational rehabilitation for musculoskeletal disorders can be cost-effective.

(Backman 2006; Burton & Waddell 2002; Franche et al. 2005b; Hanson et al. 2006; Loisel et al. 2003; Schonstein et al. 2003)

Examples

Three examples illustrate that a range of vocational rehabilitation interventions in different settings can be effective for musculoskeletal disorders.

Prevention of long-term sickness absence in primary care:

A randomised controlled trial in Sweden showed that a cognitive behavioural intervention lowered the risk of long-term sick leave nine-fold. The patients had low back pain and perceived themselves at risk of long-term problems. The intervention comprised six sessions of group treatment by a therapist to change beliefs and behaviours so they could cope better with their problems. The control group had usual care (Linton & Andersson 2000).

Population-based model to improve return to work:

A randomised controlled trial in Quebec showed that workers who received a structured intervention combining clinical and occupational interventions returned to work 2.4 times faster than usual care. The subjects in a workers compensation setting had been absent >4 weeks due to back pain. A six-year follow-up found that usual care generated some very costly cases because of long-term disability. The combination of work rehabilitation and workplace interventions at the sub-acute stage may provide important long-term savings (Loisel et al. 1997; Loisel et al. 2002).

Workplace-based intervention tackling obstacles to return to work:

A controlled trial in the UK showed that an early psychosocial intervention package, delivered at the workplace, improved return to work time from 10 days to 6 days. The subjects were workers with musculoskeletal disorders. The intervention package, delivered by occupational health nurses, addressed psychosocial obstacles to recovery through a supportive network that included advice, modified work and communication with the GP. Modest benefits can be achieved for low cost (McCluskey et al. 2006).

Interpretation

The main finding of this section is the strength of the evidence base on effective return-to-work and vocational rehabilitation interventions for musculoskeletal conditions. For many years the strongest evidence was on low back pain, but more recent evidence shows that the same principles apply to most people with most common musculoskeletal disorders, irrespective of diagnosis or cause. This can be achieved successfully across a variety of settings: in routine healthcare and workplace management; and in more structured vocational rehabilitation interventions for those who need additional help.

Healthcare must place greater emphasis on occupational outcomes, in addition to its traditional role of treatment to control symptoms/pathology. Cognitive behavioural approaches that promote helpful beliefs and behaviours should underpin both clinical and occupational management. The role of the workplace is crucial: maintaining contact and the provision of transitional work arrangements are important (and relatively inexpensive) elements to facilitate return to work. Good communication between the key players - healthcare, the worker, and the workplace - is essential. Early implementation of these principles should mean that fewer individuals will require more structured (and more costly) interventions.

MENTAL HEALTH PROBLEMS

Table 4a lays out the evidence on anxiety and depression and Table 4b on 'stress'.

At any one time, about a third of the working age population have some mental symptoms (e.g. fatigue, irritability, or worry), about one sixth would meet diagnostic criteria for a mental illness, but only 6% seek healthcare[14] (Lelliott et al. 2008). The most common mental illnesses are depression, anxiety or a combination of the two[15]. There are standard diagnostic criteria for anxiety and depression (DSM-IVR, ICD-10) and evidence-based guidelines for their clinical management (NICE 2004a; NICE 2007). Community surveys suggest that the prevalence of diagnosable psychiatric disorders has been stable over time, at least up to 2000[16] (Kessler et al. 2005; Seymour & Grove 2005; Singleton et al. 2000; Wessely 2004).

---

14   Care is required interpreting such statistics: the presence of symptoms does not necessarily mean mental illness and it is a matter of perspective where to draw the boundary of 'normal'. It is a matter of further debate how much of this is 'unmet need' or potential medicalisation of everyday symptoms (Pilgrim & Bentall 1999; Rose 2007; Wessely 2004).

15   For comparison, the lifetime prevalence of severe mental illness such as schizophrenia is about 1-2%.

16   There is no clear evidence on any significant increase in prevalence since 2000, though this remains uncertain until the results of the ONS survey undertaken in 2007 are published.

However, there has clearly been a change in diagnostic and sick certification rates of mental illness. Mental health problems are now the most common reason for sickness absence in non-manual workers in the UK (CIPD 2007). One quarter of all UK sick certificates are for mental health problems, but the average time off is about twice as long so they account for 40% of total time certified (Shiels et al. 2004). Mental health problems are the largest and fastest growing reason for Incapacity Benefits and now account for 39% of all UK Incapacity Benefit recipients (DWP administrative statistics).

The problem of 'stress' requires specific attention. There has been substantial growth in 'stress cases' with little medical basis to explain the trend (Henderson et al. 2003). The very term 'stress' is ambiguous since it is used to describe both cause and consequences. There is no scientific agreement on the conceptual basis of 'stress', its definition, assessment, or its causal relationship with work (Cox et al. 2006; Rick et al. 2001; Rick et al. 2002; Spurgeon 2007). For these reasons, 'stress' is not included as a separate category in standard diagnostic classifications of mental illness (DSM-IVR, ICD-10), and is not accepted as a Prescribed Disease (IIAC 2004; Spurgeon 2007).

There is a widespread and simplistic perception that work causes mental illness and 'stress' (NHS 1999; Sanderson & Andrews 2006), but the interactions between work and mental (ill) health are complex. On the one hand, mental health problems affect work: work participation and productivity depend on good mental health; while mental ill-health can reduce both. On the other hand, work can be harmful to mental well-being; though actual mental illness is usually multifactorial and work is only one and often not the main cause (Lelliott et al. 2008; Wessely 2004). At the same time, there is strong evidence that work is generally good for mental health and the benefits usually outweigh the risks (Lelliott et al. 2008; Waddell & Burton 2006). This leads to the important point that having a mental health problem does not necessarily preclude work (Sullivan 2005). Work has the potential to be part of the recovery process (Leff 2001; Morris & Lloyd 2004; Thomas et al. 2002), and can provide a number of protective factors for problems such as depression, including structure to the day, social contacts and self-esteem (Kirby et al. 2004; Nieuwenhuijsen et al. 2008).

Evidence Statements

References in this section are to Table 4.

MH-1   #   People with mental health problems attach a high priority to employment. There is general agreement throughout the literature that work is an appropriate goal of management for many of them. Work has potential to be part of the recovery process. Health professionals caring for patients with mental health problems have an important role in helping them to (return to) work.

Table 4a: (Boardman et al. 2003; Canadian Senate 2004; Davis & Rinaldi 2004; DHC 2006; Grove 1999; Harnois & Gabriel 2000; Leff 2001; Lelliott et al. 2008; Royal College of Psychiatrists 2002; Social Exclusion Unit 2004; Teasdale & Deahl 2007)

MH-2 # The literature on mental health problems is focused mainly on clinical management and outcomes, with much less evidence on vocational rehabilitation and work outcomes. There is a particular lack of work focus in policy documents, clinical guidelines and Cochrane Reviews on mental health problems.

Table 4a

MH-3 *** There is strong evidence that various medical and psychological treatments for anxiety and depression can improve symptoms, clinical outcomes and quality of life.

Table 4a: (Abbass et al. 2006; Churchill et al. 2001; DH 2001; DH 2007b; Gava et al. 2007; Hunot et al. 2007; Kaltenthaler et al. 2004; NICE 2004a; NICE 2006; NICE 2007; Roth & Fonagy 2005)

In principle, clinical improvement might reasonably be expected to improve participation and productivity. However, there is poor correlation between level of symptoms and workability (Lelliott et al. 2008), and limited evidence to support this proposition (MH-4 and MH-5).

MH-4 * There is limited evidence that symptomatic treatments for depression (by medication, psychotherapy or a combination of both, and including Cognitive Behavioural Therapy[17]) in themselves improve occupational outcomes and no clear evidence on the magnitude of any effect.

Table 4a: (Abbass et al. 2006; Bilsker et al. 2006; Canadian Senate 2004; Donohue & Pincus 2007; Goldner et al. 2004; Lelliott et al. 2008; Nieuwenhuijsen et al. 2008; Steffick et al. 2006; Teasdale & Deahl 2007)

MH-5 0 There is no evidence that symptomatic treatments for anxiety disorders (including PTSD) improve work outcomes.

Table 4a: (Bisson & Andrew 2007; Hunot et al. 2007; Keane et al. 2006)

MH-6 ** There is moderate evidence that stress management interventions[18] improve subjective outcomes, such as mental well-being, complaints and perceived

---

17 It is beyond the scope of this review to compare the relative merits of different pharmacological and psychological treatments for different mental illnesses. CBT is only mentioned because of recent interest (Black 2008; DH 2008; Layard 2006) and to clarify what the evidence shows about its effect on occupational outcomes.

18 Stress management interventions fall into two broad types: organizational-level and individual-level. Many organizational-level interventions aim mainly at primary prevention, which is outside the scope of this review. Individual-level interventions mainly aim to reduce symptoms or improve coping, but the particular interest of this review is whether they improve work outcomes such as sickness absence or return to work rates.

quality of work (though these are usually measured at workforce level, and not specifically in workers with mental health problems).

Table 4a: (Lelliott et al. 2008; NICE 2006)

Table 4b: (van der Klink et al. 2001)

MH-7   *   For workers who have already developed mental health problems, there is limited and conflicting evidence that stress management interventions improve sickness absence rates or return to work.

Table 4a: (Lelliott et al. 2008)

Table 4b: (Cox et al. 2000b; Damiani et al. 2004; Giga et al. 2003; van der Klink & van Dijk 2003)

MH-8   0   Recipients are generally satisfied with counselling. Counselling in primary care is associated with modest reduction in psychological symptoms in the short-term, though it offers no advantage in the longer-term. However, there is no high quality evidence that counselling or Employee Assistance Programmes in the workplace improve work outcomes for people who have mental health problems.

Table 4a: (Arthur 2000; Bower & Rowland 2006; Giga et al. 2003)

MH-9   *   There is rational argument and some consensus, and limited evidence, that people with mental health problems require additional help (over and above symptomatic treatment) in order to (return to) work.

Table 4a: (Bilsker et al. 2006; Davis & Rinaldi 2004; Dong et al. 2002; Grove 1999; Harnois & Gabriel 2000; Henderson et al. 2005; Lelliott et al. 2008; NICE 2007; Royal College of Psychiatrists 2002; Sullivan 2005; Thomas et al. 2002)

MH-10   *   There is moderate evidence that various forms of disease management and case management can improve quality of care and clinical outcomes in depression, and limited evidence that they improve work outcomes.

Table 4a: (Goetzel et al. 2005; Kates & Mach 2007; Neumeyer-Gromen et al. 2004; Pirraglia et al. 2004; Steffick et al. 2006)

MH-11   *   There is general consensus that organisation-level interventions (disability management, improved communication, early contact with absent worker, an agreed rehabilitation plan, flexibility in work organisation and return to work arrangements) are applicable to mental health problems, and limited evidence that they improve work outcomes.

Table 4a: (Egan et al. 2007; Lelliott et al. 2008; NICE 2008; Seymour & Grove 2005)

Table 4b (Cox et al. 2000b; Damiani et al. 2004; Dong et al. 2002; Giga et al. 2003; Thomson et al. 2003; van der Klink et al. 2001)

MH-12   [0]   There is no high quality evidence on the cost-effectiveness of interventions to improve work outcomes for common mental health problems[19]

Table 4a: (Donohue & Pincus 2007; Goetzel et al. 2002; Hunot et al. 2007; Löthgren 2004a; Löthgren 2004b; Seymour & Grove 2005)

Examples

Managing somatising patients in general practice

A randomised controlled trial in The Netherlands compared two or three 10-30 minute sessions of 'reattribution' with a GP to usual GP care. At two year follow-up, this reduced median sickness absence in the past six months from four weeks to zero (p<0.0001) (Blankenstein 2001).

An activating intervention in adjustment disorders

A cluster randomised controlled trial in the Netherlands compared an activating intervention by an occupational physician (4-5 sessions, total length 90 minutes) with usual occupational healthcare. At one year follow-up, this reduced median time for return to work from 51 to 37 days (p<0.001) (van der Klink et al. 2003).

Interpretation

The main finding of this section is that although there is strong evidence that various medical and psychological treatments for anxiety and depression can improve symptoms and quality of life, there is limited evidence that they improve work outcomes. There is a general lack of focus on vocational rehabilitation or on work outcomes throughout this literature.

The second main finding is the lack of scientific clarity about 'stress', with little or no evidence that any *vocational* rehabilitation interventions are effective for work outcomes.

Mental health problems are a major challenge for vocational rehabilitation (Wittchen & Jacobi 2005). There are similarities to low back pain in the 1980s (Waddell 1987): an exponential increase in sickness absence and long-term incapacity, despite no good evidence of significant change in the prevalence of mental illness; a lack of distinction between non-specific psychological symptoms and diagnosable mental illness; a debate over the provision of more healthcare set against concerns about over-medicalisation; and a focus on purely clinical rather than work outcomes. This review found limited evidence on effective return-to-work and vocational rehabilitation interventions for depression (MH-4), and even less for anxiety and stress (MH-5, MH-7, MH-8). So, sickness absence and long-term incapacity associated with mental health problems are unlikely to be improved simply by providing more healthcare (though there are of course other reasons to improve

---

19   Though that is quite separate from the question of their cost-effectiveness for symptomatic relief, clinical outcomes and healthcare costs.

the quality of clinical services for mental health problems[20]. Instead, there needs to be a fundamental shift in healthcare and workplace thinking and management. Clinicians need greater understanding of work and mental health (D-1, D-6), while employers need to be more accommodating of mental health problems (D-9). Stigma and discrimination in the workplace remain major issues (Lelliott et al. 2008; Mental Health Foundation 2002; Thomas et al. 2002; WHO 2005)[21].

CARDIO-RESPIRATORY CONDITIONS

Cardiovascular conditions

Table 5a lays out the evidence on cardiac rehabilitation.

Cardiac rehabilitation programmes are currently provided almost exclusively to patients who have had a myocardial infarction or a cardiac procedure (NACR 2007), though they can provide similar benefits to patients with heart failure and angina, and may be appropriate for patients with other cardiovascular conditions like hypertension and arrhythmia (B Lewin, personal communication).

About 30% of myocardial infarction survivors were aged <65 years and employed at the time of their cardiac event (NACR 2007). More than half of those who were previously employed do return to work, though some of them stop work again or retire early within one year (Lewin 1999; Perk & Alexanderson 2004). Of those who do not return to work, about half are considered to do so for psychosocial reasons rather than because of their (physical) cardiac condition (Lewin 1999; Mital et al. 2004; Perk & Alexanderson 2004).

About 40% of myocardial infarction survivors receive cardiac rehabilitation (Cortés & Arthur 2006; NACR 2007). There is a major problem of non-participation, particularly for women (Cooper et al. 2002; Daly et al. 2002). There is a further problem with adherence: ~50% drop out of exercise programmes by 6-12 months (Daly et al. 2002; NHS Centre for Reviews 1998), with little high quality evidence on how to improve these figures (Beswick et al. 2005; Cooper et al. 2002).

Cardiac rehabilitation generally consists of a comprehensive, long-term programme involving medical evaluation, prescribed exercise, cardiac risk factor modification, education, and counselling. These programmes are designed to limit the physiological and psychological effects of cardiac illness, reduce the risk of sudden death or re-infarction, control cardiac symptoms, stabilise or reverse the atherosclerotic process, and enhance

---

20 Dept of Health press release 26-2-08 (DH 2008)
21 But that is beyond the remit of this review.

the psychosocial and vocational status of selected patients (Balady et al. 2007; Thomas et al. 2007).

Evidence Statements

References in this section are to Table 5a.

CR-1   #   There is recognition in principle that the goals of cardiac rehabilitation should include return to work.

(Balady et al. 2007; Lewin 1999; Mital et al. 2004; Mital & Mital 2002; NZGG 2002; Thomas et al. 2007; Waddell & Burton 2006)

CR-2   #   Current cardiac rehabilitation programmes are directed to clinical outcomes and cardiac risk factor modification. Of UK patients receiving cardiac rehabilitation, <1% get any form of vocational assessment. Occupational outcomes are generally not reported in the literature, including Cochrane Reviews, NICE and SIGN guidelines, and the National Audit of Cardiac Rehabilitation.

Table 5a

CR-3   **   There is moderate evidence that current cardiac rehabilitation programmes do *not* influence return to work rates after myocardial infarction.

(Cannon et al. 2002; Lewin 1999; Mital et al. 2004; Mital & Mital 2002; NHS Centre for Reviews 1998; Perk & Alexanderson 2004)

CR-4   0   Although there is moderate evidence that cardiac rehabilitation programmes are cost-effective based on direct healthcare costs, there is no economic evidence about their indirect cost-benefits.

(Ades et al. 1997)

CR-5   0   Although Critical Pathways and Disease Management programmes improve quality of care for patients with other cardiovascular conditions and are cost-effective, there is no evidence about their impact on occupational outcomes.

(Cannon et al. 2002; Goetzel et al. 2005; Holland et al. 2005; Ofman et al. 2004)

CR-6   0   There is no high quality evidence about the effectiveness of cardiac rehabilitation programmes for occupational outcomes in patients with other cardiovascular conditions.

(ExTraMATCH Collaborative 2004; Falcone et al. 2003; Phillips et al. 2005; Reynolds et al. 2004; Smidt et al. 2005)

Examples

A randomised controlled trial of early return to work after myocardial infarction

Patients who had made a good recovery from a myocardial infarction and were at low risk were advised early return to normal activities including work at two weeks. They did just as well as those who received standard cardiac rehabilitation. Early return to work was safe for this selected group of patients and saved $300 per low risk patient (Bunker 2002; Hall et al. 2002; Kovoor et al. 2006)

Changing illness perceptions after myocardial infarction

A randomised controlled trial compared three 30-40 minute sessions with a psychologist to usual cardiac rehabilitation with a nurse. At three month follow-up, those receiving the intervention were about twice as likely to have returned to work ($P<0.05$) (Petrie et al. 2002)

Interpretation

The main finding of this section is that, despite recognition in principle that the goals of cardiac rehabilitation should include work outcomes (CR-1), current programmes focus almost entirely on clinical and disease outcomes (CR-2). Cardiac rehabilitation for people of working age needs to place greater emphasis on work outcomes and the high costs of cardiac disease provide strong economic reasons for pursuing this. Current cardiac rehabilitation programmes are generally cost-effective, based on healthcare costs (CR-4), so any additional gain in work outcomes would be a significant bonus, and it should be possible to achieve this without any major increase in programme costs.

Respiratory conditions

Table 5b lays out the evidence on respiratory conditions.

For the present purpose, respiratory disorders can be broadly divided into a) minor upper respiratory tract infections, b) occupational asthma, and c) chronic obstructive pulmonary disease (chronic bronchitis and emphysema).

Minor upper respiratory tract infections are the most common reason for GP consultation (McCormick et al. 1995) and sickness absence from work (CIPD 2007). However, these are biologically and socially self-limiting conditions, and are not a rehabilitation issue.

There are about 600 new cases of occupational asthma recorded each year but this is probably a substantial under-estimate - up to 142,000 people in the UK have 'breathing problems' which they believe to be 'work-related' (HSE 2007b). Occupational asthma may be allergic (about 90%) or irritant-induced, both of which are well-defined clinical entities (HSE 2007a; Newman Taylor et al. 2004; Nicholson et al. 2005). However, up to a quarter of all adult asthma may be aggravated by work, though that is less well understood (Banks & Jalloul 2007; Henneberger 2007; Vandenplas et al. 2003).

An estimated 3 million people in the UK have chronic obstructive pulmonary disease (COPD), though this is often undiagnosed (British Lung Foundation, www.lunguk.org). However, the literature on COPD in Table 5b focuses on more severe cases, generally in workers close to retirement age (Blanc & Torén 2007; Effing et al. 2007; Namath & Kuschmer 2006) whose medical condition is commonly severe and progressive[22] (Antó et al. 2001).

Evidence Statements

References in this section are to Table 5b.

CR-7   #   There is a strong evidence base, logical rationale and general consensus for the clinical and workplace management of occupational asthma. The basic principle (in addition to medical treatment) is to identify the cause, and to eliminate exposure (by control of the hazard or relocation of the worker[23]) as soon as possible after the diagnosis is confirmed[24].

(Banks & Jalloul 2007; Beach et al. 2005; British Thoracic Society & SIGN 2007; Cambach et al. 1999; Gibson et al. 2002; Hyman 2005; Talmage & Melhorn 2005)

(Henneberger 2007; HSE 2007a; Iqbal et al. 2002; Moscato & Rampulla 2003; Newman Taylor et al. 2004; Nicholson et al. 2005)

CR-8   ***   There is wide variation in reported symptomatic recovery rates from occupational asthma, averaging about one-third. More than 50% of patients continue to have some degree of symptoms and bronchial hyper-responsiveness. About 30% remain unemployed for periods of years.

(Ameille & Descatha 2005; Beach et al. 2005; British Thoracic Society & SIGN 2007; Lombardo & Balmes 2000; Namath & Kuschmer 2006; Nicholson et al. 2005; Peters et al. 2007; Rachiotis et al. 2007; Vandenplas et al. 2003)

CR-9   ***   There is strong evidence that disease management programmes and self-management education programmes for asthma[25] reduce sickness absence and are cost-effective.

(Gibson et al. 2002; Goetzel et al. 2005; Ofman et al. 2004; Toelle & Ram 2004; Van Weel et al. 2006)

---

22   COPD does not fit the original definition of 'common health problems' because of permanent and progressive impairment, but it is included here for completeness.

23   Depending on the type of asthma (Banks & Jalloul 2007; Henneberger 2007; Mapp et al. 2005).

24   And a similar approach applies to rhinitis (Gautrin et al. 2006; Hellgren et al. 2003) and to latex allergy (Bousquet et al. 2006)

25   Note that CR-9 is about adult asthma in general; whilst not specifically about occupational asthma, the principles are likely to apply to a greater or lesser extent.

CR-10   #   There is rational argument and general consensus that improved work outcomes for occupational asthma will require not only better clinical and workplace management, but also better compensation and retraining arrangements.

(Ameille & Descatha 2005; Henneberger 2007; Jeebhay & Quirce 2007; Malo 2005; Newman Taylor et al. 2004; Nicholson et al. 2005; Vandenplas et al. 2003)

CR-11   **   There is moderate evidence that current pulmonary rehabilitation, disease management and self-management education programmes for COPD do *not* show clinically significant effects on health-related quality of life, functional capacity or work outcomes.

(Effing et al. 2007; Ofman et al. 2004; Turnock et al. 2005)

Example

Outcome of occupational asthma after cessation of exposure

Workers with latex induced asthma were followed up for 56 months. Stopping exposure to latex was associated with improvement in symptoms, lung function and asthma severity scores. Those who remained in work (compared with those who left work) had better functional status, better quality of life and maintained their income (Vandenplas et al. 2002)

Interpretation

The main finding of this section is that there is scope to improve outcomes of occupational asthma (CR-8, CR-9). In principle, risk assessment, and control, early detection, clinical treatment, and workplace management should prevent most cases of occupational asthma going on to long-term incapacity for work. The present findings suggest that management is still often sub-optimal, particularly for early detection, clinical management directed to occupational outcomes, and the provision of modified or alternative employment (including retraining).

The other main finding is that current approaches to COPD focus on the later stages of the disease, and have little impact on work outcomes (CR-11). The high prevalence of COPD and an aging workforce suggest the need to develop better methods to support workers at an earlier stage of the disease, to enable them to continue working as long as possible.

DELIVERY

Table 6 lays out the evidence on delivery: 6a on primary healthcare interventions, 6b on workplace interventions, 6c on structured vocational rehabilitation interventions and 6d on social security and policy interventions. Evidence linking on these generic issues is also drawn from other sections of the Findings.

Primary healthcare interventions

Most people with mild/moderate musculoskeletal, mental health and cardio-respiratory conditions who seek help are managed successfully in primary healthcare and return to work relatively quickly and uneventfully. Those who do not achieve a timely return to work continue to attend primary healthcare. The advice and management given in primary care has a major and lasting impact on the individual's (and their family's and employer's) beliefs about the health condition and how it should be managed. It also has a major impact on sickness absence and return to work, so what happens in primary care is relevant to vocational rehabilitation. Primary care management can have either a positive or negative impact on occupational outcomes.

D-1   #   There is general consensus, based on background evidence, logical reasoning and clinical guidelines, that GPs and other health professionals:

- play a key role in advising and supporting patients about (return to) work

- need to understand their patients' work situation

- should appreciate that (return to) work is an important outcome for clinical management

- should help patients develop a return to work plan

- can facilitate return to work by communication and coordination with the workplace

- need better training and support (in the primary care setting) to help address work issues

Table 6a: (Black et al. 2000; FOM 2005; Frank & Sawney 2003; Kazimirski 1997; Verbeek 2006; Weevers et al. 2005)(Doctors.net 2007)

Table 6c: (Frank & Thurgood 2006)

D-2   *   There is limited evidence that primary care management following those principles leads to better occupational outcomes.

Table 3: (Breen et al. 2007; Carter & Birrell 2000)

Table 6a: (Garg et al. 2005; Goldfarb et al. 2004)

D-3   ***   Many GPs and other health professionals feel ill-equipped, and lack training and expertise on work issues.

Table 3: (Rainville et al. 2005)

Table 6a: (Breen et al. 2006; Crawford & Laiou 2005; Mowlam & Lewis 2005; Van Weel et al. 2006; Verbeek et al. 2002)(Doctors.net 2007)

D-4   **   Guideline dissemination and implementation, computerised clinical decision support systems, audit and feedback, and multifaceted interventions *can* change health professionals' behaviour, but the effects are small to moderate.

Table 6a: (Garg et al. 2005; Grimshaw et al. 2001;
Grimshaw et al. 2004; Grimshaw et al. 2005; Jamtvedt et al. 2006)

D-5   ***   Many GPs report insufficient time, resources and support to address work issues adequately.

Table 6a: (Breen et al. 2006; Mowlam & Lewis 2005;
Van Weel et al. 2006)(Doctors.net 2007)

D-6   *   Providing accurate information and advice about work and health issues is effective in changing beliefs, but there is conflicting evidence about an effect on occupational outcomes.

Table 3: (ARMA 2007; Backman 2006; Henrotin et al. 2006)

Table 6d: (Burton & Waddell 2002; Frank et al. 1998; Trevena et al. 2006)

Examples

<u>Early communication between healthcare provider, patient and the workplace</u>

187 Ontario workers with lost-time claims for back, neck or upper extremity occupational musculoskeletal injuries completed a telephone survey 17-43 days post injury. Three items of early communication were associated with a more than twofold chance of earlier return to work compared with a lack of communication: (1) giving a return to work date, (2) advice about work, (3) contact between the healthcare provider and the workplace. The healthcare provider playing an active role early in the return to work process facilitates early return (Kosny et al. 2006)

<u>Effectiveness of early physiotherapy for LBP</u>

3867 patients were seen at an occupational health service within 3 weeks of a low back injury: 1379 had their first therapy session either on the day of injury or the next day, 2005 within two to seven days, and 483 more delayed. Patients in the early intervention group had fewer physician visits, fewer restricted workdays, fewer days away from work, and shorter case duration. No formal economic analysis was performed, but the authors considered early intervention produced major cost savings (Zigenfus et al. 2000).

Interpretation

The main finding of this section is the importance of primary care management and the key role of the GP in return to work. The problem is lack of sufficient time, training and resources in primary care to address work issues adequately.

Workplace interventions

Under UK and European legislation, employers have a statutory duty to ensure the risks of harm from work are as small as reasonably practicable, and they have an equally important role in managing sickness absence (HSE 2004c). Sickness absence each year in the UK averages 7-8 days per employee and costs business £13-15 billion (CBI/AXA 2007; CIPD 2007) though the hidden costs are much higher (Bevan & Hayday 2001). The total cost to society of ill health in people of working age may be over £100 billion (Black 2008). Helping workers return to work brings a wide range of business benefits (HSE 2004c), so business has developed sickness absence and disability management policies and programmes (Table 6b).

The return to work process must involve and depends on the workplace. There is an increasing trend in recent years for vocational rehabilitation to be linked to the workplace.

D-7   ***   There is strong evidence that the return to work process and vocational rehabilitation interventions are more effective if they are closely linked to, or located in, the workplace.

Table 3: (Breen et al. 2007; Hagberg 2005; IASP 2005; Karjalainen et al. 2000; Loisel et al. 2003; Ostelo et al. 2005)

Table 6b: (Hill et al. 2007; IWH 2007; The Work Foundation 2006; WHO 1995)

D-8   #   Vocational rehabilitation cannot be considered in isolation but must be integrated into company policies for health and safety, occupational health, sickness absence management and disability management.

Table 6b: (ACOEM 2006; Boardman & Lyon 2006; CBI 2000; Curtis & Scott 2004; HSE 2004c; ILO 2002; TUC 2002)(IIAC 2007)

D-9   ***   There is strong evidence that temporary provision of modified work[26] reduces duration of sickness absence and increases return to work rates. It is often low-cost, and can be cost-effective.

Table 3: (Burton et al. 2008; Hanson et al. 2006; Talmage & Melhorn 2005; Waddell & Burton 2004; Weir & Nielson 2001)

Table 6b: (Brewer et al. 2007; Franche et al. 2005b; Greenstreet Berman Ltd 2004; Hill et al. 2007; Kumar 2001)

Table 7b: (Tompa et al. 2008)

---

26 Modified work is also referred to as transitional work arrangements, adjustments, or accommodations. These are changes to the individual's usual work tasks, equipment or organisation for the specific purpose of facilitating (early) return to work; it does not imply that work was the primary cause of the health problem. Work modification can be achieved, when required, through the use of ergonomics principles with input from the worker(s) concerned.

D-10   ***   There is strong evidence and considerable UK business experience that sickness absence and disability management is cost-effective, and may reduce sickness absence by 20-60%.

Table 3: (Franche et al. 2005b; Hanson et al. 2006)

Table 6b: (Brewer et al. 2007; CIPD 2007; Curtis & Scott 2004; Hanson et al. 2007; Marsden et al. 2004; Thornbory 2008) (IIAC 2007)

Table 7b: (Tompa et al. 2008)

D-11   #   There is considerable business experience and general consensus that effective sickness absence management should incorporate the following principles[27]:

- senior management engagement

- joint labour-management cooperation

- line managers playing a key role

- monitoring and information systems

- early, regular and sensitive contact with absent workers

- formal return to work plans and processes

- fast-tracking healthcare (if required)

- provision of modified working arrangements or adjustments (if required)

- use of case management (if required)

- use of structured vocational rehabilitation programmes (for the minority of workers who need them).

Table 6b: (EEF 2004; Employers' Forum on Disability 2008; HSE 2004b; HSE 2004c; ILO 2002; IWH 2007; James et al. 2002; James et al. 2003; Nice & Thornton 2004; NIDMAR 2000; TUC 2002)

D-12   0   There is a lack of evidence on effective occupational health and vocational rehabilitation models in small and medium enterprises[28].

Table 6b: (BOMEL Ltd 2005; Stephens et al. 2004; Tyers et al. 2007)

Table 6c: (Hanson et al. 2006)

---

27   Which of these principles are appropriate and practical will depend on the particular context.

28   Variously referred to as small and medium-sized enterprises, small and medium-sized businesses or small and medium businesses: they are companies whose headcount falls below certain limits (typically 250 employees in the European Union, 500 in the USA).

Examples

Sickness absence management policy

Rolls Royce implemented a sickness absence management policy and programme. Trade union representatives were consulted at the planning stage. All staff were trained on the new policies & procedures, explaining the responsibilities of managers, human resources and occupational health advisors. An IT programme was introduced to monitor absence, record the reasons for absence and calculate costs. Early rehabilitation was provided to anyone absent for 4+ weeks, including an action plan and physiotherapy services (for both work and non work-related injuries). The business benefits included: a reduction in staff absence from 2.9% (1999) to 2.4% (2002) of the workforce, compared with a national average of about 3.3%; a saving of around £11m; employees felt managers were positively interested in their prompt return to work; management time on absence spent more effectively (HSE 2005).

An RCT of an occupational health service

418 employees in construction, service and maintenance work, identified as being at high risk of sickness absence because of musculoskeletal or mental health problems, were randomised to an intervention group or 'usual care'. Those in the intervention group were invited to the occupational health service for a consultation, helped to construct an action plan to deal with their health problems, and referred for specialist treatment if appropriate. Mean sickness absence over the next 12 months was 19 days in the intervention group and 30 days in the usual care group. Economic evaluation showed that the intervention was cost saving and more cost-effective than usual care (Taimela et al. 2008a; Taimela et al. 2008b).

Interpretation

The main finding of this section is that proactive company approaches to sickness absence and disability management, together with accommodations and modified work, can be effective and have significant cost-benefits. Perhaps surprisingly, there is good evidence that workplace interventions can be more effective than healthcare interventions for work outcomes. There is a good business case for employers to take a proactive approach to supporting health at work, the return to work process, and vocational rehabilitation.

Another notable finding is the lack of evidence on return to work and vocational rehabilitation interventions in small and medium enterprises (SMEs) (D-12), which face particular problems in accessing and providing occupational health and vocational rehabilitation. Given the large proportion of the workforce employed by SMEs, there is pressing need to develop effective services to support them.

'Structured' vocational rehabilitation interventions

This section considers formal or 'structured' vocational rehabilitation interventions for workers who have more difficult problems, or who do not return to work quickly. The evidence covers various types of intervention, and comes from various areas.

Multidisciplinary interventions involve a number of professionals from different clinical disciplines working together. Disease management is an evidence-based, multidisciplinary approach to long-term healthcare delivery for patients with chronic conditions, and includes the use of pathways and protocols. Case management is 'a collaborative process which assesses, plans, implements, coordinates, monitors and evaluates the options and services required to meet an individual's healthcare, educational and employment needs, using communication and available resources to promote quality, cost-effective outcomes' (Case Management Society UK, www.cmsuk.org).

D-13   ***   There is strong evidence (mainly in musculoskeletal conditions) that multidisciplinary interventions that address health, personal *and* workplace factors (a 'biopsychosocial' approach), and that are linked to the workplace, *can be* effective and cost-effective for improving occupational outcomes.

> Table 3: (Burton et al. 2008; de Buck et al. 2002; Loisel et al. 2003; Schonstein et al. 2003; Selander et al. 2002; van Geen et al. 2007; Zampolini et al. 2007)
>
> Table 6c: (Dunstan & Covic 2006; Gobelet et al. 2007a; Kenyon 2003; Shaw et al. 2007; WAG 2006)
>
> Table 7a: (Waddell & Burton 2004)

D-14   *   Although disease management interventions are effective and cost-effective for health outcomes, there is limited evidence that they improve occupational outcomes for certain health conditions (e.g. depression and asthma) and the effect size is small.

> Table 4a: (Kates & Mach 2007; Neumeyer-Gromen et al. 2004)
>
> Table 5b: (Gibson et al. 2002; Goetzel et al. 2005; Ofman et al. 2004; Toelle & Ram 2004; Van Weel et al. 2006)
>
> Table 6c: (Goetzel et al. 2005)

D-15   **   There is moderate evidence that the use of case management approaches, including return to work coordinators, is effective and cost-effective for occupational outcomes.

> Table 3: (Burton et al. 2008; Cole et al. 2006; Shaw et al. 2002)
>
> Table 4: (Pirraglia et al. 2004)
>
> Table 6c: (Green-McKenzie et al. 2004; Hanson et al. 2006; Shaw et al. 2007)

Interpretation

The main finding of this section is that structured vocational rehabilitation interventions can be effective and cost-effective (the evidence being strongest for workers with musculoskeletal conditions). These interventions and 'programmes' can (but do not have to) involve significant resources and costs, but the evidence shows they can be devised and delivered in cost-effective ways. They should be reserved for individuals who are experiencing difficulty in returning to work.

Social security and policy interventions

In the UK only about 50% of adults with a limiting long-standing illness or long-term disability are employed, compared with 74% for non-disabled people. The main UK social security benefit relevant to vocational rehabilitation is Incapacity Benefit (IB)[29]. For employees, IB follows a period of Statutory Sick Pay from the employer and generally does not start till the 29th week of sickness absence. However, about 60% of recipients are not employed at the point of starting benefits. In addition to their health problem, many IB recipients have multiple disadvantages and face multiple barriers in returning to work: age (half are aged >50 years), poor work history (one-third of new recipients have already been out of work for >2 years), low skills (40% have no qualifications, 15% have basic skills problems), high local unemployment rates and employer discrimination (Waddell & Aylward 2005). Once recipients have been on IB for more than 1-2 years, they are likely to remain on benefits long-term (Waddell et al. 2003).

D-16   #   Vocational rehabilitation is one element of broader health, employment and social policies, and must be set in that context.

Table 6d: (Gründemann 1997; Leigh-Doyle & Mulvihill 2004; Scottish Executive 2004; Waddell et al. 2002; Wynne & McAnaney 2004)

D-17   **   There is moderate evidence that personal advice and support, incorporating case management approaches, is an effective method of delivering employment services to clients with a disability or chronic illness.

Table 6d: (Bambra et al. 2005; Corden & Thornton 2002; Wynne et al. 2006)(DWP-2)

D-18   **   Structured vocational rehabilitation interventions can improve work outcomes for claimants/beneficiaries in the early stages of IB (or similar benefits)[30].

Table 6d: (Leech 2004)(DWP-2)(DWP-3)

---

29 Incapacity Benefit is due to be replaced by Employment and Support Allowance from October 2008, but the recipients and their characteristics are likely to be very similar to those currently on IB. Other disability benefits include Disability Living Allowance, Income Support with disability premium and Industrial Injuries Disablement Benefit (IIDB).

30 Although these are not 'high quality scientific studies' as defined in Box 1, they are careful studies in 'the real world' which involved many thousands of benefit claimants and they compared the interventions with control data.

D-19   0   There is no high quality evidence on effective and cost-effective vocational rehabilitation interventions for people who have been on IB long-term (more than 1 year on benefits)[31]

Table 6d: (Bambra et al. 2005; Hogelund 2001; Thornton et al. 2003; Waddell et al. 2002)

Examples

DWP Job Retention and Rehabilitation Pilot

This was a randomised controlled trial in six areas of the UK. 2845 people with sickness absence of 6-28 weeks but who were still employed received a healthcare intervention, a workplace intervention, the combination, or 'usual care'. There were almost identical return-to-work rates for each of the four groups: 44% for the healthcare intervention; 45% for the workplace intervention; 44% for the combined intervention; and 45% for the control group. It had a negative impact on people with mental health problems.

The JRRP is sometimes quoted as 'proving' that vocational rehabilitation and early intervention do not work. That is contrary to all the other scientific evidence. The organization, planning and management of the JRRP were so bad they probably foredoomed it to failure. There are doubts (and no clear evidence) whether the health and workplace interventions were comparable to what current scientific evidence shows to be effective. What the JRRP proved is that *this trial was a failure - nothing more.* (See Table 6d, (DWP-1) for more detailed analysis of the JRRP).

DWP *Pathways to Work*

Pathways to work is an integrated package of support provided by DWP and the NHS and designed to help Incapacity Benefit (IB) recipients to manage their health problems and get back to work. It consists of: 1) a mandatory Work Focused Interview with a DWP Personal Adviser; 2) a Choices package of work focused support provided by DWP; 3) innovative, NHS Condition Management Programmes; and 4) Return to work Credits (financial support). Pilot studies started in October 2003 and it is being progressively rolled out across the UK.

- By March 2008, 564,570 people had taken part.

- Participants were generally satisfied with the programme and the support received.

- 35% were in paid work a year later, and a further 20% were actively looking for work or waiting to start a job.

- *Pathways* has been variously estimated to increase the number who entered work by 7-9% though it was more effective for claimants with musculoskeletal conditions and less effective for those with mental health conditions.

- Cost-benefit analysis shows that overall *Pathways* is saving the Exchequer money.

Pathways to work is one of the largest and most successful social security pilot studies in the world for clients with health problems. It has a much higher take-up rate than most social security pilots. It is one of the few to demonstrate a significant and sustained impact on work outcomes. It has received very positive publicity. (See Table 6d, (DWP-3) for more detailed analysis of *Pathways).*

---

31   There are some isolated reports of successful vocational rehabilitation interventions for long-term social security recipients (Desouza et al. 2007; Watson et al. 2004), but they reported on small numbers of selected individuals.

Interpretation

Historically, most pilot studies of individual-level vocational rehabilitation interventions for social security clients had (very) low uptake, limited effect on occupational outcomes, and doubtful cost-effectiveness (Thornton et al. 2003; Waddell et al. 2002). *Pathways to work* is the most successful social security pilot study of an individual-level vocational rehabilitation intervention for Incapacity Benefit claimants, both in terms of its high uptake and its significant and sustained impact on entering work. The only comparable success was in the Irish Renaissance Project (Leech 2004), which was solely for new claimants with low back pain.

No vocational rehabilitation interventions have been shown to be effective for benefit recipients who have been on benefits and/or out of work more than about 1-2 years. The available evidence therefore supports the rationale of providing any vocational rehabilitation intervention *before* people become trapped on benefits (OECD 2003; Thornton et al. 2003; Waddell & Aylward 2005).

TIMING AND COORDINATION

Table 7 lays out the evidence: 7a on timing and 7b on coordination. Evidence linking on these generic issues is also drawn from other sections of the Findings.

Timing

Sickness and disability are dynamic processes over time, so clinical and workplace management - and vocational rehabilitation interventions - must be tailored to suit the stage of the illness (Franche & Krause 2002; Waddell & Burton 2004; Young et al. 2005a). Anyone who stops work because of a health problem sets off on a 'patient journey' that can end in full or partial return to work (for most) or long-term incapacity (for a minority). Over the course of that journey, personal, health, and occupational factors change. Returning to work after a few days or weeks is very different from the prospect of obtaining and starting a new job after long-term incapacity. The obstacles to return to work and the clinical, workplace and vocational rehabilitation interventions required to overcome them become more complex over time (Waddell & Burton 2004). This 'timeline' can be used to guide clinical, workplace and vocational rehabilitation interventions.

The high prevalence and fluctuating nature of many common health problems makes it difficult to define the 'start' and duration of an episode. A more pragmatic approach is to focus on duration of sickness absence, which is simpler to define and identify. Time on benefits should be distinguished from time out of work; what matters is whether or not the individual is still employed and the time since they last worked, rather than time on benefits.

TC-1   #   In the absence of any clear boundary between everyday symptoms, illness and incapacity for work, medicalisation can be harmful and cause iatrogenic disability[32].

Table 3: (Talmage & Melhorn 2005; Zampolini et al. 2007)

Table 7a: (Balderson & Von Korff 2002; Frank et al. 1996; Pilgrim & Bentall 1999; Rose 2007; Von Korff 1999; Wessely 2002)

TC-2   ***   There is strong evidence that the longer the duration of sickness absence, the lower the chances of return to work, and the greater the obstacles to return to work and vocational rehabilitation[33]. Depending on context, workers who are off work for 4-12 weeks then have a 10-40% risk of still being off work at one year.

Table 3: (COST B13 Working Group 2004; IASP 2005)

Table 7a: (Joling et al. 2006; Waddell et al. 2003; Waddell & Burton 2004)

TC-3   #   Workers compensation and insurance company experience supports the use of disability duration guidelines on appropriate duration of sickness absence.

Table 7a: (Harris et al. 2001; Prezzia & Denniston 2001)

TC-4   ***   There is strong evidence that simple, inexpensive healthcare and workplace interventions in the early stages of sickness absence can be effective and cost-effective for increasing return to work rates and reducing the number of people who go on to long-term disability.

Table 3: (Breen et al. 2007; Brox et al. 2007; Burton et al. 2008; Carter & Birrell 2000; EASHAW 2007; Gross et al. 2006; Hanson et al. 2006; Mueller et al. 2003; Nash et al. 2004)

Table 7a: (DH 2004; Frank et al. 1998; Frank et al. 1996; Waddell & Burton 2004)

---

32 Medicalisation is the process by which events or conditions of everyday life come to be defined and treated as health problems and a matter for medical diagnosis and treatment. This labelling is typically associated with changed perceptions, expectations, and management of the condition.

33 This is probably largely due to 'state dependency' and also some element of 'omitted heterogeneity'. State dependence is when individuals get worse and therefore the probability of each individual returning to work declines with time. Omitted heterogeneity is when different individuals (e.g. a 25 year old and a 55 year old) each have intrinsically different rates of returning to work but for each individual that rate remains constant over time, so that as duration increases those most likely to recover and easiest to help return to work, leaving behind those who are less likely to return to work and harder to help.

TC-5   ***   There is strong evidence that structured vocational rehabilitation interventions are effective (and limited evidence that they are cost-effective) between about 1 and 6+ months sickness absence (though the exact limits are unclear).

Table 3: (Hoffman et al. 2007; Loisel et al. 2003; Schonstein et al. 2003; Seferiadis et al. 2004)

Table 7a: (Frank et al. 1998; Frank et al. 1996; Waddell et al. 2003; Waddell & Burton 2004)

TC-6   #   There is a good rational argument and general consensus that a stepped-care approach[34] provides an optimal framework for allocating finite resources most appropriately and efficiently to meet individual needs.

Table 3: (Breen et al. 2007; Burton et al. 2008; Loisel et al. 2003)

Table 7a: (DH 2004; Frank et al. 1998; Frank et al. 1996; Freud 2007; Stephens & Gross 2007; Von Korff 1999; Von Korff et al. 2002; Waddell & Burton 2004)

Interpretation

A central theme of this section is the concept of early intervention, with the rationale that it is simpler, more effective and likely to be most cost-effective to prevent people with common health problems going on to long-term incapacity. With more prolonged time off work, helping people return to work becomes progressively more complex, resource-intensive and costly, and its success rate lower. The critical question is what is 'early'?

There is strong evidence about the timing of interventions for musculoskeletal disorders (TC-2). The general principles apply equally to other conditions (TC-3; Waddell et al 2003; Waddell & Burton 2004), though further evidence is required on whether the exact timing may need to be adjusted, particularly for mental health problems.

In the first 3-6 weeks[35] of sickness absence, the likelihood of recovery and rapid return to work is high, with or without healthcare. The great majority of workers with common health problems return to work quickly and uneventfully. Intervention at this stage should be limited to good clinical and workplace management and practice; there is no need for more structured vocational rehabilitation interventions.

---

34 Stepped care is not an intervention in itself, rather an approach that guides care based on individual needs: in essence it delivers just what's needed when it's needed for the individual, whilst permitting allocation of resources to greatest effect on a population basis.

35 Various studies define a transition point at which symptoms are less likely to resolve spontaneously; there is insufficient evidence to decide precisely when that point should be, but it is generally agreed to lie between 3 and 6 weeks.

The evidence suggests that structured vocational rehabilitation interventions are most effective between about 1 and 6+ months sickness absence, though the exact boundaries for the optimal 'window of opportunity' are unclear. It depends on the context just when the window commences, but as time passes the worker's needs increase. The best evidence on the upper limit for effective interventions is between 3-6 months; there is progressively less evidence for effectiveness between 6-12 months, and very little for interventions after 12 months. That is consistent with the social security evidence about the most effective intervention being for new claimants (D-18). In principle, and on the balance of the evidence, the sooner intervention takes place within that optimal window the more effective it is likely to be, and the risks of delay generally outweigh concerns about 'deadweight'. Ideally, structured intervention should be initiated as soon as possible after about six weeks of sickness absence; every effort should be made to avoid undue delay, certainly beyond six months. There is scope for piloting the timing of structured interventions within that window to suit a particular context.

Ideally, individuals at risk of long-term incapacity might be identified early and provided with more intensive vocational rehabilitation. Unfortunately, the accuracy of such 'screening' is low (Frank et al. 1996; Waddell et al. 2003) and the most reliable proxy for identifying those who need extra help is the duration of sickness absence (Freud 2007; Waddell et al. 2003). The logical approach then is a 'stepped-care approach' (TC-6). This starts with simple, low-intensity, low-cost interventions and 'steps up' to more intensive, complex and costly interventions for people who fail to respond. It sequences and coordinates individual, healthcare and workplace interventions, based on functional outcomes. It provides a practical framework for allocating finite resources to those individuals with greatest needs and to the greatest effect on a population basis.

Coordination: 'all players onside' and communication

Many stakeholders have an interest in work and health: workers, employers, trade unions, insurers, health professionals, policy makers and government. For most short-term sickness absence, the key players[36] in the return to work process are the worker/patient, GP and employer. For longer-term sickness absence, vocational rehabilitation may involve a more extensive list of players: which may include any combination of the worker/patient, GP and primary care team, employer, occupational health, rehabilitation team, insurer, case manager, and DWP Personal Adviser. Different stakeholders have different perspectives, agendas and budgets, which are not always aligned. Vocational rehabilitation interventions will only be successful if the various players work together and not at cross-purposes. And the development of vocational rehabilitation policy depends on keeping all stakeholders onside.

---

36 The term 'players' is used to denote individuals or groups whose active participation in the return to work process is essential for its effectiveness. The term 'stakeholders' refers to individuals or groups who have an interest in the outcome of the process – but who may or may not be active players.

TC-7   ***   There is strong evidence that vocational rehabilitation is more effective if all players recognise their roles in the return to work process, take responsibility and play their parts when appropriate. However, implementing this can be difficult.

Table 3: (Bongers et al. 2006; Cole et al. 2006; Feldman 2004; Hanson et al. 2006; Kunkel & Miller 2002; MacEachen et al. 2006; Selander et al. 2002; Williams & Westmorland 2002)

Table 6c: (Frank & Thurgood 2006; IUA/ABI 2007)

Table 6d: (Leigh-Doyle & Mulvihill 2004)

Table 7b: (Franche et al. 2005a; Freeman 2004; Lerner et al. 2005; OECD 2003; Pransky et al. 2004; Pransky et al. 2005; Young et al. 2005b)

TC-8   ***   There is strong evidence that improved communication between all players leads to faster return to work and less sickness absence overall, and is cost-effective.

Table 3: (Bongers et al. 2006; Franche et al. 2005b; Gross et al. 2006; Loisel et al. 2003; MacEachen et al. 2006; Selander et al. 2002; Shaw et al. 2002)

Table 6c: (Gobelet et al. 2007a; Shaw et al. 2007; Von Korff et al. 2002)

Table 6d: (Leigh-Doyle & Mulvihill 2004)

Table 7b: (Franche et al. 2005a; Frank et al. 1998; OECD 2003; Tompa et al. 2008)

TC-9   **   There is moderate evidence that the duration of sickness absence is significantly reduced by early and sustained contact between the employer and absent workers.

Table 3: (Carter & Birrell 2000; Hagberg 2005; Hanson et al. 2006)

Table 6b: (Franche et al. 2005b; HSE 2004c)(IIAC 2007)

TC-10   ***   There is strong evidence that the duration of sickness absence is significantly reduced by contact between healthcare provider and the workplace.

Table 6b: (Franche et al. 2005b; Norwich Union Healthcare 2006)

Table 7b: (Beaumont 2003a; Beaumont 2003b; Sawney & Challenor 2003; Tompa et al. 2008)

Example

A classic example of good workplace communication

When workers were off work with back injuries their supervisor phoned to say: 'How are you? We are thinking about you. You are a vital part of the team. Your work is important and your job is waiting for you.' That simple message, and the company culture it reflected, cut the number staying off long-term from 7.1% to 1.7% (Wood 1987).

Interpretation

No single professional group or service can deliver effective vocational rehabilitation for everyone who needs it, so communication and coordination of effort is essential. Unfortunately, communication between employers and absent workers, and between GPs and employers (and occupational health professionals) is usually non-existent or inadequate. Lack of (effective) communication is a major barrier to vocational rehabilitation and the return to work process, and there is broad agreement that communication needs to be improved (Beaumont 2003a; Beaumont 2003b; MacEachen et al. 2006; Shaw et al. 2002).

Healthcare, the workplace and vocational rehabilitation

These Findings emphasise the need to reconsider the relationship between healthcare, the workplace, and vocational rehabilitation.

The primary goal of healthcare is to treat any specific pathology and to relieve symptoms. Most people sick-listed with a common health problem do return to work relatively quickly and uneventfully, but if they do not, healthcare often fails to address work outcomes (MH-2, CR-2) and may be insufficient by itself to improve work outcomes (MSD-5, MH-4, MH-5, MH-7, CR-3, CR-11). There is strong evidence that work outcomes are improved if clinical management is linked to the workplace (MSD-6, D-7, D-13).

On the other hand, current company provision of 'vocational rehabilitation' in the UK is largely about expediting healthcare (CBI/AXA 2007). Employers tend to wait passively for healthcare to 'cure' the problem. The present Findings show the limitations of this approach and suggest that what happens in the workplace itself is actually more important for work outcomes (MSD-6, MH-9, MH-11, D-7, D-10). There is strong evidence for a more proactive approach to sickness absence (D-10, D-11) and on the value of modified work and workplace accommodations (MSD-7, D-9).

Overall, the evidence in this review shows that effective return-to-work and vocational rehabilitation interventions depend on:

1. **Healthcare which includes a focus on work** (incorporating the *idea* of vocational rehabilitation, early intervention, and intervention tailored to individual needs);

and

2. **Workplaces that are accommodating** (incorporating a proactive approach to supporting return–to-work, and the temporary provision of modified work and accommodations).

Both are necessary: they are inter-dependent. To make a real and lasting difference, both need to be addressed and coordinated.

More than 90% of people with common health problems (Waddell et al. 2003) can be helped to return to work by following a few basic principles of good healthcare and workplace management (MSD-4, MSD-7, MSD-8, D-10, D-13, D-15, TC-4). Yet these simple measures, together with structured vocational rehabilitation interventions for those who need additional help, could reduce long-term sickness absence and the number of workers going on to long-term incapacity benefits by 20-60% (MSD-8, D-10, TC-4).

Improving work outcomes depends not only on the availability of effective interventions, but on whether workers receive them. The first challenge is to get health professionals and employers to change their thinking and practice to implement what the evidence shows to be effective. GPs need to be convinced that work is a vitally important health outcome; employers need to be convinced that they have a critical role in facilitating work outcomes. The second challenge is to ensure workers have universal access to appropriate help.

The benefits for the individual are obvious: better health and work outcomes, and the prevention of long-term sickness and disability with all its social and economic consequences. Health budgets could see savings from reduced healthcare consumption and the high costs of chronic illness. Employers have a good business case. Government and society stand to gain from increased employment rates and reduced social expenditure on ill-health.

This all needs to be underpinned by raised awareness and understanding of the evidence that work is generally good for health and that return to work can promote recovery (Black 2008; Waddell & Burton 2006). Public education that includes workers, employers and health professionals has the potential to support the necessary cultural change (Buchbinder et al. 2001; Waddell et al. 2007).

More specifically, it is important to address the concern that staying at work or early return to work might aggravate a worker's health condition, particularly if that condition is attributed to work (see Appendix 2). Ready access to healthcare for advice and treatment is important, but that must be balanced against the risk of medicalising everyday symptoms and causing iatrogenic disability (TC-1). Concerns about work having an adverse effect on health are often over-emphasised: various aspects of work can certainly influence symptoms, but the high prevalence of common health problems in the general population means that work has a limited role in primary causation (Appendix 2; Waddell & Burton 2004). The balance of the evidence is that (early) return to work does not make these conditions worse, and it usually *reduces* rather than increases the risks of recurrent symptoms and 're-injury' (MSD-3, MH-1). The beneficial effects of work on physical and mental health and well-being generally outweigh the risks of work and the harmful effects of prolonged sickness absence (Waddell & Burton 2006). Overall, the presumption should be that staying at or returning to work is beneficial, unless there is evidence in the individual case to the contrary (e.g. occupational asthma, where exposure to the causal hazard should be avoided). Facilitating return to work through workplace accommodation is preferable to prolonging sickness absence 'to play safe'.

Implications for policy

These Findings have implications for Government strategy to improve the health of working age people (Black 2008; HM Government 2005; HSC 2000). A more detailed discussion of the implications for healthcare and workplace practice will be published elsewhere.

This review has demonstrated that there is now strong scientific evidence for many aspects of vocational rehabilitation – *what works, for whom and when*. It has also shown that there is a good business case for vocational rehabilitation, and more evidence on cost-benefits (MSD-11, MH-12, CR-4, D-15, TC-8) than for many health and social policy areas. Insufficient evidence can no longer be used as an excuse for inaction.

This review has also demonstrated the need to give high priority to common health problems. Mild/moderate musculoskeletal, mental health and cardio-respiratory conditions are responsible for as much human suffering, morbidity, and disability as serious diseases[37]. They account for about two-thirds of long-term sickness absence, incapacity for work and ill health retirement (CBI/AXA 2007; CIPD 2007); DWP administrative statistics), which has been estimated to cost UK over £100 billion each year (Black 2008). Most important, many of these conditions should be manageable and there is good evidence that many of these consequences are preventable *if people are provided with suitable advice and effective help.*

In general, vocational rehabilitation principles and interventions should be the same whether or not the health condition is work-related, and whether it is classified as an injury or a disease (see Appendix 2).

In principle, the earlier someone with a health problem can be helped to return to work, the better for the individual, the employer and society. The evidence in this review demonstrates that early intervention can be simple, inexpensive, and effective (MSD-4, D-9, TC-4). As sickness absence becomes more prolonged, and especially once the person is no longer employed, vocational rehabilitation becomes more complex (MSD-8, D-13, D-15, TC-5). The appropriate level of care should then be provided to meet individual need, which changes over time (TC-2), so that those with simple needs receive a 'light touch' approach, and only those in greatest need receive more intensive and costly interventions. This 'stepped-care' approach permits the most efficient use of finite resources (TC-6).

---

37   Priority areas and targets in the NHS Planning Framework and the Public Service Agreement Objectives (DH 2002) centre on 'major killer diseases' such as cancer and coronary heart disease, mental health, waiting times for appointments and treatment, healthcare for older people and improving life chances for children. Although mental health is included, DH priorities and targets are about severe mental illness, psychiatric services and suicide.

The implication is that vocational rehabilitation is not a single intervention or service or the preserve of any one profession: a wide range of stakeholders have roles and responsibilities for delivery. It is as much an idea and an approach to *helping people with health problems stay at, return to and remain in work*. Help can be provided in various ways using interventions of differing intensity delivered by different stakeholders. The policy question is how to make sure that everyone receives the help they need. Logically, this should start from the needs of people with health problems (at various stages); build on the evidence about effective interventions; and finally consider potential resources and the practicalities of how these interventions might be delivered. From a policy perspective, there are three broad types of clients, who are differentiated mainly by duration out of work, and who have correspondingly different needs:

- Most newly sick or injured workers, within the first six weeks or so of sickness absence, need work-focused healthcare coupled with proactive workplace management.

- A minority of workers (possibly 5-10% (Waddell et al 2003)), who are having difficulty returning to work after about six weeks sickness absence[38], need a structured vocational rehabilitation intervention.

- The long-term incapacitated, who are more than about 6 months out of work, need an intervention that can address the substantial personal and social barriers, including help with re-employment.

All of these must be done to address the totality of need. They form an integrated package, with close coordination between the various 'services' to provide seamless case transfer so that no-one falls between the cracks.

HEALTHCARE AND WORKPLACE MANAGEMENT

The policy goal here is to promote work-focused healthcare *and* accommodating workplaces.

The healthcare professions acknowledge the need to place greater priority on working health, supporting return to work and work outcomes, e.g. in the recent Healthcare Professionals' Consensus Statement (Black 2008). Yet this still does not occur in many areas of healthcare (MH-2, CR-2, D-5). Many health professionals feel they lack expertise in this area (D-3) and have insufficient time or resources to contribute effectively (D-1, D-5).

---

38   See earlier section on Timing for discussion of when this intervention should occur. Account must also be taken of practicalities.

Good employers recognise the value of a more proactive approach to facilitating the return to work process (D-9, D-10, D-11). However, *all* employers need to be convinced that they have a crucial role, and that they have a good business case to fulfil it.

There is an urgent need to develop methods of delivering effective vocational rehabilitation support for SMEs, who are always difficult to reach and help. Other occupational groups face similar difficulties (e.g. temporary, agency, part-time and self-employed workers).

No Government department has any direct involvement with the individual in the early stage of sickness absence[39]. Nevertheless, Government has a vital interest, because success at this stage minimises the number of people who go on to longer term sickness or to disability and incapacity benefits. Government is then dependent on other stakeholders, so policy should be directed to 'shifting the culture' and to expanding the skills of health professionals and employers:

- Promoting the evidence and the business case for better healthcare and workplace management of common health problems.

- Helping to provide advice, training and support for healthcare professionals and employers to deliver this management.

- Keeping the key stakeholders on side – unions, employers, insurers and health professionals.

This can be done with existing or minimal additional resources, and is low cost or cost-neutral.

STRUCTURED VOCATIONAL REHABILITATION

No matter how much healthcare and workplace management are improved, there will always be a minority of people (possibly 5-10% (Waddell et al. 2003)) who do not return to work in a timely manner and who need additional help. And because of the prevalence of common health problems, they will add up to large numbers.

Lack of appropriate (vocational) help for these people is one of the greatest gaps in current UK services. The problem is that there are no NHS vocational rehabilitation services (BSRM 2000). Instead, patients are referred to various medical specialties, which do not meet their vocational rehabilitation needs, and this delays more appropriate intervention. At the same time, provision of vocational rehabilitation through occupational health or private providers is fragmentary and only available to a minority of workers (Black 2008).

---

39 Obviously government departments do have direct involvement with their own employees, where it may be argued that Government should set an example of best practice.

Yet there is strong evidence that structured vocational rehabilitation interventions at this stage are effective and cost-effective (MSD-8, MH-9, D-11, D-13, D-15, TC-5). The evidence on musculoskeletal conditions provides the best template: key elements include: rapid access; individualised advice, assessment and treatment; a focus on work outcomes; and close links to the workplace (MSD-6, MSD-8, D-13). Many of these principles appear generic, though they should be applied with caution and may need to be adapted for other conditions. The policy challenge is to develop ways of delivering these interventions on a national scale.

Workers with common health problems who remain sick listed after about six weeks should be considered for a more structured vocational rehabilitation intervention. Important operational issues are: (1) to identify these people promptly; and (2) to assign responsibility for ensuring that the review and referral process takes place. Every worker in this situation requires a sick certificate, so primary health care or the sick certification system could provide a universal entry point to any service. In practice, GPs may need additional tools (e.g. built into computerised medical records or sick certification systems) and support (e.g. by practice staff, therapists or work advisers). Self-referral is a further option that has been shown to be efficient in a similar context (HTA 2008).

There are examples of successful delivery models: a) within NHS services (HTA 2008); b) in business (HSE 2005); and c) integrating healthcare and workplace interventions (Loisel et al. 2003). More generally, however, the evidence in this review suggests that the delivery system:

- Should *not* consist of healthcare alone, as that is generally insufficient to improve work outcomes at this stage (MSD-5, MH-4, MH-5, MH-7, CR-3, CR-11). Following the same principle of demedicalisation, any healthcare element should be at primary care or community level, and *not* a hospital specialty.

- Should consist of *both* healthcare and workplace elements, which must be closely coordinated (MSD-6, D-7, D-13).

- Requires both healthcare and workplace elements to take a proactive approach to *helping people with health problems return to work* (rather than focusing on 'treatment' and 'sickness absence management' respectively).

Clearly, many of the principles are the same as in the previous stage. The issue now is how to provide them in a more structured form for those workers for whom routine healthcare and workplace management has not achieved return to work.

There are then linked questions of *who* might provide these structured vocational rehabilitation interventions and *where* they might be provided. As far as possible, this should build on existing resources. Healthcare possibilities include primary health care, physiotherapists, occupational therapists (when available), psychotherapists, and community mental health teams. The recent proposal to recruit an additional 3600 psychological therapists (DH 2008) offers a timely opportunity for an innovative approach. In principle, occupational health could provide an ideal bridge between healthcare and the workplace, though it is presently dispersed between the NHS, industry and private providers, and there are limitations of manpower and access. There are increasing numbers of rehabilitation providers in the UK, though many are outside the NHS, and with widely varying professional backgrounds and training. In the workplace, line managers have a key role and, ideally, any intervention should reach them. Workplace personnel who could potentially play a part in any service include union and health and safety representatives, occupational safety and health professionals, and human resources staff. The crux of the matter is striking the balance between healthcare and the focus on work – in staffing, in the location, and in the functioning of the service. It is not enough for any of these healthcare or workplace personnel to continue 'doing their thing': work outcomes will only be improved if they deliver a work-focused service in the manner outlined above. There would therefore need to be careful selection and training of suitable staff to ensure that they have the necessary skills and, most important, the fundamental shift in focus and ethos required to deliver effective vocational rehabilitation interventions.

Any system must be sufficiently flexible to provide different kinds and intensity of help according to individual needs. Many workers require relatively simple help, which may vary from individual to individual, but the obstacles to return to work change over time from six weeks to six months sickness absence. Therefore, there can never be a single, inflexible service. Coordination is then vital (TC-7 to TC-10). The key element that would need to be created afresh is a single Gateway that takes all those identified after about six weeks sickness absence and provides a) individual needs assessment, b) signposting to the appropriate help, and c) coordination of healthcare and workplace interventions to facilitate the return to work process. This is essentially a case management approach, though only the most complex cases may need formal case management (Hanson et al. 2006).

The other important issue is independent assurance of the content and quality of the interventions provided – to make sure that there is the necessary shift from a 'clinical' service to true vocational rehabilitation, and including objective assessment of standards of practice, performance indicators and outcome measures. This could well be a continuing function of the Gateway. Possible allies include HSE and health and safety inspectors, who have a strong national structure, legislative power and universal access to business. They are in a position to promote vocational rehabilitation, but that would require a major shift in focus from 'safety' to 'working health and well-being'.

Only government is in a position to provide a universal and integrated identification system, Gateway and quality assurance system for a structured vocational rehabilitation service.

Development of structured vocational rehabilitation services would require investment of resources and funding, but there is good evidence on the likely cost-benefits (MSD-11, D-10, D-13). Funding could be by various government departments, insurers and/or employers, all of whom stand to make financial savings. Consideration might also be given to the tax regime for occupational health and vocational rehabilitation provisions, for both employers and individuals.

High quality pilot studies will be required to improve the evidence base on the effectiveness and cost-benefits of service delivery model(s) in the UK context.

Mental health problems remain an ongoing challenge (MH-4, MH-5, MH-7). One of the most urgent priorities must be research and development to improve the effectiveness of vocational rehabilitation interventions for workers with mental health problems (Black 2008; Lelliott et al. 2008). Despite the present lack of evidence on cost-effectiveness (MH-12), the human, social and economic costs of mental health problems make this well worth pursuing[40] (Dewa et al. 2007; McDaid et al. 2005; Steffick et al. 2006; Sullivan 2005; The Sainsbury Centre for Mental Health 2007; WHO 2005).

Clearly, many of these issues would need to be addressed in planning the proposed *Fit for Work* service (Black 2008) and any other future developments.

HELP FOR THE LONG-TERM SICK

The evidence in this review shows that early intervention can prevent people with common health problems ever reaching the stage of disability and incapacity benefits, and is likely to be cost-effective (OECD 2003; Waddell & Burton 2004). Providing early access to effective help should be the policy imperative.

Nevertheless, provision must be made for those who do reach this stage. There will always be some inflow from the failures of healthcare and workplace management, and even of structured vocational rehabilitation services. There is also an ongoing need to try to rehabilitate the stock of long-term benefit recipients, and to assist those who have never worked due to sickness or disability. These individuals can be effectively helped to return to independence and employment. While this requires more resources than are needed at earlier stages, it can still be cost-effective.

These people face multiple obstacles to (return to) work: a health problem; long-term work absence (comparable to unemployment); and often multiple social disadvantages (Waddell & Aylward 2005). Vocational rehabilitation at this stage must extend beyond treatment to

---

40   The direct and indirect costs of mental health problems such as anxiety and depression are high, and these are borne by all stakeholders (Andlin-Sobocki & Wittchen 2005; Löthgren 2004a; Löthgren 2004b). However, it has been pointed out that benefits from improvements are spread across stakeholders and therefore diluted, which means each stakeholder perceives less incentive to invest in mental health outcomes (Dewa et al. 2007)).

condition management, and include capability to deal with problems of motivation and confidence. It must also address labour market issues including (where necessary) work trials, short training courses, and training in job seeking skills. Employers need to be engaged to provide suitable job opportunities to workers if the transition to economic independence is to be successful. Although the evidence shows that not all clients require all the elements, service provision must inevitably be multidisciplinary and designed specifically to meet complex needs.

Pathways to work is the most effective example to date of such an intervention (See Table 6d - DWP-3). *Pathways* increases the return to work rate of new claimants by 7-9% and cost-benefit analysis shows that it saves the Exchequer money. Continuing research and evaluation is required to identify the most effective and cost-effective elements of the package, the best models of service delivery, and how best to improve *Pathways* for clients with mental health problems and the stock of long-term clients.

There is scope to improve vocational rehabilitation for workers who are long-term incapacitated by occupational asthma and work-related asthma (CR-9, CR-10). Most patients with occupational asthma are medically fit for some work; for those who cannot return to their previous job, there is a good rationale and general consensus for retraining, re-placement and support into alternative employment[41] (CR-11). In view of the working life expectancy of these workers, this is likely to be a worthwhile use of resources.

The lack of good evidence on effective interventions for recipients who have been on benefits for more than 1 year (D-19) reinforces the need to intervene *before* people become trapped on benefits.

---

41 It may be argued that issues of retraining and placement could apply more generally. However, occupational asthma and similar conditions affect finite numbers of people, are objective medical conditions, and have a clear work causation; many of the other common health problems are more subjective, difficult to define or assess objectively, and potentially involve very large numbers of people.

Practical suggestions

- The fundamental principle is that everyone of working age should have access to vocational rehabilitation, at the appropriate level for their needs.

- Vocational rehabilitation should be integrated into the *Health, Work and Well-Being Strategy* and broader government policies on health, employment and occupational health.

- Common health problems – mild/moderate musculoskeletal, mental health and cardio-respiratory conditions – should get high priority in both work and health policy, and healthcare delivery.

- Return to work should be one of the key performance indicators of healthcare. Health policy, clinical guidelines, research, and audit should routinely include work outcomes. Government funded research bodies, NICE and SIGN[42], and the Cochrane Collaboration might make this mandatory.

- Employers have a key role in vocational rehabilitation and should take a proactive approach to facilitating return to work and accommodating workers with common health problems.

- ***Healthcare and workplace management***

    - Policy should be directed to persuading and supporting health professionals and employers to implement basic principles of good healthcare and workplace management.

    o *Healthcare*

        - Government should continue to support the appropriate professional bodies to enhance undergraduate and post-graduate education and training, including continuing professional education on work and health issues, and on vocational rehabilitation. This should be extended to non-health professions in and around the workplace.

        - Better methods should be developed and evaluated to support primary healthcare on work and health issues.

---

42   NICE and SIGN now recognise this.

o *Workplace*

- Government should work with employers' organisations to develop and promote the business case for vocational rehabilitation.

- Better methods should be developed and evaluated to support business on work and health issues.

- There is a particular need to develop methods of delivering effective vocational rehabilitation support for SMEs.

o *Communication*

- There is a need to develop practical and effective methods of communication between healthcare and the workplace.

- **Vocational rehabilitation services**

  - There is a need to develop systems of delivering effective vocational rehabilitation interventions for the minority of workers who need additional help to return to work. These systems should include *both* healthcare and workplace elements, with a proactive approach focused on return to work. It is vital to strike the correct balance between healthcare and the focus on work, and to coordinate these efforts. There should be a universal Gateway that a) identifies workers after about six weeks sickness absence, b) directs them to appropriate help, and c) ensures the content and quality of the interventions provided. Pilot studies will be required to improve the evidence base on the effectiveness and cost-benefits of service delivery model(s) in the UK context. This will involve investment but the potential benefits far outweigh the expenditure and the enormous costs of doing nothing.

  - There is an urgent need to improve vocational rehabilitation interventions for mental health problems. Promising approaches include healthcare which incorporates a focus on return to work, workplaces that are accommodating and non-discriminating, and early intervention to support workers to stay in work and so prevent long-term incapacity.

- **Social security benefit claimants**

  - *Pathways to work* is the most effective example to date of a vocational rehabilitation intervention for disability and incapacity benefit claimants. Continued work is required to optimise *Pathways* for claimants with mental health problems and for long-term benefit recipients.

  - Better support, including retraining, should be provided for workers with occupational asthma who are unable to return to their previous jobs.

- Vocational rehabilitation needs to be underpinned by public education (with appropriate elements directed to workers, health professionals and employers) about the value of work for health and recovery, and their part in the return to work process. Public education campaigns have the potential both to change the culture and to improve healthcare and workplace practices.

- Government cannot do this alone and it is absolutely imperative to keep the key stakeholders onside – unions, employers, insurers and health professionals.

Conclusion

There is broad consensus among all the key stakeholders on the need to improve vocational rehabilitation in the UK. This review has demonstrated that there is now a strong scientific evidence base for many aspects of vocational rehabilitation, and a good business case for action. It has identified *what works, for whom, and when* and indicated areas where further research and development is required. Vocational rehabilitation should be fundamental to Government strategy to improve the health of working age people.

References

Abbass AA, Hancock JT, Henderson J, Kisely S. 2006. Short-term psychodynamic psychotherapies for common mental disorders (Cochrane Review). In *Cochrane Database of Systematic Reviews, Issue 4* John Wiley & Sons, Ltd, Chichester.

Abenhaim L, Rossignol M, Valat JP, Nordin M, Avouac B, Blotman F, Charlot J, Dreiser RL, Legrand E, Rozenberg S, Vautravers P. 2000. The role of activity in the therapeutic management of back pain. Report of the International Paris Task Force on back pain. *Spine* 25 (4S): 1S-33S.

ACOEM. 2006. Preventing needless work disability by helping people stay employed. *JOEM* 48: 972-985.

Adam S, Bozio A, Emmerson C, Greenberg D, Knight G. 2008. *A cost-benefit analysis of Pathways to Work for new and repeat incapacity benefits claimants (DWP RR 498)*. Corporate Document Services, Leeds.

Adams N, Sim J. 2005. Rehabilitation approaches in fibromyalgia. *Disability and Rehabilitation* 27: 711-723.

Ades PA, Pashkow FJ, Nestor JR. 1997. Cost-effectiveness of cardiac rehabilitation after myocardial infarction. *Journal of Cardiopulmonary Rehabilitation* 17: 222-231.

AFOM/RACP. 2001. *Compensable injuries and health outcomes*. The Royal Australasian College of Physicians, Sydney.

Allen NB, Hetrick SE, Simmons JG, Hickie IB. 2007. Early intervention for depressive disorders in young people: the opportunity and the (lack of) evidence. *MJA* 187: S15-S17.

Ameille J, Descatha A. 2005. Outcome of occupational asthma. *Curr Opin Allergy Clin Immunol* 5: 125-128.

Andlin-Sobocki P, Wittchen H-U. 2005. Cost of anxiety disorders in Europe. *European Journal of Neurology* 12 Suppl 1: 39-44.

Antó JM, Vermeire P, Vestbo J, Sunyer J. 2001. Epidemiology of chronic obstructive pulmonary disease. *Eur Respir J* 17: 982-994.

Ara S. 2004. A literature review of cardiovascular disease management programs in managed care populations. *Journal of Managed Care Pharmacy* 10: 326-344.

ARMA. 2004. *Standards of care*. Arthritis and Musculoskeletal Alliance, London www.arma.uk.net (accessed 17 February 2006).

ARMA. 2007. *Standards of care for people with regional musculoskeletal pain*. Arthritis and Musculoskeletal Alliance, London.

Arthur AR. 2000. Employee assistance programmes: the emperor's new clothes of stress management? *British Journal of Guidance & Counselling* 28: 549-559.

Athanasou JA. 2005. Return to work following whiplash and back injury: a review and evaluation. *Med Leg J* 73: 29-33.

Backman CL. 2006. Psychosocial aspects in the management of arthritis pain. *Arthritis Research & Therapy* 8: 221.

Bailey R, Hales J, Hayllar O, Wood M. 2007. *Pathways to work: customer experience and outcomes (DWP RR 456)*. Corporate Document Services, Leeds.

Balady GJ, Williams MA, Ades PA, Bittner V, Comoss P, Foody JM, Franklin B, Sanderson B, Southard D. 2007. Core components of cardiac rehabilitation/secondary prevention programs: 2007 update: a scientific statement from the American heart association exercise, cardiac rehabilitation, and prevention committee, the council on clinical cardiology; the councils on cardiovascular nursing, epidemiology and prevention, and nutrition, physical activity, and metabolism; and the American association of cardiovascular and pulmonary rehabilitation. *Circulation* 115: 2675-2682.

Balderson BHK, Von Korff M. 2002. The stepped care approach to chronic back pain. In *New avenues for the prevention of chronic musculoskeletal pain and disability. Pain research and clinical management. Vol 12* (Ed. Linton SJ): 237-244, Elsevier Science B.V., Amsterdam.

Baldwin ML, Butler RJ. 2006. Upper extremity disorders in the workplace: Costs and outcomes beyond the first return to work. *J Occup Rehabil* 16: 303-323.

Ballard J. 2006. Job Retention and Rehabilitation Pilot. Part 1: the research. *Occupational Health [at Work]* 3: 19-22.

Bambra C, Whitehead M, Hamilton V. 2005. Does 'welfare-to-work' work? A systematic review of the effectiveness of the UK's welfare-to-work programmes for people with a disability or chronic illness. *Social Science and Medicine* 60: 1905-1918.

Banks DE, Jalloul A. 2007. Occupational asthma, work-related asthma and reactive airways dysfunction syndrome. *Curr Opin Pulm Med* 13: 131-136.

Barbui C, Tansella M. 2006. Identification and management of depression in primary care settings. A meta-review of evidence. *Epidemiologia e Psichiatria Sociale* 15: 276-283.

Beach J, Rowe BH, Blitz S, Crumley E, Hooton N, Russell K, Spooner C, Klassen T. 2005. *Diagnosis and management of work-related asthma.* Agency for Healthcare Research and Quality, Rockville, USA.

Beaumont DG. 2003a. Rehabilitation and retention in the workplace - the interaction between general practitioners and occupational health professionals: a consensus statement. *Occupational Medicine* 53: 254-255.

Beaumont DG. 2003b. The interaction between general practitioners and occupational health professionals in relation to rehabilitation for work: a Delphi study. *Occupational Medicine* 53: 249-253.

Bellamy R. 1997. Compensation neurosis: financial reward for illness as nocebo. *Clinical Orthopaedics and Related Research* 336: 94-106.

Benson K, Hartz AJ. 2000. A comparison of observational studies and randomized, controlled trials. *The New England Journal of Medicine* 342: 1878-1886.

Benz Scott LA, Ben-Or K, Allen JK. 2002. Why are women missing from outpatient cardiac rehabilitation programs? A review of multilevel factors affecting referral, enrollment, and completion. *Journal of Women's Health* 11: 773-791.

Beswick AD, Rees K, West RR, Taylor FC, Burke M, Griebsch I, Taylor RS, Victory J, Brown J, Ebrahim S. 2005. Improving uptake and adherence in cardiac rehabilitation: literature review. *Journal of Advanced Nursing* 49: 538-555.

Bevan S, Hayday S. 2001. *Costing sickness absence in the UK. Report 382.* Institute for Employment Studies, Brighton.

Bevan S, Passmore E, Mahdon M. 2007. *Fit for Work? Musculoskeletal disorders and labour market participation.* The Work Foundation, London.

Bewley H, Dorsett R, Haile G. 2007. *The impact of pathways to work (DWP RR 435).* Corporate Document Services, Leeds.

Bilsker D, Wiseman S, Gilbert M. 2006. Managing depression-related occupational disability: a pragmatic approach. *Can J Psychiatry* 51: 76-83.

Binder LM, Rohling ML. 1996. Money matters: a meta-analytic review of the effects of financial incentives on recovery after closed-head injury. *Am J Psychiatry* 153: 7-10.

Binks CA, Fenton M, McCarthy L, Lee T, Adams CE, Duggan C. 2006. Psychological therapies for people with borderline personality disorder (Cochrane Review). In *Cochrane Database of Systematic Reviews, Issue 1* John Wiley & Sons, Ltd, Chichester.

Bisson J, Andrew M. 2007. Psychological treatment of post-traumatic stress disorder (Cochrane Review). In *Cochrane Database of Systematic Reviews, Issue 3* John Wiley & Sons, Ltd, Chichester.

Bjarnason-Wehrens B, Grande G, Loewel H, Völler H, Mittag O. 2007. Gender-specific issues in cardiac rehabilitation: do women with ischaemic heart disease need specially tailored programmes? *European Journal of Cardiovascular Prevention and Rehabilitation* 14: 163-171.

Black C. 2008. *Working for a healthier tomorrow: Dame Carol Black's review of the health of Britain's working age population.* TSO, London www.workingforhealth.gov.uk (accessed 19 March 2008).

Black C, Cheung L, Cooper J, Curson-Prue S, Doupe L, Guirguis S, Haines T, Hawkins L, Helmka S, Holness L, Levitsky M, Liss G, Malcolm B, Painvin C, Wills M. 2000. *Injury/illness and return to work/function.* Workplace Safety and Insurance Board, Toronto.

Blanc PD, Torén K. 2007. Occupation in chronic obstructive pulmonary disease and chronic bronchitis: an update. *Int J Tuberc Lung Dis* 11: 251-257.

Blankenstein AH. 2001. *Somatising patients in general practice: reattribution, a promising approach [thesis].* Vrije Universiteit, Amsterdam.

Boardman J, Grove B, Perkins R, Shepherd G. 2003. Work and employment for people with psychiatric disabilities. *British Journal of Psychiatry* 182: 467-468.

Boardman J, Lyon A. 2006. *Defining best practice in corporate occupational health and safety governance (HSE RR 506).* HSE Books, London.

BOMEL Ltd. 2005. *Occupational health and safety support systems for small and medium sized enterprises: a literature review (RR 410).* HSE Books, London.

Bongers P, Ijmker S, den Heuvel Sv, Blatter B. 2006. Epidemiology of work related neck and upper limb problems: psychosocial and personal risk factors (Part I) and effective interventions from a bio behavioural perspective (Part II). *Journal of Occupational Rehabilitation* 16: 272-295.

Boocock MG, McNair PJ, Larmer PJ, Armstrong B, Collier J, Simmonds M, Garrett N. 2007. Interventions for the prevention and management of neck/upper extremity musculoskeletal conditions: a systematic review. *Occup Environ Med* 64: 291-303.

Bousquet J, Flahault A, Vandenplas O, Ameille J, Duron JJ, Pecquet C, Chevrie K, Annesi-Maesano I. 2006. Natural rubber latex allergy among health care workers: a systematic review of the evidence. *Journal of Allergy and Clinical Immunology* 118: 447-454.

Bower P, Rowland N. 2006. Effectiveness and cost effectiveness of counselling in primary care (Cochrane Review). In *Cochrane Database of Systematic Reviews, Issue 3* John Wiley & Sons, Ltd, Chichester.

Bradley J, Moran F, Greenstone M. 2002. Physical training for bronchiectasis (Cochrane Review). In Cochrane *Database of Systematic Reviews, Issue 2* John Wiley & Sons, Ltd, Chichester.

Breen A, Langworthy J, Baghust J. 2007. *Improved early pain management for musculoskeletal disorders: (HSE RR 399).* HSE Books, London.

Breen AC, van Tulder MW, Koes BW, Jensen I, Reardon R, Bronfort G. 2006. Mono-disciplinary or multidisciplinary back pain guidelines? How can we achieve a common message in primary care? *European Spine Journal* 15: 641-647.

Brewer S, King E, Amick B, Delclos G, Spear J, Irvin E, Mahood Q, Lee L, Lewis C, Tetrick L, Gimeno D, Williams R. 2007. *A systematic review of injury/illness prevention and loss control programs (IPC).* Institute for Work & Health, Toronto www.iwh.on.ca/sr/wi_ipc_programs.php (accessed 23 April 2008).

British Thoracic Society, SIGN. 2007. *British guideline on the management of asthma: a national clinical guideline.* British Thoracic Society and Scottish Intercollegiate Guidelines Network, www.brit-thoracic. org.uk www.sign.ac.uk (accessed 12 March 2008).

Brox JJ, Storheim K, Grotle M, Tveito TH, Indahl A, Eriksen HR. 2007. Systematic review of back schools, brief education, and fear-avoidance training for chronic low back pain. *The Spine Journal* In Press.

BSRM. 2000. *Vocational rehabilitation. The way forward.* British Society of Rehabilitation Medicine, London.

BSRM. 2003. *Vocational rehabilitation. The way forward - 2nd Edition.* British Society of Rehabilitation Medicine, London www.bsrm.co.uk/Publications/Summary-Voc-Rehab.pdf (accessed 12 March 2008).

BSRM. 2004. *Musculoskeletal rehabilitation. Report of a working party convened by the British Society of Rehabilitation Medicine.* British Society of Rehabilitation Medicine, London www.bsrm.co.uk/ Publications/Publications.htm (accessed 12 March 2008).

Buchbinder R, Jolley D, Wyatt M. 2001. Population based intervention to change back pain beliefs and disability: three part evaluation. *BMJ* 322: 1516-1520.

Bültmann U, Franche R-L, Hogg-Johnson S, Côté P, Lee H, Severin C, Vidmar M, Carnide N. 2007. Health status, work limitations, and return-to-work trajectories in injured workers with musculoskeletal disorders. *Quality of Life Research* 16: 1167-1178.

Bunker S. 2002. Cardiac rehabilitation after acute myocardial infarction: for the many or the few? *Heart, Lung and Circulation* 11: 7.

Burkhauser RV, Butler JS, Weathers II RR. 2001. How policy variables influence the timing of applications for social security disability insurance. *Social Security Bulletin* 64: 52-83.

Burton AK. 1997. Back injury and work loss: biomechanical and psychosocial influences. *Spine* 22: 2575-2580.

Burton AK, Kendall NAS, Pearce BG, Birrell LN, Bainbridge LC. 2008. *Management of upper limb disorders and the biopsychosocial model.* HSE Books, London.

Burton AK, Waddell G. 2002. Educational and informational approaches. In *New avenues for the prevention of chronic musculoskeletal pain and disability. Pain research and clinical management. Vol 12* (Ed. Linton SJ): 245-258, Elsevier Science B.V., Amsterdam.

Butler RJ, Durbin DL, Helvacian NM. 1996. Increasing claims for soft tissue injuries in workers' compensation: cost shifting and moral hazard. *Journal of Risk and Uncertainty* 13: 73-87.

Butterfield TM, Ramseur JH. 2004. Research and case study findings in the area of workplace accommodations including provisions for assistive technology: a literature review. *Technology and Disability* 16: 201-210.

Cambach W, Wagenaar RC, Koelman TW, van Keimpema T, Kemper HCG. 1999. The long-term effects of pulmonary rehabilitation in patients with asthma and chronic obstructive pulmonary disease: a research synthesis. *Arch Phys Med Rehabil* 80: 103-111.

Camp PG, Dimich-Ward H, Kennedy SM. 2004. Women and occupational lung disease: sex differences and gender influences on research and disease outcomes. *Clinics in Chest Medicine* 25: 269-279.

Campbell J, Wright C, Moseley A, Chilvers R, Richards S, Stabb L. 2007. *Avoiding long-term incapacity for work: developing an early intervention in primary care.* Peninsula Medical School, Universities of Exeter and Plymouth, Exeter.

Canadian Senate. 2004. *Mental health, mental illness and addiction: issues and options for Canada.* Standing Senate Committee on Social Affairs, Science and Technology: Senate Can, Ottawa www.parl. gc.ca (accessed 02 April 2008).

Cannon CP, Hand MM, Bahr R, Boden WE, Christenson R, Gibler B, Eagle K, Lambrew CT, Lee TH, MacLeod B, Ornato JP, Selker HP, Steele P, Zalenski RJ. 2002. Critical pathways for management of patients with acute coronary syndromes: an assessment by the National Heart Attack Alert Program. *American Heart Journal* 143: 777-789.

CARF. 2007. *Medical rehabilitation standards*. Commission on Accreditation of Rehabilitation Facilities, Tucson, USA.

Carter JT, Birrell LN. 2000. *Occupational health guidelines for the management of low back pain at work - principle recommendations*. Faculty of Occupational Medicine, London.

Caulfield N, Chang D, Dollard MF, Elshaug C. 2004. A review of occupational stress interventions in Australia. *International Journal of Stress Management* 11: 149-166.

CBI. 2000. *Their health in your hands: focus on occupational health partnerships*. Confederation of British Industry, London.

CBI/AXA. 2007. *Attending to absence: CBI/AXA absence and labour turnover survey 2007: a summary*. Confederation of British Insurers, London.

Cherry N. 1999. Occupational disease. *BMJ* 318: 1397-1399.

Churchill R, Hunot V, Corney R, Knapp M, McGuire H, Tylee A, Wessely S. 2001. A systematic review of controlled trials of the effectiveness and cost-effectiveness of brief psychological treatments for depression. *Health Technology Assessment* 5: (35).

CIPD. 2007. *Absence management: annual survey report 2007*. Chartered Institute of Personnel and Development, London www.cipd.co.uk (accessed 04 April 2008).

Clark AM, Hartling L, Vandermeer B, McAlister FA. 2005a. Meta-analysis: secondary prevention programs for patients with coronary artery disease. *Ann Intern Med* 143: 659-672.

Clark AM, McAlister FA, Hartling L, Vandermeer B. 2005b. *Randomized trials of secondary prevention programs in coronary artery disease: a systematic review*. Agency for Healthcare Research and Quality, Rockville, USA.

Cole DC, Van Eerd D, Bigelow P, Rivilis I. 2006. Integrative interventions for MSDs: nature, evidence, challenges & directions. *J Occup Rehabil* 16: 359-374.

Concato J, Shah N, Horwitz RI. 2000. Randomized, controlled trials, observational studies, and the hierarchy of research designs. *The New England Journal of Medicine* 342: 1887-1892.

Contaldo M. 2007. *Building the evidence base: third sector values in the delivery of public services*. HM Treasury, London www.hm-treasury.gov.uk (access 23 April 2008).

Cooper A, Skinner J, Nherera L, Feder G, Ritchie G, Kathoria M, Turnbull N, Shaw G, MacDermott K, Minhas R, Packham C, Squires H, Thomson D, Timmis A, Walsh J, Williams H, White A. 2007. *Clinical guidelines and evidence review for post myocardial infarction: secondary prevention in primary and secondary care for patients following a myocardial infarction*. National Collaborating Centre for Primary Care and Royal College of General Practitioners, London.

Cooper AF, Jackson G, Weinman J, Horne R. 2002. Factors associated with cardiac rehabilitation attendance: a systematic review of the literature. *Clinical Rehabilitation* 16: 541-552.

Corden A, Nice K. 2006. *Pathways to work: findings from the final cohort in a qualitative longitudinal panel of incapacity benefits recipients (DWP RR 398)*. Corporate Document Services, Leeds.

Corden A, Thornton P. 2002. *Employment programmes for disabled people: Lessons from research evaluations. (DWP In-house report 90)*. Her Majesty's Stationery Office, London.

Cortés O, Arthur HM. 2006. Determinants of referral to cardiac rehabilitation programs in patients with coronary artery disease: a systematic review. *Am Heart J* 151: 249-256.

COST B13 Working Group. 2004. *Low back pain: guidelines for its management.* European Commission Research Directorate General, www.backpaineurope.org (accessed 12 March 2008).

Coudeyre E, Givron P, Vanbiervliet W, Benaïm C, Hérisson C, Pelissier J, Poiraudeau S. 2006. The role of an information booklet or oral information about back pain in reducing disability and fear-avoidance beliefs among patients with subacute and chronic low back pain. A randomized controlled trial in a rehabilitation unit. *Annales de réadaption et de médecine physique* 49: 600-608.

Cox T, Griffiths A, Barlowe C, Randall R, Thomson L, Rial-Gonzalez E. 2000a. *Organisational interventions for work stress. A risk management approach (HSE CRR 286).* HSE Books, London.

Cox T, Griffiths A, Houdmont J. 2006. *Defining a case of work-related stress (HSE RR 449).* HSE Books, London.

Cox T, Griffiths A, Rial-Gonzalez E. 2000b. *Research on work-related stress.* European Agency for Safety and Health at Work, Luxembourg.

Crawford JO, Laiou E. 2005. *Effective management of upper limb disorders by general practitioners and trainee occupational physicians (HSE RR 380).* HSE Books, London.

Crawford JO, Laiou E. 2007. Conservative treatment of work-related upper limb disorders - a review. *Occupational Medicine* 57: 4-17.

CSAG. 1994. *Back pain: report of a CSAG committee on back pain.* HMSO, London.

Curran C, Knapp M, McDaid D, Tómasson K. 2007. Mental health and employment: an overview of patterns and policies across Western Europe. *Journal of Mental Health* 16: 195-209.

Curtis J, Scott LR. 2004. Integrating disability management into strategic plans: creating health organizations. *AAOHN Journal* 52: 298-301.

Daly J, Sindone AP, Thompson DR, Hancock K, Chang E, Davidson P. 2002. Barriers to participation in and adherence to cardiac rehabilitation programs: a critical literature review. *Progress in Cardiovascular Nursing* 17: 8-17.

Damiani G, Federico B, Pinnarelli L, Ricciardi G. 2004. Do occupational stress management programmes affect absenteeism rates? *Occupational Medicine* 54: 58-59.

Datta D, ZuWallack R. 2004. High versus low intensity exercise training in pulmonary rehabilitation: is more better? *Chronic Respiratory Disease* 1: 143-149.

Davis A, Davis S, Moss N, Marks J, McGrath J, Hovard L, Axon J, Wade D. 1992. First steps towards an interdisciplinary approach to rehabilitation. *Clinical Rehabilitation* 6: 237-244.

Davis M, Rinaldi M. 2004. Using an evidence-based approach to enable people with mental health problems to gain and retain employment, education and voluntary work. *British Journal of Occupational Therapy* 67: 319-322.

Day W. 2003. Women and cardiac rehabilitation: a review of the literature. *Contemporary Nurse* 16: 92-101.

de Buck PDM, Schoones JW, Allaire SH, Vliet Vlieland TPM. 2002. Vocational rehabilitation in patients with chronic rheumatic diseases: a systematic literature review. *Seminars in Arthritis and Rheumatism* 32: 196-203.

de Gaudemaris R. 2000. Clinical issues: return to work and public safety. *Occupational Medicine: State of the Art Reviews* 15: 223-230.

de Vries JS, Krips R, Sierevelt IN, Blankevoort L, van Dijk CN. 2006. Interventions for treating chronic ankle instability (Cochrane Review). In *Cochrane Database of Systematic Reviews, Issue 4* John Wiley & Sons, Ltd, Chichester.

DeGood DE, Kiernan B. 1996. Perception of fault in patients with chronic pain. *Pain* 64: 153-159.

Dembe AE. 2001. The social consequences of occupational injuries and illnesses. *American Journal of Industrial Medicine* 40: 403-417.

den Boer PCAM, Wiersma D, Russo S, van den Bosch RJ. 2005. Paraprofessionals for anxiety and depressive disorders (Cochrane Review). In *Cochrane Database of Systematic Reviews, Issue 2* John Wiley & Sons, Ltd, Chicester.

Dersh J, Polatin PB, Leeman G, Gatchel RJ. 2004. The management of secondary gain and loss in medicolegal settings: strengths and weaknesses. *Journal of Occupational Rehabilitation* 14: 267-279.

Desouza M, Sycamore M, Little S, Kirker SGB. 2007. The Papworth Early Rehabilitation Programme: vocational outcomes. *Disability and Rehabilitation* 29: 671-677.

Dewa CS, McDaid D, Ettner SL. 2007. An international perspective on worker mental health problems: who bears the burden and how are costs addressed? *Can J Psychiatry* 52: 346-356.

DH. 2001. *Treatment choice in psychological therapies and counselling: evidence based clinical practice guideline.* Department of Health, London www.dh.gov.uk/en/index.htm (accessed 26 March 2008).

DH. 2002. *Improvement, expansion and reform: the next 3 years: priorities and planning framework 2003 - 2006.* Department of Health, London www.dh.gov.uk (accessed 09 June 2008).

DH. 2004. *Improving chronic disease management.* Department of Health, London www.dh.gov.uk/organisation (accessed 09 April 2008).

DH. 2007a. *Commissioning a brighter future: improving access to psychological therapies - positive practice guide.* Department of Health, London www.dh.gov.uk/en/index.htm (accessed 26 March 2008).

DH. 2007b. *Improving access to psychological therapies (IAPT) programme: computerised cognitive behavioural therapy (cCBT) implementation guidance.* Department of Health, London www.dh.gov.uk/en/index.htm (accessed 26 March 2008).

DH. 2008. *Major new training program to expand psychological therapies workforce: press release 26 February 2008.* Department of Health, London http://nds.coi.gov.uk/environment/dh (accessed 14 May 2008).

DHC. 2006. *A vision for change: report of the expert group on mental health policy.* The Stationery Office Dublin (on behalf of Department for Health and Children), Dublin www.dohc.ie (accessed 26 March 2008).

Dong A, Doupe L, Ross M, Gardiner E, Mendel J, on behalf of OMA Committee on Work & Health. 2002. *Mental illness and workplace absenteeism: exploring risk factors and effective return to work strategies.* Ontario Medical Association, Ontario http://oma.org/pcomm/OMR/apr/02returnwork.htm (accessed 12 March 2008).

Donohue JM, Pincus HA. 2007. Reducing the societal burden of depression: a review of economic costs, quality of care and effects of treatment. *Pharmaeconomics* 25: 7-24.

Druss BG, von Esenwein SA. 2006. Improving general medical care for persons with mental and addictive disorders: systematic review. *General Hospital Psychiatry* 28: 145-153.

Dunstan DA, Covic T. 2006. Compensable work disability management: a literature review of biopsychosocial perspectives. *Australian Occupational Therapy Journal* 53: 67-77.

Durand MJ, Vézina N, Loisel P, Baril R, Richard MC, Diallo B. 2007. Workplace interventions for workers with musculoskeletal disabilities: A descriptive review of content. *J Occup Rehabil* 17: 123-136.

DWP. 2004. *Building capacity for work: a UK framework for vocational rehabilitation.* The Department for Work and Pensions, London.

DWP. 2007. *In work, better off: next steps to full employment.* Department for Work and Pensions (HMSO), London.

EASHAW. 2007. *Work-related musculoskeletal disorders: Back to work report.* Office for Official Publications of The European Communities, Luxembourg.

Edwards D, Burnard P. 2003a. A systematic review of stress and stress management interventions for mental health nurses. *Journal of Advanced Nursing* 42: 169-200.

Edwards D, Burnard P. 2003b. A systematic review of the effects of stress and coping strategies used by occupational therapists working in mental health settings. *British Journal of Occupational Therapy* 66: 345-355.

EEF. 2004. *Fit for work: the complete guide to managing sickness absence and rehabilitation.* EEF, London www.eef.org.uk (accessed 04 April 2008).

Effing TW, Monninkhof EM, van der Valk PDLPM, Zielhuis GA, van Herwaarden CLA, Partridge MR, Walters EH, van der Palen J. 2007. Self-management education for patients with chronic obstructive pulmonary disease (Cochrane Review). In *Cochrane Database of Systematic Reviews, Issue 4* John Wiley & Sons, Ltd, Chichester.

EFILWC. 2007. *Managing musculoskeletal disorders.* European Foundation for the Improvement of Living and Working Conditions, Dublin www.eurofound.europa.eu/ewco/studies/tn0611018s/index.htm (accessed 12 March 2008).

Egan M, Bambra C, Thomas S, Petticrew M, Whitehead M, Thomson H. 2007. The psychosocial and health effects of workplace reorganisation. 1. A systematic review of organisational-level interventions that aim to increase employee control. *J Epidemiol Community Health* 61: 945-954.

Egger M, Juni P, Bartlett C, Holenstein F, Sterne J. 2003. How important are comprehensive literature searches and the assessment of trial quality in systematic reviews? Empirical study. *Health Technol Assess* 7: 1-76.

Elders LAM, van der Beek AJ, Burdorf A. 2000. Return to work after sickness absence due to back disorders - a systematic review on intervention strategies. *International Archives of Occupational and Environmental Health* 73: 339-348.

Employers' Forum on Disability. 2008. *Attendance management and disability: line manager guide.* Employers' Forum on Disability, London.

Engel GL. 1977. The need for a new medical model: a challenge for biomedicine. *Science* 196: 129-136.

Epping-Jordan JE, Pruitt SD, Bengoa R, Wagner EH. 2004. Improving the quality of health care for chronic conditions. *Qual Saf Health Care* 13: 299-305.

ExTraMATCH Collaborative. 2004. Exercise training meta-analysis of trials in patients with chronic heart failure (ExTraMATCH). *BMJ* doi:10.1136/bmj.37938.645220.EE.

Faber E, Kuiper JI, Burdorf A, Miedema HS, Verhaar JAN. 2006. Treatment of impingement syndrome: a systematic review of the effects on functional limitations and return to work. *Journal of Occupational Rehabilitation* 16: 7-25.

Falcone RA, Hirsch AT, Regensteiner JG, Treat-Jacobson D, Williams MA, Hiatt WR, Stewart KJ. 2003. Peripheral arterial disease rehabilitation. *Journal of Cardiopulmonary Rehabilitation* 23: 170-175.

Farrell C, Nice K, Lewis J, Sainsbury R. 2006. *Experiences of the job retention and rehabilitation pilot* (DWP RR 339). Corporate Document Services, Leeds.

Feldman JB. 2004. The prevention of occupational low back pain disability: evidence-based reviews point in a new direction. *Journal of Surgical Orthopaedic Advances* 13: 1-14.

Feuerstein M, Harrington CB. 2006. Secondary prevention of work-related upper extremity disorders: recommendations from the annapolis conference. *J Occup Rehabil* 16: 401-409.

Fishbain DA, Rosomoff HL, Cutler RB, Rosomoff RS. 1995. Secondary gain concept: a review of the scientific evidence. *Clinical Journal of Pain* 11: 6-21.

FOM. 2005. *The health and work handbook.* Faculty of Occupational Medicine, Royal College of General Practitioners, Society of Occupational Medicine, London. www.facoccmed.ac.uk/library/docs/h&w.pdf (accessed 9 December 2005).

Fordyce WE. 1995. *Back pain in the workplace: management of disability in nonspecific conditions.* IASP Press, Seattle.

Foreman P, Murphy G, Swerissen H. 2006. *Barriers and facilitators to return to work: a literature review.* Australian Institute for Primary Care, La Trobe University, Melbourne www.workcover.com/documents. aspx#B%20 (accessed 16 April 2008).

Franche RL, Baril R, Shaw W, Nicholas M, Loisel P. 2005a. Workplace-based return-to-work interventions: optimizing the role of stakeholders in implementation and research. *Journal of Occupational Rehabilitation* 15: 525-542.

Franche RL, Cullen K, Clarke J, Irvin E, Sinclair S, Frank J, The Institute for Work & Health (IWH) Workplace-Based RTW Intervention Literature Review Research Team. 2005b. Workplace-based return-to-work interventions: a systematic review of the quantitative literature. *J Occup Rehabil* 15: 607-631.

Franche RL, Krause N. 2002. Readiness for return to work following injury or illness: conceptualizing the interpersonal impact of health care, workplace, and insurance factors. *Journal of Occupational Rehabilitation* 12: 233-256.

Frank AO, Sawney P. 2003. Vocational rehabilitation. *J Royal Soc Med* 96: 522-524.

Frank AO, Thurgood J. 2006. Vocational rehabilitation in the UK: opportunities for health-care professionals. *Int J Ther Rehabil* 13: 126-134.

Frank J, Sinclair S, Hogg-Johnson S, Shannon H, Bombardier C, Beaton D, Cole D. 1998. Preventing disability from work-related low-back pain: new evidence gives new hope - if we can just get all the players onside. *Canadian Medical Association Journal* 158: 1625-1631.

Frank JW, Brooker A-S, DeMaio SE, Kerr MS, Maetzel A, Shannon HS, Sullivan TJ, Norman RW, Wells RP. 1996. Disability resulting from occupational low back pain. Part II: What do we know about secondary prevention? A review of the scientific evidence on prevention after disability begins. *Spine* 21: 2918-2929.

Freeman EJ. 2004. Union-management solutions for preventing workplace injury of older workers. *Work* 22: 145-151.

Freud D. 2007. *Reducing dependency, increasing opportunity: options for the future of welfare to work.* Corporate Document Services, Leeds.

Furukawa TA, Watanabe N, Churchill R. 2007. Combined psychotherapy plus antidepressants for panic disorder with or without agoraphobia (Cochrane Review). In *Cochrane Database of Systematic Reviews, Issue 1* John Wiley & Sons, Ltd, Chichester.

GAO. 2007. *Vocational rehabilitation: report to congressional requesters.* United States Government Accountability Office, Washington www.gao.gov/new.items/d07332.pdf (accessed 16 April 2008).

Garg AX, Adhikari NKJ, McDonald H, Rosas-Arellano MP, Devereaux PJ, Beyene J, Sam J, Haynes RB. 2005. Effects of computerized clinical decision support systems on practitioner performance and patient outcomes: a systematic review. *JAMA* 293: 1223-1238.

Gatchel RJ, Adams L, Polatin PB, Kishino ND. 2002. Secondary loss and pain-associated disability: theoretical overview and treatment implications. *Journal of Occupational Rehabilitation* 12: 99-110.

Gates LB. 2000. Workplace accommodation as a social process. *Journal of Occupational Rehabilitation* 10: 85-98.

Gautrin D, Desrosiers M, Castano R. 2006. Occupational rhinitis. *Curr Opin Allergy Clin Immunol* 6: 77-84.

Gava I, Barbui C, Aguglia E, Carlino D, Churchill R, De Vanna M, McGuire HF. 2007. Psychological treatments versus treatment as usual for obsessive compulsive disorder (OCD) (Cochrane Review). In *Cochrane Database of Systematic Reviews, Issue 2* John Wiley & Sons, Ltd, Chichester.

Gibson PG, Powell H, Coughlan J, Wilson AJ, Abramson M, Haywood P, Bauman A, Hensley MJ, Walters EH. 2002. Self-management education and regular practitioner review for adults with asthma (Cochrane Review). In *Cochrane Database of Systematic Reviews, Issue 3* John Wiley & Sons, Ltd, Chicester.

Giga SI, Noblet AJ, Faragher B, Cooper CL. 2003. The UK perspective: a review of research on organisational stress management interventions. *Australian Psychologist* 38: 158-164.

Glasziou P, Vandenbroucke J, Chalmers I. 2004. Assessing the quality of research. *BMJ* 328: 39-41.

Gobelet C, Luthi F, Al-Khodairy AT, Chamberlain MA. 2007a. Vocational rehabilitation: a multidisciplinary intervention. *Disability and Rehabilitation* 29: 1405-1410.

Gobelet C, Luthi F, Al-Khodairy AT, Chamberlain MA. 2007b. Work in inflammatory and degenerative joint diseases. *Disability and Rehabilitation* 29: 1331-1339.

Goetzel RZ, Ozminkowski RJ, Sederer LI, Mark TL. 2002. The business case for quality mental health services: why employers should care about the mental health and well-being of their employees. *J Occup Environ Med* 44: 320-330.

Goetzel RZ, Ozminkowski RJ, Villagra VG, Duffy J. 2005. Return on investment in disease management: a review. *Health Care Financing Review* 26: 1-19.

Goldfarb N, Weston C, Hartmann CW, Sikirica M, Crawford A, Howell J, Maio V, Clarke J, Nuthulaganti B, Cobb N. 2004. Impact of appropriate pharmaceutical therapy for chronic conditions on direct medical costs and workplace productivity: a review of the literature. *Disease Management* 7: 61-75.

Goldner E, Bilsker D, Gilbert M, Myette L, Corbière M, Dewa CS. 2004. Disability management, return to work and treatment. *Healthcare Paper* 5: 76-90.

Goldsmith MR, Bankhead CR, Austoker J. 2007. Synthesising quantitative and qualitative research in evidence based patient information. *J Epidemiol Community Health* 61: 262-270.

Grant HJ, Arthur A, Pichora DR. 2004. Evaluation of interventions for rotator cuff pathology: a systematic review. *J Hand Ther* 17: 274-299.

Green S, Buchbinder R, Hetrick S. 2003. Physiotherapy interventions for shoulder pain (Cochrane Review). In *Cochrance Database of Systematic Reviews 2003, Issue 2* John Wiley & Sons, Ltd, Chicester.

Green-McKenzie J, Kiselica D, Watkins M. 2004. Managing workers' compensation costs: success of initiatives to change outcomes. *Clin Occup Environ Med* 4: 295-308.

Greenberg D, Davis A. 2007. *Evaluation of the new deal for disabled people: the cost and cost-benefit analyses (DWP RR 431).* Corporate Document Services, Leeds.

Greenstreet Berman Ltd. 2004. *Cost and benefits of return to work and vocational rehabilitation in the UK. Summary report for the Association of British Insurers. Evidence from overseeas and UK case studies.* Greenstreet Berman Ltd, Reading www.abi.org.uk/Bookshop (accessed 16 February 2006).

Griffith R. 2006. Compensation for psychiatric injury: evolution of a law of nervous shock. *British Journal of Community Nursing* 11: 396-401.

Grimshaw JM, Shirran L, Thomas R, Mowatt G, Fraser C, Bero L, Grilli R, Harvey E, Oxman A, O'Brien MA. 2001. Changing provider behavior: an overview of systematic reviews of interventions. *Medical Care* 39: II-2-II-45.

Grimshaw JM, Thomas RE, MacLennan G, Fraser C, Ramsay CR, Vale L, Whitty P, Eccles MP, Matowe L, Shirran L, Wensing M, Dijkstra R, Donaldson C. 2004. Effectiveness and efficiency of guideline dissemination and implementation strategies. *Health Technology Assessment* 8: http://www.hta.ac.uk/project/994.asp (accessed 12 March 2008).

Grimshaw JM, Winkens RAG, Shirran L, Cunningham C, Mayhew A, Thomas A, Fraser C. 2005. Interventions to improve outpatient referrals from primary care to secondary care (Cochrane Review). In *Cochrance Database of Systematic Reviews, Issue 3* John Wiley & Sons, Ltd, Chicester.

Gross D, Lowe A, LaRocque D, Muir I. 2006. *Disability management of injured workers. A best practices resource guide for physical therapists.* College of Physical Therapists of Alberta, Edmonton, Canada www.cpta.ab.ca/resources/publications_disabilitymanagement_guide.pdf.

Grove B. 1999. Mental health and employment: shaping a new agenda. *J Mental Health* 8: 131-140.

Gründemann R. 1997. *Preventing absenteeism at the workplace: research summary.* European Foundation for the Improvement of Living and Working Conditions, Dublin www.eurofound.eu.int (accessed 09 April 2008).

Guthrie R, Jansz J. 2006. Women's experience in the workers' compensation system. *J Occup Rehabil* 16: 485-499.

Guzmán J, Esmail R, Karjalainen K, Malmivaara A, Irvin E, Bombardier C. 2001. Multidisciplinary rehabilitation for chronic low back pain: systematic review. *BMJ* 322: 1511-1516.

Haafkens J, Moerman C, Schuring M, van Dijk F. 2006. Searching bibliographic databases for literature on chronic disease and work participation. *Occup Med* 56: 39-45.

Haddon WJr. 1973. Energy damage and the ten countermeasure strategies. *J Trauma* 13: 321-331.

Hadler NM, Tait RC, Chibnall JT. 2007. Back pain in the workplace. *JAMA* 297: 1594-1596.

Hagberg M. 2005. Clinical assessment, prognosis and return to work with reference to work related neck and upper limb disorders. *G Ital Med Lav Erg* 27: 51-57.

Hall JP, Wiseman VL, King MT, Ross DL, Kovoor P, Zecchin RP, Moir FM, Denniss AR. 2002. Economic evaluation of a randomised trial of early return to normal activities versus cardiac rehabilitation after acute myocardial infarction. Heart, Lung and *Circulation* 11: 10-18.

Hamm RM, Reiss DM, Paul RK, Bursztajn HJ. 2007. Knocking at the wrong door: insured workers' inadequate psychiatric care and workers' compensation claims. *International Journal of Law & Psychiatry* 30: 416-426.

Hannigan B, Edwards D, Burnard P. 2004. Stress and stress management in clinical psychology: findings from a systematic review. *Journal of Mental Health* 13: 235-245.

Hanson M, Murray K, Wu O. 2007. *Evaluation of OHSxtra, a pilot occupational health case management programme within NHS Fife and NHS Lanarkshire.* The Scottish Government, Edinburgh.

Hanson MA, Burton AK, Kendall NAS, Lancaster RJ, Pilkington A. 2006. *The costs and benefits of active case management and rehabilitation for musculoskeletal disorders (HSE RR 493).* HSE Books, London.

Haralson RHI. 2005. Working with common lower extremity problems. In *A Physician's Guide to Return to Work* (Ed. Talmage JB, Melhorn JM): 215-231, American Medical Association, Chicago.

Harnois G, Gabriel P. 2000. *Mental health and work: impact, issues and good practices.* World Health Organization, Geneva (WHO/MSD/MPS/00.2).

Harris GR, Susman JL. 2002. Managing musculoskeletal complaints with rehabilitation therapy: Summary of the Philadelphia Panel evidence-based clinical practice guidelines on musculosksletal rehabilitation interventions. *The Journal of Family Practice* 51: 1042-1046.

Harris JS, Bengle AL, Makens PK. 2001. *Returning to work: an examination of existing disability duration guidelines and their applicability to the Texas Workers' Compensation system.* Research and Oversight Council on Workers' Compensation, Austin.

Hasluck C, Green AE. 2007. *What works for whom? A review of evidence and meta-analysis for the Department for Work and Pensions (DWP RR 407).* Corporate Document Services, Leeds.

Hayden C, Boaz A, Taylor F. 1999. *Attitudes and aspirations of older people: a qualitative study (DWP RR 102).* Corporate Document Services, Leeds www.dwp.gov.uk/asd/asd5/report_abstracts/rr_abstracts/rra_102.asp#startcontent (accessed 09 May 2008).

Hayden JA, van Tulder MW, Malmivaara A, Koes BW. 2005. Exercise therapy for treatment of non-specific low back pain (Cochrane Review). In *Cochrane Database of Systematic Reviews, Issue 3* John Wiley & Sons, Ltd, Chichester.

Hellgren J, Karlsson G, Torén K. 2003. The dilemma of occupational rhinitis. Management options. *Am J Respir Med* 2: 333-341.

Henderson M, Glozier N, Elliott KH. 2005. Long term sickness absence is caused by common conditions and needs managing. *BMJ* 330: 802-803.

Henderson M, Hotopf M, Wessely S. 2003. Workplace counselling. An appeal for evidence. *Occupational and Environmental Medicine* 60: 899-900.

Henneberger PK. 2007. Work-exacerbated asthma. *Curr Opin Allergy Clin Immunol 7:* 146-151.

Henrotin YE, Cedraschi C, Duplan B, Bazin T, Duquesnoy B. 2006. Information and low back pain management: a systematic review. *Spine* 15: E326-E334.

Hestbaek L, Leboeuf-Yde C, Manniche C. 2003. Low back pain: what is the long-term course? A review of studies of general patient populations. *Eur Spine J* 12: 149-165.

Heymans MW, van Tulder MW, Esmail R, Bombardier C, Koes BW. 2004. Back schools for non-specific low-back pain (Cochrane Review). In *Cochrane Database of Systematic Reviews, Issue 4* John Wiley & Sons, Ltd, Chichester.

Hill D, Lucy D, Tyers C, James L. 2007. *What works at work?* Corporate Document Services, Leeds.

Hirsch BT. 1997. Incentive effects of workers compensation. *Clinical Orthopaedics and Related Research* 336: 33-41.

Hlobil H, Staal JB, Spoelstra M, Ariëns GAM, Smid T, van Mechelen W. 2005. Effectiveness of a return-to-work intervention for subacute low-back pain. *Scand J Work Environ Health* 31: 249-257.

HM Government. 2005. *Health, work and well-being - caring for our future.* Department for Work and Pensions, London www.dwp.gov.uk/publications/dwp/2005/health_and_wellbeing.pdf (accessed 18 January 2006).

Hoffman BM, Papas RK, Chatkoff DK, Kerns RD. 2007. Meta-analysis of psychological interventions for chronic low back pain. *Health Psychology* 26: 1-9.

Hogelund J. 2001. Work incapacity and reintegration: a literature review. In *Who returns to work and why: a six country study on work incapacity and reintegration* (Ed. Bloch FS, Prins R): 27-50, Transaction Publishwers, New Brunswick.

Holland R, Battersby J, Harvey I, Lenaghan E, Smith J, Hay L. 2005. Systematic failure of multidisciplinary interventions in heart failure. *Heart* 91: 899-906.

HSA. 2008. *Workplace health and well-being strategy: report of expert group.* Health and Safety Authority, Dublin http://publications.hsa.ie/index.asp?locID=32&docID=289 (accessed 28 May 2008).

HSC. 1992. *Management of health and safety at work: approved code of practice.* HMSO, London.

HSC. 2000. *Securing health together: a long-term occupational health strategy for England, Scotland and Wales.* HSE Books, London.

HSE. 2002. *Initiative evaluation report back to work.* (HSE CRR 441/2002). HSE Books, London [out of print].

HSE. 2004a. *Management standards for work-related stress.* Health & Safety Executive, London http://www.hse.gov.uk/stress/standards/ (accessed 13 December 2005).

HSE. 2004b. *Managing sickness absence in the public sector: a joint review by the Ministerial Task Force for Health, Safety and Productivity and the Cabinet Office.* HSE Books, London www.hse.gov.uk/gse/sickness.pdf (accessed 04 April 2008).

HSE. 2004c. *Managing sickness and return to work. An employers' and managers' guide (HSG249).* HSE Books, London.

HSE. 2005. *The business case for health and safety: Better Business - Rolls-Royce plc.* Health & Safety Executive, London www.hse.gov.uk/betterbusiness/large/casestudies_rolls.htm (accessed 09 June 2008).

HSE. 2007a. *Asthma.* Health & Safety Executive, www.hse.gov.uk/asthma (accessed 05 March 2008).

HSE. 2007b. *Occupational asthma.* Health & Safety Executive, www.hse.gov.uk/statistics/causdis/asthma/index.htm (accessed 05 March 2008).

HTA. 2008. *Service delivery organisation for acute low back pain. Health Technology Assessment Report 12.* NHS Quality Improvement Scotland, Edinburgh.

Huibers MJH, Beurskens AJHM, Bleijenberg G, van Schayck CP. 2007. Psychosocial interventions by general practitioners (Cochrane Review). In *Cochrane Database of Systematic Reviews, Issue 3* John Wiley & Sons, Ltd, Chichester.

Huisstede BMA, Bierma-Zeinstra SMA, Koes BW, Verhaar JAN. 2006. Incidence and prevalence of upper-extremity musculoskeletal disorders. a systematic appraisal of the literature. *BMC Musculoskeletal Disorders* doi:10.1186/1471-2474-7-7.

Hunot V, Churchill R, Teixeira V, Silva de Lima M. 2007. Psychological therapies for generalised anxiety disorder (Cochrane Review). In *Cochrane Database of Systematic Reviews, Issue 1* John Wiley & Sons, Ltd, Chichester.

Hyman MH. 2005. Working with common cardiopulmonary problems. In *A Physician's Guide to Return to Work* (Ed. Talmage JB, Melhorn JM): 233-266, American Medical Association, Chicago.

IASP. 2005. Work rehabilitation. In *Core curriculum for professional education in pain* (Ed. Charlton EJ) International Association for the Study of Pain, Seattle.

IIAC. 2004. *Stress at work as a prescribed disease and post-traumatic stress disorder. Position Paper No.13.* Industrial Injuries Advisory Council, London www.iiac.org.uk/papers.shtml (accessed 18 January 2006).

IIAC. 2006. *Work-related upper limb disorders: report by the Industrial Injuries Advisory Council.* Her Majesty's Stationery Office, London.

IIAC. 2007a. *Back and neck pain: Industrial Injuries Advisory Council Postion Paper 18.* Industrial Injuries Advisory Council, London www.iiac.org.uk/pdf/reports/IIAC_Pospaper.pdf (accessed 12 March 2008).

IIAC. 2007b. *IIAC Proceedings of the 6th Public Meeting, Belfast.* Industrial Injuries Advisory Council, London www.iiac.org.uk/pdf/reports/BelfastPublicMeeting190607.pdf (accessed 07 May 2008).

ILO. 1998. *Occupational injuries.* International Labour Organization, Geneva.

ILO. 2002. *Managing disability in the workplace: ILO code of practice.* International Labour Organization, Geneva.

Innvær S, Vist G, Trommald M, Oxman A. 2002. Health policy-makers' perceptions of their use of evidence: a systematic review. *Journal of Health Services Research & Policy* 7: 239-244.

Iqbal A, Schloss S, George D, Isonaka S. 2002. Worldwide guidelines for chronic obstructive pulmonary disease: a comparison of diagnosis and treatment recommendations. *Respirology* 7: 233-239.

Irving A, Chang D, Sparham I. 2004. *Developing a framework for vocational rehabilitation: qualitative research (DWP RR 224).* Corporate Document Services, Leeds.

Isernhagen SJ. 2006. Job matching and return to work: occupational rehabilitation as the link. *Work* 26: 237-242.

IUA/ABI. 2007. *The 2007 Rehabilitation Code.* IUA-ABI, London www.rehabcode.org (accessed 12 March 2008).

IWH. 2007. *Seven 'principles' for successful return to work.* Institute for Work & Health, Toronto www.iwh.on.ca (accessed 12 March 2008).

James P, Cunningham I, Dibben P. 2002. Absence management and the issues of job retention and return to work. *Human Resource Management Journal* 12: 82-94.

James P, Cunningham I, Dibben P. 2003. *Job retention and vocational rehabilitation: The development and evaluation of a conceptual framework (RR 106).* HSE Books, London.

Jamtvedt G, Young JM, Kristoffersen DT, O'Brien MA, Oxman AD. 2006. Audit and feedback: effects on professional practice and health care outcomes (Cochrane Review). In *Cochrane Database of Systematic Reviews, Issue 2* John Wiley & Sons, Ltd, Chichester.

Jeebhay MF, Quirce S. 2007. Occupational asthma in the developing and industrialised world: a review. *Int J Tuberc Lung Dis* 11: 122-133.

Johnston M, Sherer M, Whyte J. 2006. Applying evidence standards to rehabilitation research. *Am J Phys Med Rehabil* 85: 292-309.

Joling C, Groot W, Janssen PPM. 2006. Duration dependence in sickness absence: how can we optimize disability management intervention strategies? *JOEM* 48: 803-814.

Jolliffe JA, Rees K, Taylor RS, Thompson D, Oldridge N, Ebrahim S. 2001. Exercise-based rehabilitation for coronary heart disease (Cochrane Review). In *Cochrane Database of Systematic Reviews, Issue 1* John Wiley & Sons, Ltd, Chichester.

Jolly K, Taylor RS, Lip GYH, Stevens A. 2006. Home-based cardiac rehabilitation compared with centre-based rehabilitation and usual care: a systematic review and meta-analysis. *International Journal of Cardiology* 111: 343-351.

Kaltenthaler E, Parry G, Beverley C. 2004. Computerized cognitive behaviour therapy: a systematic review. *Behavioural and Cognitive Psychotherapy* 32: 31-55.

Karjalainen K, Malmivaara A, van Tulder M, Roine R, Jauhiainen M, Hurri H, Koes B. 2000. Multidisciplinary biopsychosocial rehabilitation for subacute low back pain among working age adults (Cochrane review). In *The Cochrane Library, Issue 3* Update Software, Oxford.

Karjalainen K, Malmivaara A, van Tulder M, Roine R, Jauhiainen M, Hurri H, Koes B. 2003a. Biopsychosocial rehabilitation for upper limb repetitive strain injuries in working age adults (Cochrane Review). In *The Cochrane Library, Issue 3* Update Software, Oxford.

Karjalainen K, Malmivaara A, van Tulder M, Roine R, Jauhiainen M, Hurri H, Koes B. 2003b. Multidisciplinary biopsychosocial rehabilitation for neck and shoulder pain among working age adults (Cochrane Review). In *The Cochrane Library, Issue 3* Update Software, Oxford.

Karjalainen K, Malmivaara A, van Tulder M, Roine R, Jauhiainen M, Hurri H, Koes B. 2003c. Multidisciplinary rehabilitation for fibromyalgia and musculoskeletal pain in working age adults (Cochrane Review). In *The Cochrane Library, Issue 3* Update Software, Oxford.

Kates N, Mach M. 2007. Chronic disease management for depression in primary care: a summary of the current literature and implications for practice. *The Canadian Journal of Psychiatry* 52: 77-85.

Kay TM, Gross A, Goldsmith C, Santaguida PL, Hoving J, Bronfort G. 2005. Exercises for mechanical neck disorders (Cochrane Review). In *Cochrane Database of Systematic Reviews, Issue 3* John Wlley & Sons, Ltd, Chichester.

Kazimirski JC. 1997. CMA Policy Summary. The physician's role in helping patients return to work after an illness or injury. *Can Med Assoc J* 156: 680A-680C.

Keane TM, Marshall AD, Taft CT. 2006. Posttraumatic stress disorder: etiology, epidemiology, and treatment outcome. *Annual Review of Clinical Psychology* 2: 161-197.

Kendall E, Muenchberger H, Gee T. 2006. Vocational rehabilitation following traumatic brain injury: a quantitative synthesis of outcome studies. *Journal of Vocational Rehabilitation* 25: 149-160.

Kendall N. 2006. *Management and governance of occupational safety and health in five countries (United Kingdom, United States of America, Finland, Canada, Australia). Technical Report prepared for the National Occupational Health and Safety Advisory Committee: NOHSAC Technical Report 8.* National Occupational Health and Safety Advisory Committee, Wellington.

Kendall NAS, Thompson BF. 1998. A pilot programme for dealing with the comorbidity of chronic pain and long-term unemployment. *Journal of Occupational Rehabilitation* 8: 5-26.

Kenyon P. 2003. *Cost benefit analysis of rehabilitation services provided by CRS Australia.* The Institute for Research into International Competitiveness at Curtin University of Technology, Perth.

Kessler RC, Demler O, Frank RG, Olfson M, Pincus HA, Walters EE, Wang P, Wells KB, Zaslavsky AM. 2005. Prevalence and treatment of mental disorders, 1990 to 2003. *The New England Journal of Medicine* 352: 2515-2523.

Kirby MJI, Keon WJ, on behalf of the Standing Senate Committee on Social Affairs SaT. 2004. *Report 3: Mental health, mental illness and addiction: issues and options for Canada (interim report).* Parliament of Canada, Ottawa www.parl.gc.ca (accessed 12 March 2008).

Kool J, de Bie R, Oesch P, Knüsel O, van den Brandt P, Bachmann S. 2004. Exercise reduces sick leave in patients with non-acute non-specific low back pain: a meta-analysis. *J Rehabil Med* 36: 49-62.

Kornfeld R, Rupp K. 2000. The net effects of the Project NetWork return-to-work case management experiment on participant earnings, benefit receipt, and other outcomes. *Social Security Bulletin* 63: 12-33.

Kosny A, Franche R-L, Pole J, Krause N, Côté P, Mustard C. 2006. Early healthcare provider communication with patients and their workplace following a lost-time claim for an occupational musculoskeletal injury. *Journal of Occupational Rehabilitation* 16: 25-37.

Kovoor P, Lee AKY, Carrozzi F, Wiseman V, Byth K, Zecchin R, Dickson C, King M, Hall J, Ross DL, Uther JB, Denniss AR. 2006. Return to full normal activities including work at two weeks after acute myocardial infarction. *Am J Cardiol* 97: 952-958.

Krause N, Frank JW, Dasinger LK, Sullivan TJ, Sinclair SJ. 2001. Determinants of duration of disability and return-to-work after work-related injury and illness: challenges for future research. *American Journal of Industrial Medicine* 40: 464-484.

Krause N, Ragland DR. 1994. Occupational disability due to low back pain: a new interdisciplinary classification based on a phase model of disability. *Spine* 19: 1011-1020.

Krupa T. 2007. Interventions to improve employment outcomes for workers who experience mental illness. *Can J Psychiatry* 52: 339-345.

Kumar S. 2001. Disability, injury and ergonomics intervention. *Disability and Rehabilitation* 23: 805-814.

Kunkel M, Miller SD. 2002. Return to work after foot and ankle injury. *Foot Ankle Clin N Am* 7: 421-428.

Kupper A, Mackenzie S, Heasman T. 2004. *The challenge of managing upper limb disorders - how can health professionals become more effective? (HSE RR 215).* Health & Safety Executive, London.

Lacasse Y, Goldstein R, Lasserson TJ, Martin S. 2006. Pulmonary rehabilitation for chronic obstructive pulmonary disease (Cochrane Review). In *Cochrane Database of Systematic Reviews, Issue 4* John Wiley & Sons, Ltd, Chichester.

Langley J, Brenner R. 2004. What is an injury? *Injury Prevention* 10: 69-71.

Layard R. 2006. *The depression report: a new deal for depression and anxiety disorders.* Mental Health Policy Group, Centre for Economic Performance, London School of Economics, London http://cep.lse.ac.uk/research/mentalhealth (accessed 26 March 2008).

Leavitt F. 1992. The physical exertion factor in compensable work injuries: a hidden flaw in previous research. *Spine* 17: 307-310.

Lee AJ, Strickler GK, Shepard DS. 2007. The economics of cardiac rehabilitation and lifestyle modification. A review of literature. *Journal of Cardiopulmonary Rehabilitation and Prevention* 27: 135-142.

Leech C. 2004. *Renaissance Project - preventing chronic disability from low back pain.* The Stationery Office (Government of Ireland), Dublin (Government Publications Office).

Leff J. 2001. The state of the evidence: mental health services and barriers to implementation. In *Mental health: a call for action by world health ministers: ministerial round tables 2001: 54th World Health Assembly* (Ed. WHO) World Health Organization, Geneva.

Leigh-Doyle S, Mulvihill R. 2004. *Illness and employment: retaining the link to work: summary.* European Foundation for the Improvement of Living and Working Conditions, Dublin www.eurofound.eu.int (accessed 09 April 2008).

Lelliott P, Boradman J, Harvey S, Hendersen M, Knapp M, Tulloch S. 2008. *Mental health and work: a report for the National Director for Work and Health.* Royal College of Psychiatrists, London.

Leng GC, Fowler B, Ernst E. 2000. Exercise for intermittent claudication (Cochrane Review). In *Cochrane Database of Systematic Reviews, Issue 2* John Wiley & Sons, Ltd, Chichester.

Leonesio MV. 1996. The economics of retirement: a nontechnical guide. *Social Security Bulletin* 59: 29-50.

Lerner D, Allaire SH, Reisine ST. 2005. Work disability resulting from chronic health conditions. *JOEM* 47: 253-264.

Levack WMM, Dean SG, Siegert RJ, McPherson KM. 2006. Purposes and mechanisms of goal planning in rehabilitation: the need for a critical distinction. *Disability and Rehabilitation* 28: 741-749.

Lewin R. 1999. Return to work after MI, the roles of depression, health beliefs and rehabilitation. *International Journal of Cardiology* 72: 49-51.

Linton SJ. 2002. Cognitive behavioral therapy in the prevention of musculoskeletal pain: description of a program. In *New avenues for the prevention of chronic musculoskeletal pain and disability. Pain research and clinical management. Vol 12* (Ed. Linton SJ): 269-276, Elsevier Science B.V., Amsterdam.

Linton SJ, Andersson T. 2000. Can chronic disability be prevented? a randomized trial of a cognitive-behavior intervention and two forms of information for patients with spinal pain. *Spine* 25: 2825-2831.

Loeser JD, Henderlite SE, Conrad DA. 1995. Incentive effects of workers' compensation benefits: a literature synthesis. *Medical Care Research and Review* 52: 34-59.

Loisel P, Abenhaim L, Durand P, Esdaile JM, Suissa S, Gosselin L, Simard R, Turcotte J, Lemaire J. 1997. A population-based, randomized clinical trial on back pain management. *Spine* 15: 2911-2918.

Loisel P, Buchbinder R, Hazard R, Keller R, Scheel I, van Tulder M, Webster B. 2005. Prevention of work disability due to musculoskeletal disorders: the challenge of implementing evidence. *Journal of Occupational Rehabilitation* 15: 507-521.

Loisel P, Durand MJ, Berthelette D, Vézina N, Baril R, Gagnon D, Larivière C, Tremblay C. 2001. Disability prevention: new paradigm for the management of occupational back pain. *Dis Manage Health Outcomes* 9: 351-360.

Loisel P, Durand MJ, Diallo B, Vachon B, Charpentier N, Labelle J. 2003. From evidence to community practice in work rehabilitation: the Quebec experience. *The Clinical Journal of Pain* 19: 105-113.

Loisel P, Lemaire J, Poitras S, Durand M-J, Champagne F, Stock S, Diallo B, Tremblay C. 2002. Cost-benefit and cost-effectiveness analysis of a disability prevention model for back pain management: a six year follow up study. *Occup Environ Med* 59: 807-815.

Lombardo LJ, Balmes JR. 2000. Occupational asthma: a review. *Environmental Health Perspectives* 108: 697-704.

Löthgren M. 2004a. Economic evidence in affective disorders: a review. *Eur J Health Econom* 5 Suppl 1: S12-S20.

Löthgren M. 2004b. Economic evidence in anxiety disorders: a review. *Eur J Health Econom* 5 Suppl 1: S20-S25.

Lotters F, Meerding W-J, Burdorf A. 2005. Reduced productivity after sickness absence due to musculoskeletal disorders and its relation to health outcomes. *Scand J Work Environ Health* 31: 367-374.

Lunt J, Bowen J, Lee R. 2005. *HSE review of the risk prevention approach to occupational health: applying models to 21st century occupational health needs: health models information pack (HSL/2005/57).* Health & Safety Executive/Health & Safety Laboratory, London.

Macdonald EB, Docherty G. 2007. Healthy working lives: the Scottish strategy for improving health in the workplace. In *Supporting health at work: international perspectives on occupational health services* (Ed. Westerholm P, Walters D) IOSH Services Limited, Wigston, Leicestershire www.iosh.co.uk/policyandpractice (accessed 09 April 2008).

MacEachen E, Clarke J, Franche RL, Irvin E. 2006. Systematic review of the qualitative literature on return to work after injury. *Scand J Work Environ Health* 32: 257-269.

Mahalik J, Shigaki CL, Baldwin D, Johnstone B. 2006. A review of employability and worksite interventions for persons with rheumatoid arthritis and osteoarthritis. *Work* 26: 303-311.

Main CJ, Sullivan MJL, Watson PJ. 2008. *Pain management: practical applications of the biopsychosocial perspective in clinical and occupational settings.* Churchill Livingstone, Edinburgh.

Malo J-L. 2005. Future advances in work-related asthma and the impact on occupational health. *Occupational Medicine* 55: 606-611.

Mancuso LL. 1990. Reasonable accommodation for workers with psychiatric disabilities. *Psychosocial Rehabilitation Journal* 14: 3-19.

Mannino DM, Braman S. 2007. The epidemiology and economics of chronic obstructive pulmonary disease. *Proc Am Thor Soc* 4: 502-506.

Mannino DM, Buist AS. 2007. Global burden of COPD: risk factors, prevalence, and future trends. *Lancet* 370: 765-773.

Mapp CE, Boschetto P, Maestrelli P, Fabbri LM. 2005. Occupational asthma. *American Journal of Respiratory and Critical Care Medicine* 172: 280-305.

Marhold C, Linton SJ, Melin L. 2002. Identification of obstacles for chronic pain patients to return to work: evaluation of a questionnaire. *Journal of Occupational Rehabilitation* 12: 65-75.

Marsden S, Beardwell C, Shaw J, Wright M, Green N, McGurry B. 2004. *The development of case studies that demonstrate the business benefit of effective management of occupational health and safety (RR 249).* HSE Books, London.

Martimo KP, Verbeek J, Karppinen J, Furlan AD, Kuijer PPFM, Viikari-Juntura E, Takala E-P, Jauhiainen M. 2007. Manual material handling advice and assistive devices for preventing and treating back pain in workers (Cochrane Review). In *Cochrane Database of Systematic Reviews, Issue 3* John Wiley & Sons, Ltd, Chichester.

Mays N, Pope C, Popay J. 2005. Systematically reviewing qualitative and quantitative evidence to inform management and policy-making in the health field. *Journal of Health Services Research & Policy* 10 Suppl 1: 6-20.

MBWDC. 2000. *Report of the task force on vocational rehabilitation in workers' compensation.* Michigan Bureau of Workers' Disability Compensation, Lansing http://michigan.gov/documents/wca_vr_task_rprt_2000_147281_7.pdf (accessed 30 April 2008).

McAlister FA, Stewart S, Ferrua S, McMurray JJJV. 2004. Multidisciplinary strategies for the management of heart failure patients at high risk for admission. A systematic review of randomized trials. *J Am Coll Cardiol* 44: 810-819.

McCluskey S, Burton AK, Main CJ. 2006. The implementation of occupational health guidelines principles for reducing sickness absence due to musculoskeletal disorders. *Occupational Medicine* 56: 237-242.

McCormick A, Fleming D, Charlton J. 1995. *Morbidity statistics from general practice: fourth national study 1991-1992 (Office of population censuses and surveys Series MB5 no. 3).* HMSO, London.

McDaid D, Curran C, Knapp M. 2005. Promoting mental well-being in the workplace: a European policy perspective. *International Review of Psychiatry* 17: 365-373.

McIntosh A, Cohen A, Turnbull N, Esmonde L, Dennis P, Eatock J, Feetam C, Hague J, Hughes I, Kelly J, Kosky N, Lear G, Owens L, Ratcliffe J, Salkovskis P. 2004. *Clinical guidelines and evidence review for panic disorder and generalised anxiety disorder.* University of Sheffield/National Collaborating Centre for Primary Care, Sheffield/London.

McLeod J. 2001. *Counselling in the workplace: the facts. A systematic study of the research evidence.* British Association for Counselling and Psychotherapy, Warwickshire.

McLeod J, Henderson M. 2003. Does workplace counselling work? *British Journal of Psychiatry* 182: 103-104.

McLeod J, McLeod J. 2001. How effective is workplace counselling? A review of the research literature. *Counselling and Psychotherapy Research* 1: 184-190.

Meijer EM, Sluiter JK, Frings-Dresen MHW. 2005. Evaluation of effective return-to-work treatment programs for sick-listed patients with non-specific musculoskeletal complaints: a systematic review. *Int Arch Occup Environ Health* 78: 523-532.

Melhorn JM. 2005. Working with common upper extremity problems. In *A Physician's Guide to Return to Work* (Ed. Talmage JB, Melhorn JM): 181-213, American Medical Association, Chicago.

Melhorn JM, Hegmann KT. 2008. Methodology. In *Guides to the evaluation of disease and injury causation* (Ed. Melhorn JM, Ackerman WE) American Medical Association, Chicago.

Mental Health Foundation. 2002. *Out at work: A survey of the experiences of people with mental health problems within the workplace.* The Mental Health Foundation, London.

Menz FE, Botterbusch K, Hagen Foley D, Johnson PT. 2003. *Achieving quality outcomes through community-based rehabilitation programmes: the results are in.* Presented to NISH National Training Conference, April 7, Denver, Colorado.

Merrill AP. 1997. Worker's compensation, litigation, and employment factors in return to work. *Work* 9: 245-253.

Merry SN. 2007. Prevention and early intervention for depression in young people - a practical possibility? *Curr Opin Psychiatry* 20: 325-329.

Michie S, Williams S. 2003. Reducing work related psychological ill health and sickness absence: a systematic literature review. *Occup Environ Med* 60: 3-9.

Mimura C, Griffiths P. 2003. The effectiveness of current approaches to workplace stress management in the nursing profession: an evidence based literature review. *Occup Environ Med* 60: 10-15.

Mital A, Desai A, Mital A. 2004. Return to work after a coronary event. *Journal of Cardiopulmonary Rehabilitation* 24: 365-373.

Mital A, Mital A. 2002. Returning coronary heart disease patients to work: a modified perspective. *Journal of Occupational Rehabilitation* 12: 31-42.

Moffett J, McLean S. 2006. The role of physiotherapy in the management of non-specific back pain and neck pain. *Rheumatology* 45: 371-378.

Mondloch MV, Cole DC, Frank JW. 2001. Does how you do depend on how you think you'll do? A systematic review of the evidence for a relation between patients' recovery expectations and health outcomes. *Canadian Medical Association Journal* 165: 174-179.

Montori VM, Wilczynski NL, Morgan D, Haynes RB. 2005. Optimal search strategies for retrieving systematic reviews from Medline: analytical survey. *BMJ* 330: 68.

Morris P, Lloyd C. 2004. Vocational rehabilitation in psychiatry: a re-evaluation. *Australian and New Zealand Journal of Psychiatry* 38: 490-494.

Moscato G, Rampulla C. 2003. Costs of occupational asthma and of occupational chronic obstructive pulmonary disease. *Curr Opin Allergy Clin Immunol* 3: 109-114.

Mowlam A, Lewis J. 2005. *Exploring how General Practitioners work with patients on sick leave (DWP RR 257)*. Corporate Document Services, Leeds.

Mueller G, Bendix T, Bendix A. 2003. What have physicians learned about returning chronically disabled back patients to work? *Seminars in Spine Surgery* 15: 44-53.

Murta SG, Sanderson K, Oldenburg B. 2007. Process evaluation in occupational stress management programs: a systematic review. *Am J Health Promot* 21: 248-254.

NACR. 2007. *The National Audit of Cardiac Rehabilitation: annual statistical report 2007*. British Heart Foundation, London.

Namath A, Kuschmer W. 2006. Work-related airways disease. *Clinical Pulmonary Medicine* 13: 169-177.

Nash CE, Mickan SM, Del Mar CB, Glasziou PP. 2004. Resting injured limbs delays recovery: a systematic review. *The Journal of Family Practice* 53: 706-712.

NCCC. 2006. *Hypertension: management in adults in primary care: pharmacological update*. Royal College of Physicians, London.

Neumeyer-Gromen A, Lampert T, Stark K, Kallischnigg G. 2004. Disease management programs for depression. A systematic review and meta-analysis of randomized controlled trials. *Med Care* 42: 1211-1221.

Newman Taylor A. 2006. *The prescription of disease*. Industrial Injuries Advisory Council, London www.iiac.org.uk/pdf/reports/PrescriptionOfDisease.pdf (accessed 12 March 2008).

Newman Taylor AJ, Nicholson PJ, Cullinan P, Boyle C, Burge PS. 2004. *Guidelines for the prevention, identification and management of occupational asthma: evidence review and recommendations*. British Occupational Health Research Foundation, London.

NHMRC. 2004. *Evidence-based management of acute musculoskeletal pain: a guide for clinicians*. National Health and Medical Research Council, Australian Academic Press pty ltd, Bowen Hills, Queensland.

NHS. 1999. *Mental health: modern standards and service models: National Service Framework*. Department of Health, London.

NHS. 2000. Cardiac rehabilitation. In *Coronary heart disease: National Service Frameworks* Department of Health, London.

NHS Centre for Reviews. 1998. Cardiac rehabilitation. *Effective Health Care* 4: 1-12.

NICE. 2003. *Chronic heart failure: national clinical guideline for diagnosis and management in primary and secondary care*. Royal College of Physicians, London.

NICE. 2004a. *Depression: management of depression in primary and secondary care. National Clinical Practice Guideline Number 23.* National Institute for Clinical Excellence, London www.nice.org.uk/nicemedia/pdf/cg023fullguideline.pdf (accessed 02 April 2008).

NICE. 2004b. Managing stable COPD. *Thorax* 59 (Suppl 1): 39-130.

NICE. 2006. *Computerised cognitive behaviour therapy for depression and anxiety: Review of Technology Appraisal 51.* National Institute for Health and Clinical Excellence, London www.nice.org.uk/nicemedia/pdf/TA097guidance.pdf (accessed 02 April 2008).

NICE. 2007. *Depression (amended): management of depression in primary and secondary care. NICE Clinical Guideline 23 (amended).* National Institute for Health and Clinical Excellence, London www.nice.org.uk/nicemedia/pdf/CG23NICEguidelineamended.pdf (accessed 02 April 2008).

NICE. 2008. *Workplace interventions that are effective for promoting mental wellbeing: synopsis of the evidence of effectiveness and cost-effectiveness.* National Institute for Health and Clinical Excellence, London www.nice.org.uk/nicemedia/pdf/WorkplaceMentalHealthSynopsisOfEvidence.pdf. (accessed 05 March 2008).

Nice K, Thornton P. 2004. *Job retention and rehabilitation pilot: employers' management of long-term sickness absence (DWP RR 227).* Corporate Document Services, Leeds.

Nicholson PJ, Cullinan P, Newman Taylor AJ, Burge PS, Boyle C. 2005. Evidence based guidelines for the prevention, identification, and management of occupational asthma. *Occup Environ Med* 62: 290-299.

NIDMAR. 2000. *Code of practice for disability management: describing effective benchmarks for the creation of workplace-based disability management programs.* National Institute of Disability Management and Research, Ottowa, Canada.

Nieuwenhuijsen K, Bültmann U, Neumeyer-Gromen A, Verhoeven AC, Verbeek JHAM, van der Feltz-Cornelis CM. 2008. Interventions to improve occupational health in depressed people (Cochrane Review). In *Cochrane Database of Systematic Reviews, Issue 2* John Wiley & Sons, Ltd, Chichester.

Nocon A, Baldwin S. 1998. *Trends in rehabilitation policy. a review of the literature.* Kings Fund, London.

Nordin M, Balagué F, Cedraschi C. 2006. Nonspecific lower-back pain: surgical versus nonsurgical treatment. *Clinical Orthopaedics and Related Research* 443: 156-167.

Norwich Union Healthcare. 2006. *Health of the workplace report.* Norwich Union Healthcare Limited, Norwich www.norwichunion.com/healthcare (accessed 12 March 2008).

NZGG. 2002. *Cardiac Rehabilitation: summary and resource kit.* New Zealand Guidelines Group, Wellington.

O'Donnell C. 2000. Will Australian workers' compensation insurance management get better soon? *Work* 15: 177-188.

O'Donnell ML, Creamer M, Elliott P, Atkin C, Kossmann T. 2005. Determinants of quality of life and role-related disability after injury: impact of acute psychological responses. *J Trauma* 59: 1328-1335.

OECD. 2003. *Transforming disability into ability: policies to promote work and income security for disabled people.* Organisation for Economic Co-operation and Development, Paris.

Ofman JJ, Badamgarav E, Henning JM, Knight K, Gano ADJr, Levan RK, Gur-Arie S, Richards MS, Hasselblad V, Weingarten SR. 2004. Does disease management improve clinical and economic outcomes in patients with chronic diseases? A systematic review. *Am J Med* 117: 182-192.

Olsheski JA, Rosenthal DA, Hamilton M. 2002. Disability management and psychosocial rehabilitation: considerations for integration. *Work* 19: 63-70.

Orr LL, Bell SH, Lam K. 2007. *Long-term impacts of the new deal for disabled people (DWP RR 432).* Corporate Document Services, Leeds.

Ostelo RWJG, van Tulder MW, Vlaeyen JWS, Linton SJ, Morley SJ, Assendelft WJJ. 2005. Behavioural treatment for chronic low-back pain (Cochrane Review). In *Cochrane Database of Systematic Reviews, Issue 1* John WIley & Sons, Ltd, Chichester.

Palmer KT, Reading I, Calnan M, Coggon D. 2007. How common is RSI? *Occup Environ Med* doi:10.1136/oem.2007.035378.

Pawson R, Greenhalgh T, Harvey G, Walshe K. 2005. Realist review - a new method of systematic review designed for complex policy interventions. *Journal of Health Services Research & Policy* 10 Suppl 1: 21-34.

Pengel HM, Maher CG, Refshauge KM. 2002. Systematic review of conservative interventions for subacute low back pain. *Clinical Rehabilitation* 16: 811-820.

Perk J, Alexanderson K. 2004. Sick leave due to coronary artery disease or stroke. *Scand J Public Health* 32 (Suppl 63): 181-206.

Peters J, Pickvance S, Wilford J, MacDonald E, Blank L. 2007. Predictors of delayed return to work or job loss with respiratory ill-health: a systematic review. *Journal of Occupational Rehabilitation* 17: 317-326.

Petrie KJ, Cameron LD, Ellis CJ, Buick D, Weinman J. 2002. Changing illness perceptions after myocardial infarction: an early intervention randomized controlled trial. *Psychosomatic Medicine* 64: 580-586.

Phillips L, Harrison T, Houck P. 2005. Return to work and the person with heart failure. *Heart & Lung* 34: 79-88.

Pickvance S. 2006. Too little too late. Part 2: what went wrong with the Job Retention and Rehabilitation Pilot? *Occupational Health [at Work]* 3: 23-25.

Pilgrim D, Bentall R. 1999. The medicalisation of misery: a critical realist analysis of the concept of depression. *Journal of Mental Health* 8: 261-274.

Pirraglia PA, Rosen AB, Hermann RC, Olchanski NV, Neumann P. 2004. Cost-utility analysis studies of depression management: a systematic review. *Am J Psychiatry* 161: 2155-2162.

Poiraudeau S, Rannou F, Revel M. 2007. Functional restoration programs for low back pain: a systematic review. *Annales de réadaptation et de médecine physique* 50: 425-429.

Post MWM, de Witte LP, Schrijvers AJP. 1999. Quality of life and the ICIDH: towards an integrated conceptual model for rehabilitation outcomes research. *Clinical Rehabilitation* 13: 5-15.

Pransky G, Robertson MM, Moon SD. 2002. Stress and work-related upper extremity disorders: implications for prevention and management. *American Journal of Industrial Medicine* 41: 443-455.

Pransky G, Gatchel R, Linton SJ, Loisel P. 2005. Improving return to work research. *Journal of Occupational Rehabilitation* 15: 453-457.

Pransky G, Shaw W, Franche RL, Clarke A. 2004. Disability prevention and communication among workers, physicians, employers, and insurers - current models and opportunities for improvement. *Disability and Rehabilitation* 26: 625-634.

Prezzia C, Denniston P. 2001. The use of evidence-based duration guidelines. *The Journal of Workers Compensation* 10: 43-53.

PriceWaterhouseCoopers LLP. 2008. *Building the case for wellness.* PricewaterhouseCoopers LLP, London www.workingforhealth.gov.uk/Carol-Blacks-Review (accessed 16 April 2008).

Purdon S, Stratford N, Taylor R, Natarajan L, Bell S, Wittenburg D. 2006. *Impacts of the job retention and rehabilitation pilot (DWP RR 342).* Corporate Document Services, Leeds.

Rachiotis G, Savani R, Brant A, MacNeill SJ, Newman Taylor A, Cullinan P. 2007. Outcome of occupational asthma after cessation of exposure: a systematic review. *Thorax* 62: 147-152.

Rainville J, Pransky G, Indahl A, Mayer EK. 2005. The physician as disability advisor for patients with musculoskeletal complaints. *Spine* 30: 2579-2584.

Ram FSF, Robinson SM, Black PN, Picot J. 2005. Physical training for asthma (Cochrane Review). In *Cochrane Database of Systematic Reviews, Issue 4* John Wiley & Sons, Ltd, Chicester.

Rees K, Taylor RS, Singh S, Coats AJS, Ebrahim S. 2004. Exercise based rehabilitation for heart failure (Cochrane Review). In *Cochrane Database of Systematic Reviews, Issue 3* John Wiley & Sons, Ltd, Chichester.

Reynolds MW, Frame D, Scheye R, Rose ME, George S, Watson JB, Hlatky MA. 2004. A systematic review of the economic burden of chronic angina. *Am J Manag Care* 10: S347-S357.

Rick J, Briner RB, Daniels K, Perryman S, Guppy A. 2001. *A critical review of psychosocial hazard measures (HSE CRR 356).* HSE Books, London.

Rick J, O'Regan S, Kinder A. 2006. *Early intervention following trauma: a controlled longitudinal study at Royal Mail Group.* Institute for Employment Studies, Brighton www.employment-studies.co.uk/pubs/index.php (accessed 16 April 2008).

Rick J, Thomson L, Briner RB, O'Regan S, Daniels K. 2002. *Review of existing supporting scientific knowledge to underpin standards of good practice for key work-related stressors - phase 1 (HSE RR 024).* HSE Books, London.

Rinaldi M, Perkins R. 2007. Vocational rehabilitation for people with mental health problems. *Psychiatry* 6: 373-376.

Rohling ML, Binder LM, Langhinrichsen-Rohling J. 1995. Money matters: a meta-analytic review of the association between financial compensation and the experience and treatment of chronic pain. *Health Psychology* 14: 537-547.

Rose J. 2006. A model of care for managing traumatic psychological injury in a workers' compensation context. *Journal of Traumatic Stress* 19: 315-326.

Rose N. 2007. Beyond medicalisation. *Lancet* 369: 700-701.

Roth A, Fonagy P. 2005. *What works for whom? A critical review of psychotherapy research.* Guildford Press, New York.

Royal College of Psychiatrists. 2002. *Employment opportunities and psychiatric disability. Council Report CR111.* Royal College of Psychiatrists, London.

Ruotsalainen JH, Verbeek JH, Salmi JA, Jauhiainen M, Laamanen I, Pasterneck I, Husman K. 2006. Evidence on the effectiveness of occupational health interventions. *American Journal of Industrial Medicine* 49: 865-872.

Saeki S, Okazaki T, Hachisuka K. 2006. Concurrent validity of the Community Integration Questionnaire in patients with traumatic brain injury in Japan. *Journal of Rehabilitation Medicine* 38: 333-335.

Sainsbury R. 2008. *Employment Advisers in GP surgeries (DWP Research Report).* Department for Work and Pensions, London (In press).

Sanderson K, Andrews G. 2006. Common mental disorders in the workplace: recent findings from descriptive and social epidemiology. *Can J Psychiatry* 51: 63-75.

Sawney P, Challenor J. 2003. Poor communication between health professionals is a barrier to rehabilitation. *Occupational Medicine* 53: 246-248.

Schneider J. 2003. *Employment for people with mental health problems.* Department of Health / National Institute for Mental Health in England (NIMHE), London / Leeds www.nimhe.org.uk/whatshapp/item_display_publications.asp?id=324 (accessed 2003).

Schonstein E, Kenny J, Keating J, Koes BW. 2003. Work conditioning, work hardening and functional restoration for workers with back and neck pain (Cochrane Review). In *The Cochrane Library, Issue 3* Update Software, Oxford.

Schultz AB, Edington DW. 2007. Employee health and presenteeism: A systematic review. *Journal of Occupational Rehabilitation* 17: 547-579.

SCMH. 2007. *Mental health at work: developing the business case. Policy Paper 8*. The Sainsbury Centre for Mental Health, London www.scmh.org.uk/employment/index.aspx (accessed 15 April 2008).

Scottish Executive. 2004. *Healthy working lives: a plan for action.* Scottish Executive, Edinburgh www.scotland.gov.uk/Resource/Doc/924/0034156.pdf (accessed 07 May 2008).

Seddon ME, Marshall MN, Campbell SM, Roland MO. 2001. Systematic review of studies of quality of clinical care in general practice in the UK, Australia and New Zealand. *Quality in Health Care* 10: 152-158.

Seferiadis A, Rosenfeld M, Gunnarsson R. 2004. A review of treatment interventions in whiplash-associated disorders. *Eur Spine J* 13: 387-397.

Selander J, Marnetoft S-U, Bergroth A, Ekholm J. 2002. Return to work following vocational rehabilitation for neck, back and shoulder problems: risk factors reviewed. *Disability and Rehabilitation* 24: 704-712.

Semmer NK. 2006. Job stress interventions and the organization of work. *Scand J Work Environ Health* 32: 515-527.

Seymour L, Grove B. 2005. *Workplace interventions for people with common mental health problems: evidence review and recommendations.* British Occupational Health Research Foundation, London.

Shaw W, Hong Q, Pransky G, Loisel P. 2007. A literature review describing the role of return-to-work coordinators in trial programs and interventions designed to prevent workplace disability. *J Occup Rehabil* DOI: 10.1007/s10926-007-9115-y.

Shaw WS, Feuerstein M, Huang GD. 2002. Secondary prevention and the workplace. In *New avenues for the prevention of chronic musculoskeletal pain and disability. Pain research and clinical management. Vol 12* (Ed. Linton SJ): 215-236, Elsevier Science B.V., Amsterdam.

Shaw WS, Linton SJ, Pransky G. 2006. Reducing sickness absence from work due to low back pain: how well do intervention strategies match modifiable risk factors? *J Occup Rehabil* 16: 591-605.

Shaw WS, Pransky G, Fitzgerald TE. 2001. Early prognosis for low back disability: intervention strategies for health care providers. *Disability and Rehabilitation* 23: 815-828.

Sheldon TA. 2005. Making evidence synthesis more useful for management and policy-making. *Journal of Health Services Research & Policy* 10 Suppl 1: 1-5.

Sherrer YS. 2005. Working with common rheumatologic disorders. In *A Physician's Guide to Return to Work* (Ed. Talmage JB, Melhorn JM): 289-304, American Medical Association, Chicago.

Shiels C, Gabbay MB, Ford FM. 2004. Patient factors associated with duration of certified sickness absence and transition to long-term incapacity. *British Journal of General Practice* 54: 86-91.

Siegert RJ, Taylor WJ. 2004. Theoretical aspects of goal-setting and motivation in rehabilitation. *Disability and Rehabilitation* 26: 1-8.

SIGN. 2002. *Cardiac rehabilitation: a national clinical guideline.* Scottish Intercollegiate Guidelines Network, Edinburgh.

SIGN. 2007a. *Management of stable angina: a national clinical guideline.* Scottish Intercollegiate Guidelines Network, Edinburgh.

SIGN. 2007b. *Risk estimation and the prevention of cardiovascular disease: a national clinical guideline.* Scottish Intercollegiate Guidelines Network, Edinburgh.

Silverstein R, Julnes G, Nolan R. 2005. What policymakers need and must demand from research regarding the employment rate of persons with disabilities. *Behav Sci Law* 23: 399-448.

Simon GE. 2003. Social and economic burden of mood disorders. *Biol Psychiatry* 54: 208-215.

Simon GE, Barber C, Birnbaum HG, Frank RG, Greenberg PE, Rose RM, Wang PS, Kessler RC. 2001. Depression and work productivity: The comparative costs of treatment versus nontreatment. *J Occup Environ Med* 43: 2-9.

Simpson E, Pilote L. 2003. Quality of life after acute myocardial infarction: a systematic review. *Can J Cardiol* 19: 507-511.

Sinclair S, Hogg-Johnson S. 2002. Early rehabilitation: the Ontario experience. In *New avenues for the prevention of chronic musculoskeletal pain and disability. Pain research and clinical management. Vol 12* (Ed. Linton SJ): 259-268, Elsevier Science B.V., Amsterdam.

Singleton N, Bumpstead R, O'Brien M, Lee A, Meltzer H. 2000. *Psychiatric morbidity among adults living in private households, 2000: summary report.* Office for National Statistics, London www.statistics.gov.uk/statbase/Product.asp?vlnk=8258 (accessed 13 May 2008).

Sirvastava S, Chamberlain MA. 2005. Factors determining job retention and return to work for disabled employees: a questionnaire study of opinions of disabled people's organizations in the UK. *J Rehabil Med* 37: 17-22.

Slavin R. 1995. Best evidence synthesis: an intelligent alternative to met-analysis. *J Clin Epidemiol* 48: 9-18.

Smidt N, De Vet HCW, Bouter LM, Dekker J. 2005. Effectiveness of exercise therapy: a best-evidence summary of systematic reviews. *Australian Journal of Physiotherapy* 51: 71-85.

Smith GS, Sorock GS, Wellman HM, Courtney TK, Pransky GS. 2006. Blurring the distinctions between on and off the job injuries: similarities and differences in circumstances. *Injury Prevention* 12: 236-241.

Smith JR, Mugford M, Holland R, Candy B, Noble MJ, Harrison BDW, Koutantji M, Upton C, Harvey I. 2005. A systematic review to examine the impact of psycho-educational interventions on health outcomes and costs in adults and children with difficult asthma. *Health Technology Assessment* 9: (23).

Snashall D. 2003. Hazards of work. In *ABC of occupational and environmental medicine* (Ed. Snashall D, Patel D): 1-5, BMJ Books, London.

Social Exclusion Unit. 2004. *Mental health and social exclusion.* The Office of The Deputy Prime Minister, London http://archive.cabinetoffice.gov.uk/seu/docs/mental_health.pdf (accessed 02 April 2008).

Spurgeon A. 2007. Stress as an occupational disease. In *The Industrial Injuries Advisory Council. Proceedings of the 6th Public Meeting* Industrial Injuries Advisory Council, London www.iiac.org.uk/reports/index.asp (accessed 02 April 2008).

Staal JB, Hlobil H, van Tulder MW, Waddell G, Burton AK, Koes BW, van Mechelen W. 2003. Occupational health guidelines for the management of low back pain: an international comparison. *Occupational and Environmental Medicine* 60: 618-626.

Staal JB, Rainville J, Fritz J, van Mechelen W, Pransky G. 2005. Physical exercise interventions to improve disability and return to work in low back pain: current insights and opportunities for improvement. *Journal of Occupational Rehabilitation* 15: 491-502.

Stafford B. 2007. *New deal for disabled people: third synthesis report - key findings from the evaluation (DWP RR 430).* Corporate Document Services, Leeds.

Steffick DE, Fortney JC, Smith JL, Pyne JM. 2006. Worksite disease management programs for depression: potential employer benefits. *Dis Manage Health Outcomes* 14: 13-26.

Stephens B, Gross DP. 2007. The influence of a continuum of care model on the rehabilitation of compensation claimants with soft tissue disorders. *Spine* 32: 2898-2904.

Stephens P, Hickling N, Gaskell L, Burton M, Holland D. 2004. *Occupational health and SMEs: focused intervention strategies (RR 257)*. HSE Books, London.

Stratford N, Taylor R, Legard R, Natarajan L, Purdon S, Shaw A. 2005. *The job retention and rehabilitation pilot: reflections on running a randomised controlled trial (DWP RR 305)*. Corporate Document Services, Leeds.

Stucki G, Stier-Jarmer M, Grill E, Melvin J. 2005. Rationale and principles of early rehabilitation care after an acute injury or illness. *Disability and Rehabilitation* 27: 353-359.

Sullivan MJL, Feuerstein M, Gatchel R, Linton SJ, Pransky G. 2005. Integrating psychosocial and behavioral interventions to achieve optimal rehabilitation outcomes. *Journal of Occupational Rehabilitation* 15: 475-489.

Sullivan S. 2005. Promoting health and productivity for depressed patients in the workplace. *Journal of Managed Care Pharmacy* 11(3 suppl): S12-S15.

Svensson T, Mussener U, Alexanderson K. 2006. Pride, empowerment, and return to work: on the significance of promoting positive social emotions among sickness absentees. *Work* 27: 57-65.

Taimela S, Justen S, Aronen P, Sintonen H, Läärä E, Malmivaara A, Tiekso J, Aro T. 2008a. An occupational health intervention program for workers at high risk for sickness absence: cost-effectiveness analysis based on a randomised controlled trial. *Occup Environ Med* 65: 242-248.

Taimela S, Malmivaara A, Justen S, Laara E, Sintonen H, Tiekso J, Aro T. 2008b. The effectiveness of two occupational health intervention programs in reducing sickness absence among employees at risk. Two randomised controlled trials. *Occup Environ Med* 65: 236-241.

Talmage JB, Melhorn JM. 2005. *A physician's guide to return to work*. American Medical Association, Chicago.

Taylor R, Lewis J. 2008. *Understanding the impact of JRRP for people with mental health conditions (DWP Working Paper No 45)*. Her Majesty's Stationery Office, Norwich.

Taylor RS, Brown A, Ebrahim S, Jolliffe J, Noorani H, Rees K, Skidmore B, Stone JA, Thompson DR, Oldridge N. 2004. Exercise-based rehabilitation for patients with coronary heart disease: systematic review and meta-analysis of randomized controlled trials. *Am J Med* 116: 682-692.

Taylor SJC, Candy B, Bryar RM, Ramsay J, Vrijhoef HJM, Esmond G, Wedzicha JA, Griffiths CJ. 2005. Effectiveness of innovations in nurse led chronic disease management for patients with chronic obstructive pulmonary disease: systematic review of evidence. *BMJ* doi:10.1136/bmj.38512.664167.8F .

Teasdale EL, Deahl MP. 2007. Mental health and psychiatric disorders. In *Fitness for work: the medical aspects* (Ed. Palmer KT, Cox RAF, Brown I) Oxford University Press, Oxford.

Teasell RW, Bombardier C. 2001. Employment-related factors in chronic pain and chronic pain disability. *The Clinical Journal of Pain* 17: S39-S45.

The Sainsbury Centre for Mental Health. 2007. *Mental health at work: developing the business case*. The Sainsbury Centre for Mental Health, London.

The Work Foundation. 2006. *The well managed organisation: diagnostic tools for handling sickness absence*. Ministerial Task Force on Health, Safety and Productivity, London www.hse.gov.uk/services/pdfs/diagnostictools.pdf (accessed 16 April 2008).

Thomas RJ, King M, Lui K, Oldridge N, Pina IL, Spertus J. 2007. AACVPR/ACC/AHA 2007 Performance measures on cardiac rehabilitation for referral to and delivery of cardiac rehabilitation/secondary prevention services. *Circulation* 116: 1611-1642.

Thomas T, Secker J, Grove B. 2002. *Job retention & mental health: a review of the literature*. Institute for Applied Health & Social Policy, London.

Thomson L, Neathey F, Rick J. 2003. *Best practice in rehabilitating employees following absence due to work-related stress (HSE RR 138).* Health & Safety Executive, London.

Thornbory G. 2008. *Occupational Health 2008: making the business case - special report.* Workplace Law Publishing, Cambridge.

Thornton P, Zietzer I, Bruyère SM, Golden T, Houtenville A. 2003. *What works and looking ahead: a comparative study of UK and US policies and practices facilitating return to work for people with disabilities.* Cornell University, New York http://works.bepress.com/susanne_bruyere/92/ (accessed 30 April 2008).

Timbie JW, Horvitz-Lennon M, Frank RG, Normand S-LT. 2006. A meta-analysis of labor supply effects of interventions for major depressive disorder. *Psychiatric Services* 57: 212-218.

Toelle BG, Ram FSF. 2004. Written individualised management plans for asthma in children and adults (Cochrane Review). In *Cochrane Database of Systematic Reviews, Issue 1* John Wiley & Sons, Ltd, Chicester.

Tompa E, de Oliveira C, Dolinschi R, Irvin E. 2008. A systematic review of disability management interventions with economic evaluations. *J Occup Rehabil* 18: 16-26.

Trevena LJ, Davey HM, Barratt A, Butow P, Caldwell P. 2006. A systematic review on communicating with patients about evidence. *Journal of Evaluation in Clinical Practice* 12: 13-23.

Trikalinos TA, Raman G, Kupelnick B, Chew PW, Lau J. 2006. *Pulmonary rehabilitation for COPD and other lung diseases.* Agency for Healthcare Research and Quality, Rockville, USA.

Tse SS, Walsh AES. 2001. How does work work for people with bipolar affective disorder? *Occupational Therapy International* 8: 210-225.

TUC. 2000. *Consultation document on rehabilitation. Getting better at getting back.* Trades Union Congress, London.

TUC. 2002. *Rehabilitation and retention - what works is what matters.* Trades Union Congress, London.

Turnock AC, Walters EH, Walters JAE, Wood-Baker R. 2005. Action plans for chronic obstructive pulmonary disease (Cochrane Review). In *Cochrane Database of Systematic Reviews, Issue 4* John Wiley & Sons, Ltd, Chicester.

Tveito TH, Hysing M, Eriksen HR. 2004. Low back pain interventions at the workplace: a systematic literature review. *Occupational Medicine* 54: 3-13.

Tyers C, Gifford J, Gordon-Dseagu V, Lucy D, Usher T, Wilson S. 2007. *Workplace health connect. January 2007 progress report.* HSE Books, London www.hse.gov.uk/workplacehealth/whcreportjan07.pdf (accessed 09 April 2008).

van der Klink JJL, Blonk RWB, Schene AH, van Dijk FJH. 2001. The benefits of interventions for work-related stress. *J Public Health* 91: 270-276.

van der Klink JJL, Blonk RWB, Schene AH, van Dijk FJH. 2003. Reducing long term sickness absence by an activating intervention in adjustment disorders: a cluster randomised controlled design. *Occup Environ Med* 60: 429-437.

van der Klink JJL, van Dijk FJH. 2003. Dutch practice guidelines for managing adjustment disorders in occupational and primary health care. *Scand J Work Environ Health* 29: 478-487.

van Dixhoorn J, White A. 2005. Relaxation therapy for rehabilitation and prevention in ischaemic heart disease: a systematic review and meta-analysis. *Eur J Cardiovasc Prev Rehabil* 12: 193-202.

van Egmond JJ. 2003. The multiple meanings of secondary gain. *The American Jounal of Psychoanalysis* 63: 137-147.

van Geen JW, Edelaar MJ, Janssen M, van Eijk JT. 2007. The long-term effect of multidisciplinary back training: a systematic review. *Spine* 15: 249-255.

van Tulder M, Koes B, Bombardier C. 2002. Low back pain. *Best Practice & Research Clinical Rheumatology* 16: 761-775.

Van Weel C, Orbon K, Van Der Gulden J, Buijs P, Folgering H, Thoonen B, Schermer T. 2006. Occupational health and general practice: from opportunities lost to opportunities capitalised? *Medicina del Lavoro* 97: 288-294.

Vandenplas O, Jamart J, Delwiche J-P, Evrard G, Larbanois A. 2002. Occupational asthma caused by natural rubber latex: outcome according to cessation or reduction of exposure. *J Allergy Clin Immunol* 109: 125-130.

Vandenplas O, Toren K, Blanc PD. 2003. Health and socioeconomic impact of work-related asthma. *Eur Respir J* 22: 689-697.

Varekamp I, Verbeek JHAM, van Dijk FJH. 2006. How can we help employees with chronic diseases to stay at work? A review of interventions aimed at job retention and based on an empowerment perspective. *Int Arch Occup Environ Health* 80: 87-97.

Verbeek JH. 2006. How can doctors help their patients to return to work? *PLoS Med* 3: e88.

Verbeek JH, van Dijk FJ, Malmivaara A, Hulshof CT, Räsänen K, Kankaanpää EE, Mukala K. 2002. Evidence-based medicine for occupational health. *Scand J Work Environ Health* 28: 197-204.

Verbeek JHAM. 2001. Vocational rehabilitation of workers with back pain. *Scand J Work Environ Health* 27: 346-352.

Verhagen AP, Karels C, Bierma-Zeinstra SMA, Burdorf L, Feleus A, Dahaghin S, De Vet HCW, Koes BW. 2006. Ergonomic and physiotherapeutic interventions for treating work-related complaints of the arm, neck or shoulder in adults. In *Cochrane Database of Systematic Reviews, Issue 3* John Wiley & Sons, Ltd, Chichester.

Verhagen AP, Karels C, Bierma-Zeinstra SMA, Feleus A, Dahaghin S, Burdorf A, Koes BW. 2007. Exercise proves effective in a systematic review of work-related complaints of the arm, neck, or shoulder. *Journal of Clinical Epidemiology* 60: 110-117.

Von Korff M. 1999. Pain management in primary care: an individualized stepped-care approach. In *Psychosocial factors in pain: clinical perspectives* (Ed. Gatchel RJ, Turk DC) Guildford Press, New York.

Von Korff M, Glasgow RE, Sharpe M. 2002. Organising care for chronic illness. *BMJ* 325: 92-94.

Von Korff M, Moore JC. 2001. Stepped care for back pain: activating approaches for primary care. *Ann Intern Med* 134: 911-917.

VRA. 2007. *Vocational rehabilitation standards of practice.* Vocational Rehabilitation Association, Glasgow.

Waddell G. 1987. A new clinical model for the treatment of low back pain. *Spine* 12: 632-644.

Waddell G. 2004. *Compensation for chronic pain.* The Stationery Office, London.

Waddell G, Aylward M. 2005. *The scientific and conceptual basis of incapacity benefits.* The Stationery Office, London.

Waddell G, Aylward M, Sawney P. 2002. *Back pain, incapacity for work and social security benefits: an international literature review and analysis.* Royal Society of Medicine Press ltd, London.

Waddell G, Burton AK. 2000. *Occupational health guidelines for the management of low back pain at work - evidence review.* Faculty of Occupational Medicine, London.

Waddell G, Burton AK. 2004. *Concepts of rehabilitation for the management of common health problems.* The Stationery Office, London.

Waddell G, Burton AK. 2006. *Is work good for your health and well-being?* The Stationery Office, London.

Waddell G, Burton AK, Main CJ. 2003. *Screening to identify people at risk of long-term incapacity for work.* Royal Society of Medicine Press, London.

Waddell G, O'Connor M, Boorman S, Torsney B. 2007. Working Backs Scotland: a public and professional health education campaign for back pain. *Spine* 32: 2139-2143.

Waddell G, Watson PJ. 2004. Rehabilitation. In *The Back Pain Revolution* (Ed. Waddell G): 371-399, Churchill Livingstone, Edinburgh.

Wade DT, de Jong BA. 2000. Recent advances in rehabilitation. *BMJ* 320: 1385-1388.

WAG. 2006. *Improving health and the management of chronic conditions in Wales. Self management and independence: a report by the Task and Finish Group.* Welsh Assembly Government, Cardiff.

Walker-Bone K, Cooper C. 2005. Hard work never hurt anyone: or did it? A review of occupational associations with soft tissue musculoskeletal disorders of the neck and upper limb. *Ann Rheum Dis* 64: 1391-1396.

Wasiak R, Young AE, Roessler RT, McPherson KM, van Poppel MNM, Anema JR. 2007. Measuring return to work. *J Occup Rehabil* 17: 766-781.

Waterman L. 2007. The future for occupational health in the United Kingdom. In *Supporting health at work: international perspectives on occupational health services* (Ed. Westerholm P, Walters D) IOSH Services Limited, Wigston, Leicestershire www.iosh.co.uk/policyandpractice (accessed 09 April 2008).

Watson PJ, Booker CK, Moores L, Main CJ. 2004. Returning the chronically unemployed with low back pain to employment. *European Journal of Pain* 8: 359-369.

WCRCWA. 2001. *Stress, compensation and the general practitioner.* WorkCover Western Australia, Shenton Park www.workcover.wa.gov.au (accessed 12 March 2008).

Weevers H-JA, van der Beek AJ, Anema JR, van der Wal G, van Mechelen W. 2005. Work-related disease in general practice: a systematic review. *Family Practice* 22: 197-204.

Weingarten SR, Henning JM, Badamgarav E, Knight K, Hasselblad V, Gano ADJr, Ofman JJ. 2002. Interventions used in disease management programmes for patients with chronic illness - which ones work? Meta-analysis of published reports. *BMJ* 325: 925-928.

Weir R, Nielson WR. 2001. Interventions for disability management. *The Clinical Journal of Pain* 17: S128-S132.

Wessely S. 2002. Pros and cons of medicalisation. *BMJ* 324: 912.

Wessely S. 2004. Mental health issues. In *What about the workers? Proceedings of an RSM Symposium* (Ed. Holland-Elliot K): 41-46, Royal Society of Medicine Press, London.

Wewiorski NJ, Fabian ES. 2004. Association between demographic and diagnostic factors and employment outcomes for people with psychiatric disabilities: a synthesis of recent research. *Mental Health Services Research* 6: 9-21.

WHO. 1995. *Global strategy on occupational health for all: the way to health at work.* World Health Organisation, Geneva www.who.int/occupational_health/globstrategy/en (accessed 04 April 2008).

WHO. 2001. *International classification of functioning, disability and health.* World Health Organization, Geneva www.who.int/classifications/icf/site/onlinebrowser/icf.cfm (accessed 12 March 2008).

WHO. 2005. *Mental health policies and programmes in the workplace: mental health policy and service guidance package.* World Health Organization, Geneva.

Wilczynski NL, Haynes RB, Lavis JN, Ramkissoonsingh R, Arnold-Oatley AE. 2004. Optimal search strategies for detecting health services research studies in MEDLINE. *CMAJ* 171: 1179-1185.

Williams RM, Westmoreland MG, Lin CA, Schmuck G, Creen M. 2007. Effectiveness of workplace rehabilitation interventions in the treatment of work-related low back pain: a systematic review. *Disability and Rehabilitation* 29: 607-624.

Williams RM, Westmorland M. 2002. Perspectives on workplace disability management: a review of the literature. *Work* 19: 87-93.

Williams RM, Westmorland MG, Schmuck G, MacDermid JC. 2004. Effectiveness of workplace rehabilitation interventions in the treatment of work-related upper extremity disorders: a systematic review. *J Hand Ther* 17: 267-273.

Wise M. 2001. *Does workers' compensation influence recovery rates? A critical review of the literature. (A report prepared for the Workers' Compensation and Rehabilitation Commission by the School of Occupational Therapy, Curtin University of Technology, Western Australia).* WorkCover WA, Perth www.workcover. wa.gov.au (accessed 26 March 2008).

Wittchen H-U, Jacobi F. 2005. Size and burden of mental disorders in Europe - a critical review and appraisal of 27 studies. *European Neuropsychopharmacology* 15: 357-376.

Wood DJ. 1987. Design and evaluation of a back injury prevention program within a geriatric hospital. *Spine* 12: 77-82.

Wynne R, Fleming P, McAnaney D, O'Kelly C. 2006. *Employment guidance services for people with disabilities: summary.* European Foundation for the Improvement of Living and Working Conditions, Dublin www.eurofound.eu.int (accessed 09 April 2008).

Wynne R, McAnaney D. 2004. *Employment and disability: back to work strategies.* European Foundation for the Improvement of Living and Working Conditions, Dublin www.eurofound.eu.int (accessed 09 April 2008).

Yorke J, Fleming SL, Shuldham CM. 2006. Psychological interventions for adults with asthma (Cochrane Review). In *Cochrane Database of Systematic Reviews, Issue 1* John WIley & Sons, Ltd, Chichester.

Young AE, Roessler RT, Wasiak R, McPherson KM, van Poppel MNM, Anema JR. 2005a. A developmental conceptualization of return to work. *Journal of Occupational Rehabilitation* 15: 557-568.

Young AE, Wasiak R, Roessler RT, McPherson KM, Anema JR, van Poppel MNM. 2005b. Return-to-work outcomes following work disability: stakeholder motivations, interests and concerns. *Journal of Occupational Rehabilitation* 15: 543-556.

Zampolini M, Bernardinello M, Tesio L. 2007. RTW in back conditions. *Disability and Rehabilitation* 29: 1377-1385.

Zigenfus GC, Yin J, Giang GM, Fogarty WT. 2000. Effectiveness of early physical therapy in the treatment of acute low back musculoskeletal disorders. *J Occup Environ Med* 42: 35-39.

Appendix 1: Review methodology

By the nature of vocational rehabilitation, this review must cover a wide range of evidence of different types and quality. That makes the standard systematic review methodology unsuitable, because it is designed primarily for homogeneous sets of studies on specific treatments for clinical outcomes. Moreover, it relies largely on randomised controlled trials, which are inappropriate or impractical for many clinical, scientific and policy questions, where other types of evidence may be equally valid (Benson & Hartz 2000; Concato et al. 2000; Glasziou et al. 2004; Johnston et al. 2006). As a result, when applied to policy questions, systematic reviews often focus too narrowly and simply conclude that there is insufficient evidence to draw any firm conclusions (Mays et al. 2005; Pawson et al. 2005; Sheldon 2005). Actually, policy involves complex social interventions on complex social systems with sometimes unpredictable outcomes. Different stages of the process may require different *kinds* of evidence. Policy decisions must consider alternative interventions and their likely effectiveness, but also their practicality, cost, acceptability and the likely reaction of key stakeholders. Thus, policy is at the nexus between scientific evidence, practicalities and politics (Innvær et al. 2002; Mays et al. 2005; Pawson et al. 2005).

To provide a more useful evidence base for policy, this review is a 'best evidence synthesis', incorporating the available scientific evidence (background and direct, quantitative and qualitative), logical reasoning, evidence-based guidance and examples of best practice (Goldsmith et al. 2007; Silverstein et al. 2005; Slavin 1995). It summarises the relevant literature and draws conclusions about the balance of evidence, based on its quality, quantity and consistency. It sets the conclusions in context. This provides the flexibility to tackle heterogeneous evidence and complex socio-medical issues, together with quality assurance. The potential for selection and personal bias is acknowledged, but efforts were made to minimise this, and the strengths and weaknesses of the evidence and the arguments are laid out as explicitly as possible. This is a further development of the methodology used in previous reviews (Waddell & Burton 2004; Waddell & Burton 2006).

In view of the range and amount of evidence, and the time and resources available, the only manageable approach was to use existing scientific literature reviews. To reflect current knowledge, material published between January 2000 and December 2007 was eligible for inclusion, though on some fundamental issues (Tables 1, 2, 6, 7) that period was extended back to 1990 and a few more recent papers on key issues were also included.

The process for the review involved six key steps:

1.   Working definitions for the project
2.   Literature search and selection

3. Data extraction
4. Generate evidence statements
5. Grade strength of evidence
6. Peer review

Working definitions for the project

Much of the terminology relevant to this review has been used in a variety of ways, often with different meanings. To reduce the likelihood of ambiguity, and enhance the usefulness of the review, it was necessary to establish working definitions for key terminology. These were sought from a number of pertinent sources and duly tabulated (Table 1). For practical purposes some boundaries needed to be placed around 'common health problems' – these were taken to be the common cardio-respiratory, mental health, and musculoskeletal conditions that account for most sickness absence as used in previous reviews (Waddell & Burton 2004; Waddell & Burton 2006). In addition to information concerning vocational rehabilitation interventions for the three groups of common health problems, generic information concerning aspects of the delivery and timing of interventions was also gathered.

Literature Search

Throughout the review, broad and inclusive search strategies were used to retrieve as much material as possible, pertinent to the basic question: 'what helps people with common health problems return to work?' The focus was on *what* works, rather than *how* it works.

International evidence (published in English) concerning interventions and their effectiveness was included, but UK epidemiological and economic data, evidence on practice, policy reports, and examples were highlighted where possible. The population of interest was adults of working age (generally 16-65 years). The focus was on interventions directed to improving occupational outcomes (including sickness absence, job retention, return to work and the secondary prevention of long-term sickness and incapacity). The definition of vocational rehabilitation excluded 'health promotion' and the primary prevention of ill health. Ill-health retirement was also excluded because that is an end-point after rehabilitation has failed, and is complicated by social issues around retirement (Hayden et al. 1999; Leonesio 1996).

Search methods

A comprehensive and systematic literature search was conducted using five strategies: (1) searching electronic databases; 2) internet searches; (3) hand searches of relevant journals and other reports and documents; (4) personal databases; and (5) citation tracking.

Electronic databases were searched using appropriate search strings (such as those published by SIGN) and Boolean search terms from January 2000 to December 2007 to identify published literature (Montori et al. 2005; Wilczynski et al. 2004). Open search approaches were used to capture the widest possible range of articles. This resulted in large data sets that were carefully searched for relevant material. Limits applied were (i) publication from the year 2000 and (ii) English language (Egger et al. 2003). The databases searched were:

AMED (Allied and Complementary Medicine Database, which is a unique bibliographic database produced by the Health Care Information Service of the British Library. It covers a selection of journals in complementary medicine, palliative care, and several professions allied to medicine); CINAHL (Cumulative Index to Nursing & Allied Health Literature Database. The database includes citations from nearly 3,000 journals that cover nursing, allied health, biomedicine, alternative/complementary medicine, consumer health and health sciences librarianship); EMBASE (Excerpta Medica database is a major biomedical and pharmaceutical database indexing over 3,500 international journals in the following fields: drug research, pharmacology, pharmaceutics, toxicology, clinical and experimental human medicine, health policy and management, public health, occupational health, environmental health, drug dependence and abuse, psychiatry, forensic medicine, and biomedical engineering/instrumentation); MEDLINE, MEDLINE Daily Update, and MEDLINE Pending, (MEDLINE is the United States National Library of Medicine's premier bibliographic database providing information from the following fields: medicine; nursing; dentistry; veterinary medicine; allied health; and, pre-clinical sciences); and PsycINFO (a bibliographic database providing abstracts and citations to the scholarly literature in the psychological, social, behavioural, and health sciences).

Internet searches were conducted to identify relevant literature, reports, policy documents, etc. A range of relevant keywords were used including, but not limited to, the following: "vocational rehabilitation"; "occupational rehabilitation"; "work rehabilitation"; "return to work"; "RTW"; "work retention" (Haafkens et al. 2006). Searches were also conducted using relevant authors' names, with search engines such as PubMed and Google. In addition to standard search engines, a wide variety of specific databases and internet search systems was also deployed including:

Database of International Rehabilitation Research, run by the Centre for International Rehabilitation Research Information and Exchange (CIRRIE) at University at Buffalo the State University of New York, http://cirrie.buffalo.edu; NIOSHTIC-2, a searchable bibliographic database containing 41,797 citations of occupational safety and health publications, documents, grant reports, and other communication products supported in whole or in part by the National Institute for Occupational Safety and Health (U.S.), www2a.cdc.gov/nioshtic-2; Physiotherapy Evidence Database (PEDro), run by the Centre for Evidence-Based Physiotherapy (CEBP) and developed to give rapid access to bibliographic details and abstracts of randomised controlled trials, systematic reviews and evidence-based clinical practice guidelines in physiotherapy, www.pedro.fhs.usyd.edu.au; Intute: UK based search service created by a network of UK universities and partners of UK research, university lectures, scholarly reports etc, www.intute.ac.uk; Turning Research Into Practice (TRIP) database that is designed to enable health professionals to find the high quality evidence-based medicine material, www.tripdatabase.com; Education Resources Information Centre (ERIC) is a digital library of education research and information sponsored by the Institute of Education Sciences (IES) of the U.S. Department of Education, www.eric.ed.gov; NHS Economic Evaluation Database (NHS EED) is a database designed to systematically identify and describe economic evaluations, www.crd.york.ac.uk/crdweb/; Social Care Online is a UK database of social care information that includes research briefings, reports, government documents, and journal articles, www.scie-socialcareonline.org.uk; The Cochrane Collaboration disseminates systematic reviews of healthcare interventions and promotes the search for evidence in the form of clinical trials and other studies of interventions, www.cochrane.org.

Hand searches of the contents pages of several journals were conducted, covering the period from 2000 to December 2007. These included the following:

American Journal of Occupational Therapy; Archives of Physical Medicine & Rehabilitation; Case Manager; Disability & Rehabilitation; European Journal of Pain; International Journal of Rehabilitation Research; Journal of Occupational Health Psychology; Journal of Occupational Psychology; Journal of Occupational Rehabilitation; Journal of Occupational Research; Journal of Social Policy; Journal of Vocational Rehabilitation; Lippincott's Case Management; Pain; Professional Case Management; Psychiatric Rehabilitation Journal; Spine; Work & Stress.

Hand searches were also conducted through publications available from professional organisations, specific government departments and international organisations. These included:

CRS Australia (the Australian Government provider of vocational rehabilitation services), www.crsaustralia.gov.au; DWP Research Reports and In House Reports, www.dwp.gov.ul/asd/asd5/; HSE Research Reports, www.hse.gov.uk/research/rrhtm/; HSE Contract Research Reports, www.hse.gov.uk/research/crr_htm; Social Security Bulletin, www.ssa.gov/policy/docs/ssb/; European Foundation for the Improvement of Living and Working Conditions, www.eurofound.europa.eu; International Labour Organisation, www.ilo.org; International Social Security Association (ISSA), http://www.issa.int/engl/homef.htm; National Institute for Health and Clinical Excellence (NICE), www.nice.org.uk; National Institute for Health Research (NIHR), www.ncchta.org; New Zealand Guidelines Group (NZGG), www.nzgg.org.nz; Occupational Safety and Health Administration (OSHA), www.osha.gov; Organisation for Economic Cooperation and Development (OECD), www.oecd.org; Scottish Intercollegiate Guidelines Network (SIGN), www.sign.ac.uk; Social Science Information Gateway (SOSIG), www.sosig.ac.uk; UK College of Occupational Therapists bibliography on vocational rehabilitation (2006).

Citation tracking within retrieved articles was also used.

Exclusion criteria

A priori inclusion/exclusion criteria were used for article selection, and confirmed with the commissioners of the review.

Although the scope of common health problems as defined for this project is wide, it was necessary to exclude many specific medical conditions in order to maintain a practicable focus:

Allergy; amputations; ankylosing spondylitis (AS) & other inflammatory arthropathies; burns; cancer; chronic fatigue syndrome (CFS); culture and ethnicity; dermatitis; diabetes; eczema; epilepsy; irritable bowel syndrome; mental retardation; mild traumatic brain injury (MTBI)/ post-concussion syndrome (PCS); neurological conditions; obesity; post-surgery/ post-operative rehabilitation; rheumatoid arthritis (RA); severe mental illness (includes schizophrenia, bipolar disorder, personality disorder); sleep disorders; spinal cord injury (SCI); traumatic brain injury (TBI). Issues around disability discrimination were excluded because that is principally a social issue. Issues around ill-health retirement were excluded because that is an end-point after rehabilitation has failed, and is complicated by social factors around retirement. 'Presenteeism' was also excluded, because of uncertainties about the concept, its measurement and available evidence (Schultz & Edington 2007).

Under our definition of vocational rehabilitation, 'health promotion' and the primary prevention of ill health (interventions aimed at primary prevention of injury or disease) are outside the scope of this review, though their potential contribution to lowering sickness absence and improving safety is recognised.

Literature selection

A very large pool of several thousand citations was retrieved during the systematic search, and these were managed with bibliographic software. It was neither possible nor practical to review all studies, articles, or reports that were retrieved. Therefore, careful selection was performed against the a priori criteria for relevance. Systematic reviews, extensive narrative reviews, reports, and professional guidance were the primary focus, and individual studies were only selected if they added additional essential information not covered in the reviews.

The citations retrieved from the searches were grouped under the three main health condition areas and various generic categories. Tables consisting of titles and abstracts (when available) were circulated to the three reviewers (GW; KB; NK), and each indicated which should be obtained for possible inclusion in the review. Based on this voting system, the full papers of those selected for possible inclusion were obtained and scrutinised by at least two of the reviewers. Where there was disagreement, and that was only rare, it was remedied by discussion and consensus. Of the articles obtained and circulated, some 450 were considered relevant for inclusion in the review; copies were duly archived.

Data extraction and synthesis

Information from some 450 included articles was extracted, summarised and entered into evidence tables (in alphabetical order for ease of reference). Data on work-related issues is given in Table 2. Data on vocational rehabilitation interventions are presented under the three main health condition areas (cardio-respiratory, mental health, musculoskeletal - Tables 3, 4 and 5), with sub-grouping within each of the tables as appropriate. Furthermore, relevant generic information on delivery issues was tabulated in Table 6 and 7. Links between relevant information were given where applicable.

Scientific evidence on cost-effectiveness was incorporated when available. Further evidence was gathered from the policy and business literature on cost-benefit analyses (considering 'reasonable' / 'acceptable' resources and costs with evidence on likely benefits and taking account of issues such as deadweight[43] and value-added[44]) and on the business case for vocational rehabilitation.

Generate evidence statements

Building on each section of the evidence tables, themes were identified within the evidence and evidence statements were developed, refined and agreed by the three reviewers. This was an iterative process until consensus among the reviewers was reached. These were high level statements reflecting the balance of the evidence on effectiveness of interventions; it was beyond the scope of this review to assess specific treatments or providers. Each statement was explicitly linked to the underlying supportive evidence. Where appropriate, the text of the evidence statements was used to expand on the nature or limitations of the underlying evidence, and to offer any caveats or cautions. Where the evidence statements were insufficient to convey complex underlying ideas, important issues were discussed in narrative text.

---

43 Deadweight loss is a measure of economic inefficiency. In this context, it is taken to be the number of people who receive the intervention who would have returned to work anyway, without the intervention.

44 Value added: the net increase in the number who return to work because of receiving the intervention.

High level evidence statements may not fully convey the details of effective interventions, so boxed examples were selected to help illustrate what is possible; these are given in the various findings sections.

Grade strength of evidence

Detailed evidence linking was provided and the strength of the evidence supporting each statement was rated using the system outlined in Box A1 (adapted from Waddell & Burton 2006).

	Evidence Grade	Definition
Box A1: Ratings for the strength of the scientific evidence on effectiveness		
***	**Strong**	Generally consistent findings provided by (systematic) review(s) of multiple high quality studies.
**	**Moderate**	Generally consistent findings provided by review(s) of fewer and/or methodologically weaker studies.
*	**Weak**	<u>Limited evidence</u> – provided by a single high quality study <u>Conflicting evidence</u> – inconsistent findings provided by (review(s) of) multiple studies.
0	-	No high quality **scientific** evidence

In a review of this nature, some important issues are inappropriate for scientific experiment or a 'scientific' answer, which is different from saying that there is 'no evidence available'. For these issues, however, it may be possible to construct a reasoned statement based on various other criteria (Box A2). In appropriate cases this structured approach, which extends beyond consensus, can produce Statements that are just as valid as those based on scientific evidence.

Box A2: Criteria used for non-scientific evidence	
#	Background scientific evidence (e.g. epidemiology, indirect or related evidence) Logical reasoning Worthwhile use of resources Direct and indirect evidence on likely benefits

Peer review

Quality assurance was provided through oversight at various stages by members of the Vocational Rehabilitation Task Group and the Industrial Injuries Advisory Council. Individual sections of the review were commented upon by experts in each area.

Limitations of the review methodology

Compared with a systematic review, this method of evidence synthesis inevitably involves a greater degree of judgement about which articles were included or excluded, how the data were extracted and the evidence statements developed. Nevertheless, it is the most appropriate method for the present purpose. The precautions taken to minimise this risk and to make the process as explicit as possible are described above.

The focus on *what* works excluded a lot of evidence on mechanisms and on *how* to improve clinical and workplace practice.

The reliance on reviews and the general cut-off date of December 2007 could lead to the omission of some more recent studies, though some important 2008 reviews were included. Whilst it is unlikely that any single studies would overturn the main Findings, articles reporting recent and innovative vocational rehabilitation interventions will be missing. Limitation to English publications was unlikely to have any significant effect, as most major reviews and all Cochrane Reviews are published in English and many of them include individual studies from other languages. Although the scientific evidence was international, it included many individual UK studies. UK epidemiological and economic data, evidence on practice, policy reports, and examples were used wherever possible.

Appendix 2: Work-related conditions

Can vocational rehabilitation be equally effective for work injuries, or for work-related and compensable health conditions, as non work-related conditions? Or does it need to differ in any way? Synthesis of the evidence took three areas into consideration:

1)   Is there is any theoretical reason why vocational rehabilitation should be different? (Tables 1 & 2a).

2)   Does the literature on workers compensation (Table 2b) provide evidence that effective vocational rehabilitation differs for patients with compensable work injuries? The workers compensation setting provides the best available evidence on compensable work injuries, and is most similar to IIDB[45]. However, it is mainly from North America and Australia and any extrapolation to UK must be made with care.

3)   More generally, does the evidence on vocational rehabilitation interventions throughout this review (Tables 3-7) differ for work-related and non work-related conditions?

Theoretical principles

Several concepts are fundamental to this discussion (Table 2a). 'Work-related' means different things to different people. Many of the common health problems in this review are work-related, in the sense that they occur in adults of working age, symptoms are often work-relevant (precipitated or aggravated at work), and capacity for work may be affected. Some can be *caused* by work or 'arise out of or in the course of employment' (Social Security Administration Act 1992; Newman Taylor 2006). However, self-reported attributions are often unreliable and over-estimate work as the cause of any health condition (Melhorn & Hegmann 2008; Palmer et al. 2007).

An *accident* is a sudden, unexpected, and unplanned event, which causes loss, damage, or harm.

An *occupational, industrial* or *work* accident is one arising out of or in the course of employment.

An *injury* is harm or damage to a person caused by an external agent or force, with a close temporal relationship between that application and the onset of symptoms.

---

45   Industrial Injury Disablement Benefit

An *occupational, industrial* or *work* injury is one arising out of or in the course of employment.

An *occupational disease* (also called *industrial disease*) is a disease caused by exposure to a hazard[46] at work.

The problem is that legislative definitions and usage of these terms vary with the context and needs of each system (Kendall 2006). For example, in UK only 39% of work-related health problems are classified as injuries and 61% as work-related ill health, whereas in US 94% are termed injuries and only 6% occupational diseases.

These are primarily social and legal conventions, for which the medical evidence is conflicting. First, epidemiological and clinical evidence shows that most common health problems are common whether in or out of work, risk factors are multifactorial, and cause-effect relationships ambiguous (Sanderson & Andrews 2006; Waddell & Burton 2006). Work is usually only one, and often not the most important, causal factor (Carter & Birrell 2000; Henneberger 2007; Spurgeon 2007). Second, there is no clear pathological distinction between occupational 'injury' and 'disease': in practice, that distinction is often based largely on speed of onset. Conditions of sudden onset are more likely to be called 'injuries'; those which develop over time, with a latent period and gradual onset, are more likely to be called disease. Third, there is little epidemiological, pathological or clinical basis to describe most common health problems as 'injuries' (Burton 1997; Hadler et al. 2007; Hamm et al. 2007). Fourth, scientific evidence for the concept of 'cumulative trauma' producing many 'repetitive injuries' is limited and conflicting (Burton et al. 2008). Finally, the issue of work-relatedness can be extended to any form of 'harm', including mental injury or illness (Griffith 2006). There is no doubt that mental health problems are common, can be incapacitating, and can be obstacles to return to work and vocational rehabilitation (O'Donnell et al. 2005). However, there are difficulties with the measurement of psychosocial hazards at work, diagnosis based largely on subjective symptoms, and establishing a causal relationship between occupational hazard and personal harm (Industrial Injuries Advisory Council, www.iiac.org.uk). Indeed, these difficulties apply to many common health problems.

Whatever the tensions between social and legal conventions and the medical evidence, the issue of work-relatedness underpins health and safety at work, and entitlement to certain forms of compensation (Langley & Brenner 2004; Snashall 2003).

---

46 Classically a noxious substance

WR-1   #   In principle, vocational rehabilitation deals with the health condition and return to work, whatever the original cause. There is no clear conceptual or clinical distinction between many work 'injuries' and comparable 'non-specific' health conditions. There is no clear evidence of biological difference in causation, or of different needs in clinical management. Therefore, in principle, vocational rehabilitation principles and interventions should be the same, whether or not the health condition is work-related.

Tables 1 & 2a

Nevertheless, work-relatedness can affect vocational rehabilitation in several ways:

- in many jurisdictions, acceptance of work-relatedness determines entitlement to funding and resources for vocational rehabilitation

- any question of occupational causation raises the issue of safety for return to work.

- perceptions of work-relatedness, occupational attributions and secondary gain, can hinder return to work, and so affect the process and outcome of vocational rehabilitation.

WR-2   #   There are strong moral and legislative reasons to identify hazards and control risks to health and safety. Even more, vocational rehabilitation should take account of the worker's health condition and work demands, and any mismatch that may form an obstacle for return to work.

(Griffith 2006; HSE 2004b)

In addition to safety issues, beliefs that a health condition is work-related can be a major obstacle to continuing or returning to that job, *irrespective of whether they are correct* (Box 3). The 'injury model' and attribution to work dominate contemporary thinking, and this is reinforced by compensation (Bellamy 1997; Burton 1997; Hadler et al. 2007). Yet the above analysis demonstrates the tensions between the scientific evidence and popular beliefs, and suggests that many of these beliefs are unfounded. Furthermore, there is extensive clinical evidence that such beliefs, together with other psychosocial factors, are often more important than the underlying health problem in the development of long-term incapacity (DeGood & Kiernan 1996; Main et al. 2008). They form powerful obstacles to return to work (Box 3). Vocational rehabilitation must take account of individual, health professional and employer beliefs.

> **Box 3: Beliefs about work that may form obstacles to return to work**
> (Marhold et al. 2002; Waddell & Burton 2004)
>
> - Belief that the health condition was caused by work (whether an accident/injury or the physical and mental demands of work)
> - Belief that work is harmful, and that (return to) work will do further damage
> - Fear of re-injury
> - Belief that sickness absence and rest are necessary for recovery
> - Belief that no one can or should return to work until the health condition is completely 'cured'
> - Low expectations about return to work
> - Attribution of blame

WR-3   ***   Unhelpful beliefs about work-relatedness (including occupational attributions, compensation and secondary gain issues) form obstacles to return to work, and should be addressed in vocational rehabilitation (whether or not the health condition is a work 'injury', actually attributable to work or compensable).

Table 2b: (AFOM/RACP 2001; Burton 1997; DeGood & Kiernan 1996; Dersh et al. 2004; Fordyce 1995; Gatchel et al. 2002; Merrill 1997; Waddell et al. 2002)

Table 3: (Burton et al. 2008; IASP 2005; MacEachen et al. 2006; Rainville et al. 2005; Sullivan et al. 2005; Waddell & Watson 2004)

Table 5a: (Lewin 1999; Mital et al. 2004; NHS Centre for Reviews 1998; Perk & Alexanderson 2004)

Workers compensation literature

Table 2b presents the evidence from a systematic search of the workers compensation literature [47].

WR-4   #   The workers compensation literature advocates the same vocational rehabilitation principles and interventions for compensable work injuries as found in the general vocational rehabilitation literature.

Table 2b: (AFOM/RACP 2001; Burton et al. 2008; Fordyce 1995; Hadler et al. 2007; Leavitt 1992; O'Donnell 2000; Waddell 2004)

WR-5   ***   There is strong evidence that vocational rehabilitation interventions can be effective for compensable work injuries (in a workers compensation setting).

Table 2b: (Dersh et al. 2004; Leavitt 1992; Merrill 1997; Smith et al. 2006; Waddell et al. 2002)

Table 3: (Kunkel & Miller 2002; Loisel et al. 2003)

---

47   This was extended back to 1990 as there is much more evidence in the previous decade.

WR-6   ***   Workers compensation injuries have somewhat less favourable clinical outcomes, slightly higher frequency and duration of sickness absence, and slightly lower return to work rates than comparable non work-related conditions.

Table 2b: (AFOM/RACP 2001; Bellamy 1997; Binder & Rohling 1996; Dersh et al. 2004; Leavitt 1992; Loeser et al. 1995; Merrill 1997; O'Donnell 2000; Rohling et al. 1995; Waddell et al. 2002)

Table 3: (Grant et al. 2004)

There is conflicting evidence on the size of this association, ranging from 'inconclusive' (Fishbain et al. 1995; Merrill 1997) up to a maximum of about 25% (Binder & Rohling 1996; Rohling et al. 1995; Waddell et al. 2002). It is also unclear to what extent these different outcomes are direct effects of compensation (moral hazard), or due to the context and control mechanisms, to employment-related factors, or to the different characteristics of these workers (case selection) (AFOM/RACP 2001; Dersh et al. 2004; Fishbain et al. 1995; Gatchel et al. 2002; Leavitt 1992; Merrill 1997; van Egmond 2003). People injured at work are more often male, with less education and skills, smokers, in heavier manual jobs, and with less freedom to control their work and the return to work process (Fishbain et al. 1995; Leavitt 1992; Waddell et al. 2002). Overall, any direct effect of work-related 'injury' and compensation on clinical and occupational outcomes is probably quite modest and does not invalidate vocational rehabilitation for these people (AFOM/RACP 2001; Bellamy 1997; Dersh et al. 2004; Fishbain et al. 1995; Fordyce 1995; Gatchel et al. 2002; O'Donnell 2000; Waddell et al. 2002). Moreover, there are questions whether all workers receive optimal vocational rehabilitation and whether these results could be improved by better vocational rehabilitation (BSRM 2003).

WR-7   **   Adversarial legal or appeal proceedings can be a major obstacle to vocational rehabilitation, with significantly longer duration of sickness absence and significantly lower return to work rates.

Table 2b: (AFOM/RACP 2001; Bellamy 1997; Dersh et al. 2004; Hadler et al. 2007; Merrill 1997; O'Donnell 2000; Waddell et al. 2002; Wise 2001)

Vocational rehabilitation literature

At least a quarter of the IIDB caseload (>80,000 people) are of working age and out of work – and potential candidates for vocational rehabilitation (IIAC statistics)[48]. 80% of that 80,000 have had work accidents, of which 80% (>50,000 people) are unspecified musculoskeletal or soft tissue injuries. The other 20% of the 80,000 have Prescribed Diseases, of which many have poor prognosis in older patients (e.g. chronic obstructive airways disease) but ~5000 are people of working age with conditions such as work-related upper limb disorders or occupational asthma. The IIDB scheme covers small numbers of people with mental health conditions arising from an identifiable accident, but consultations have raised the question

---

48   About half the caseload is over working age and many others are working.

whether the scheme might be extended to other work-related musculoskeletal conditions or 'stress', which could potentially be much larger numbers (IIAC 2004; IIAC 2006; IIAC 2007b). These are exactly the 'common health problems' covered by the vocational rehabilitation literature in this review (Tables 3-5).

WR-8   #   Most of the literature on return to work and vocational rehabilitation does not distinguish between nor present separate data on work vs. non-work injuries, injuries vs. non-specific health conditions, or compensable vs. non-compensable conditions. Vocational rehabilitation principles, interventions, and guidelines are broadly the same for work-related and other comparable health conditions.

Table 2b: (Wise 2001)

Tables 3-7

Conclusions

1. In principle, with general consensus, and on the balance of the available evidence, vocational rehabilitation for work-related and compensable conditions should follow the same principles and use the same interventions as for other comparable health conditions (WR-1, WR-4, WR-8).

2. All vocational rehabilitation should take account of the psychosocial context, but vocational rehabilitation for work-related and compensable conditions needs to pay particular attention to unhelpful beliefs (including occupational attributions, compensation and secondary gain issues) across the players (WR-3, WR-7).

3. Vocational rehabilitation is effective for many work-related and compensable conditions, though the results are slightly poorer than for non work-related conditions (WR-6). Intervention is likely to be a worthwhile use of resources, in view of the age and working life expectancy of many of these workers, and the good medical prognosis of many of these conditions (WR-5).

Vocational rehabilitation for work-related and compensable conditions (whether caused by work, attributed to work, or expressed as work-relevant symptoms) can reasonably draw on the wider evidence about vocational rehabilitation for common health problems. Because there is scope for optimising both content and delivery for specific conditions in specific contexts, further research is justified.

Appendix 3: Further research and development

It is a truism that we can always benefit from more research, and the purpose of this section is to draw on the findings of the current review to provide some guidance on potential research priorities. There is a considerable body of evidence to support many aspects of vocational rehabilitation for numerous common health problems but, inevitably, there are some gaps in the evidence, as well as questions over how to optimise implementation of the findings in given contexts. Process issues are a priority area. A number of aspects of the process of delivering vocational rehabilitation need additional clarification, especially to enhance efficiency and matching provision of resources to actual needs in a timely fashion. While it is clear that the best efficiency will come from delivering a 'stepped-care' approach to services, there remains much to learn about specific features of this. This includes the timeframe for each step, how to discourage the delivery of serial ineffective therapies, how to trigger referral and progression from one step to the next, and how to coordinate vocational rehabilitation services with the workplace and healthcare. There is also need for investigating methods of improving communication between key players: workers, GPs and employers.

More generally, it is important that occupational outcomes (such as return-to-work and stay-at-work measures) are incorporated into *all* relevant research projects involving working age participants. This applies equally to primary and secondary studies[49]. It requires something of a 'culture change', so that work outcomes are considered as valid as those focusing on symptoms and diagnoses. Ideally, research funding decisions (and possibly ethical approval) should be contingent on including work outcomes in each relevant project. The outcome measures should be comprehensive enough to fully capture the spectrum of possible outcomes (e.g. ranging from return to same job at same workplace, partial return to work, return to functional independence without return to work, retraining into different job tasks at a different workplace, etc.). Development work to obtain a consensus on suitable categories for measuring such outcomes should be completed, disseminated, and promoted as a standard research variable. This will provide the major benefit of being able to more easily compare results between studies.

An ensuing research imperative is to improve knowledge about the cost-effectiveness of specific types of approach and interventions. This is because the uptake of all types of vocational rehabilitation strategies by both the public and private sectors of our society appears to be contingent on establishing a rationale *and* a business case.

---

49   Primary studies are the individual scientific primary articles, for example, randomised clinical trials or cohort studies. Secondary studies are systematic reviews and assessments of published material, e.g. HTA reports, clinical guidelines and systematic reviews.

Specific research issues:

A number of specific research issues can be identified, some to do with overall vocational rehabilitation strategy and others involving the process of delivery and implementation. Strategic issues include mental health, older workers and the ageing population, gender issues, long-term claimants.

Mental health: In view of the recent and current trends in both sickness absence and IB claims, mental health problems should be a major priority area for research on vocational rehabilitation. This should occur across a spectrum of areas: employers and the workplace; delivery of healthcare; and, services such as disability/case management. It seems the assumption that mental health problems preclude participation in work or other productive activity needs to be challenged, and effective methods of doing this need to be developed. There is an important need to develop a consensus about what constitutes reasonable workplace accommodations for people with mental health problems. The problem of 'stress' deserves special attention due to its inordinate problems (lack of clarity over defining a case; potential for inappropriate medicalisation and over-treatment; uncertainty about prevention and effective treatment). It would be prudent to slow the rush toward inventing a new spectrum of occupational disease, until further information and evidence becomes available. This underscores the need to fund high quality research in this field.

Older workers, ageing population: Older workers are known to have a higher prevalence of long-term incapacity and are considered most likely to require additional help in return to work, yet there is little known about the impact of age on vocational rehabilitation. Older workers may differ in their socio-economic situation, health, workability, and response to rehabilitation. Furthermore, selection bias may exclude older workers from rehabilitation programmes, and most studies do not present separate data on older workers; the few studies that do, suggest that their results may be less favourable. Many of the principles of vocational rehabilitation are likely to be the same for older workers, but further evidence is required.

Gender issues: Women are an increasing proportion of the labour force, and the question occurs whether they may differ in their vocational rehabilitation needs and responses. Furthermore, whether there are differences for men and women with specific types of health problem, at various stages of these problems, and/or between different workplaces or types of work.

Long-term claimants: While it is clear that people who are off work long-term can be helped to re-engage in work, more information is needed about enhancing the efficiency of this. Important questions include whether specific types of structured intervention are more successful, and whether these need to be tailored to specific conditions. It is not yet clear whether interventions are more effective and acceptable when aimed at the health problem, or overcoming labour market and workplace obstacles to return to work, or a mixture of both.

Small and medium enterprises: Large numbers of people work in SMEs or for agencies, yet the effectiveness and applicability of many of the vocational rehabilitation approaches are not fully understood in these environments. Important questions include how to provide access to appropriate occupational services for these workers, and what specific types of support and encouragement may be required to enhance work outcomes in this important sector of the economy.

It is therefore recommended that all key stakeholders (government, insurers, employers, unions, etc) should encourage and support research, according to these priorities.

TABLE 1: DEFINITIONS, DESCRIPTIONS, AND CONCEPTS OF REHABILITATION

TABLE 1: DEFINITIONS, DESCRIPTIONS AND CONCEPTS OF REHABILITATION

Authors	Key features *(Reviewers' comments in italic)*
(BSRM 2000)	**British Society of Rehabilitation Medicine** Rehabilitation is a process whereby those disadvantaged by illness or disability can be enabled to access, maintain or return to employment or other useful occupation (p 5). - - - Effective rehabilitation - - - enables employees to return to work more quickly. For maximum effect, medical, social and vocational rehabilitation should occur concurrently rather than sequentially (p 12). *(They expanded upon this in their Glossary (p 81)):* An active process by which people disabled by injury or disease regain their former abilities or, if full recovery is impossible, achieve their optimum physical, mental, social and vocational capacity and are integrated into the most appropriate environment of their choice. • The use of all means aimed at reducing the impact of disabling and handicapping conditions and at enabling disabled people to achieve optimal social integration. • A process of active change by which a person who has become disabled acquires the knowledge and skills needed for optimal physical, psychological and social function. This process may involve rehabilitation, (re)-training and resettlement.
(BSRM 2003)	**British Society of Rehabilitation Medicine - 2ⁿᵈ edition** Rehabilitation has many definitions, but following injury or illness it is a process of active change arriving at an improvement in functional ability and greater participation in society. In the present context, it is usually a process whereby an individual engages in an active partnership with health professionals to achieve desired goals. Vocational rehabilitation aims to maximise the ability of an individual to return to meaningful employment. Best rehabilitation practice: • Improves work and activity tolerance • Avoids illness behaviour • Prevents deconditioning • Prevents chronicity • And reduces pain and the effects of illness or disability. Successfully rehabilitated individuals feel confident about their work abilities and general well-being. Physical and biomechanical approaches should be complemented with organisational management policy and psychosocial factors such as participation, job discretion and social interaction. Attention to risk factors and workstation design require ergonomic assessment. Rehabilitation programmes that do not address changes to these conditions that have contributed to the development of the disorder are unlikely to produce positive results. Rehabilitation from acute illness or injury requires a continuum from a health-oriented specific programme - - to working full-time in the work environment. Best practice considers the employment requirements of individuals as well as their health and social rehabilitation needs. Rehabilitation in the USA has shifted from work hardening programmes, based away from the work site, to the delivery of services on site. This has the advantage of maintaining the employee in a worker role, even if on modified duties. (pp 11-12) *(There is overlap between use of the terms rehabilitation and vocational rehabilitation).*

TABLE 1: DEFINITIONS, DESCRIPTIONS AND CONCEPTS OF REHABILITATION

(CARF 2007)	**US Commission on Accreditation of Rehabilitation Facilities** An Occupational Rehabilitation Program is individualised, focused on return to work, and designed to minimise risk to and optimise the work capability of the persons served. These services are integrative in nature, with the capability of addressing the work, health, and rehabilitation needs of those served. Such a program provides for service coordination and proactive management of those persons served with injuries or illnesses. An Occupational Rehabilitation Program identifies, addresses, and reduces, when possible, risks of injury, re-injury, disease, and illness. Information about these processes is communicated to relevant stakeholders. An Occupational Rehabilitation Program encourages the persons served to assume responsibility for the self-management of their own healthcare plans in collaboration with relevant stakeholders. Information about the scope of the services and the outcomes achieved is shared by the program with stakeholders. The program may be provided as a hospital-based program, a freestanding program, or a private or group practice, or it may be provided in a work environment (at the job site). *General Occupational Rehabilitation Programs* A General Occupational Rehabilitation Program is a work-related, outcomes-focused, individualised treatment program. Such a program is usually offered at the onset of injury/ illness but may be offered at any time throughout the recovery phase. The program focuses on functional restoration and return to work. Goals of the program include, but are not limited to, improvement of cardiopulmonary and neuromusculoskeletal functions (strength, endurance, movement, flexibility, stability, and motor control functions), education of the persons served, and symptom relief. The services may include the time-limited use of passive modalities with progression to active treatment and/or simulated/real work. *Comprehensive Occupational Rehabilitation Programs* A Comprehensive Occupational Rehabilitation Program is an interdisciplinary, outcomes-focused, and individualised program. Through the comprehensive assessment and treatment provided by occupational rehabilitation specialists, the program addresses the medical, psychological, behavioral, physical, functional, and vocational components of employability and return to work. The simulated/real work used in the program addresses the complexities of the persons served and their work environments.
CMS(UK) 2008	[Case Management Society UK] ***Case management:*** a collaborative process which assesses, plans, implements, coordinates, monitors and evaluates the options and services required to meet an individual's health care, educational and employment needs, using communication and available resources to promote quality, cost-effective outcomes. www.cmsuk.org
(DWP 2004)	**Building capacity for work: a UK framework for vocational rehabilitation** *(Discussion document).* Highlighted that vocational rehabilitation means different things to different stakeholders. Vocational rehabilitation is a term used by many people to describe an approach whereby those who have a health condition, injury or disability are helped to access, maintain or return to employment *(Also gave a more detailed 'working description'):* vocational rehabilitation is a process to overcome barriers an individual faces when accessing, remaining or returning to work following injury, illness or impairment. This process includes the procedures in place to support the individual and/or employer or others (e.g. family and carers), including help to access vocational rehabilitation and to practically manage the delivery of vocational rehabilitation.

TABLE 1: DEFINITIONS, DESCRIPTIONS AND CONCEPTS OF REHABILITATION

Encyclopedia of mental disorders	Vocational rehabilitation is a set of services offered to individuals with mental or physical disabilities. These services are designed to enable participants to attain skills, resources, attitudes, and expectations needed to compete in the interview process, get a job, and keep a job. Services offered may also help an individual retrain for employment after an injury or mental disorder has disrupted previous employment. www.minddisorders.com
Google 2007	**Definitions of vocational rehabilitation on the Web:** Vocational rehabilitation is a program of services designed to enable people with disabilities to become or remain employed. Originally mandated by the Rehabilitation Act of 1973, VR programs are carried out by individually created state agencies. In order to be eligible for VR, a person must have a physical or mental disability that results in a substantial handicap to employment. ... www.zdmu.ac.ir/learn/msc/ms03.htm An entitlement of an injured employee to receive prompt medical rehabilitation and/or retraining or job placement, as may be reasonably necessary to restore him or her to useful employment. www.personal-injury-help-center.org/Glossary_of_Terms.html [SCOPE NOTE: Provision of coordinated services appropriate to the needs of persons with disabilities, and designed to achieve objectives directed toward the realization of the individuals' maximum vocational potentials; use only for the vocational rehabilitation process in general, otherwise use more particular terms such as COUNSELING, EVALUATION, or PLACEMENT] Broader terms: Programs; Rehabilitation Related terms: Client assistance programs; Employment success; Private sector ... www.cirrie.buffalo.edu/thesv.html the process of retraining an injured worker retrain and helping them find a new job. www.lieberson.com/en/neurgosurgery_glossary/v.htm Training to return to work following personal injury. Following an accident, an injured plaintiff may require vocational rehabilitation to return to work. www.millerlawinc.com/leagal_d.htm providing training in a specific trade with the aim of gaining employment www.wordnet.princeton.edu/perl/webwn
Greenstreet Berman Ltd 2004)	**Costs and benefits of return to work and vocational rehabilitation in the UK** [Association of British Insurers] 'Return to work' and 'rehabilitation' form a continuum of complementary activities, applied to match the needs of each case. The authors considered that in the employers' literature, these terms are often understood to reflect a different emphasis on aspects of helping people injured at work. The term **'return to work'** (RTW) tends to be used in the context of the more workplace oriented (employer controlled) practices, such as return to work interviews, workplace adaptations, reduced hours, light and alternative duties. The term **'rehabilitation'** tends to be used in the context of clinically oriented care delivered by health care professionals, such as physiotherapists and occupational physicians. It is also used for vocational activities such as retraining, job counselling and assistance with job seeking. It can also include subsidised job placements aimed at re-integrating people into work.

TABLE 1: DEFINITIONS, DESCRIPTIONS AND CONCEPTS OF REHABILITATION

(Hanson et al. 2006)	Vocational rehabilitation involves multi-dimensional methods to produce work retention and return to work outcomes for employees with injuries or diseases that have led to time off work. These methods include on-site workplace interventions. There has been a change in the understanding of how to achieve effective rehabilitation, with recognition that the workplace is the key place for the employee to recover. Rehabilitation therefore needs to be focused on the tasks that are required for work; with appropriate treatment and activities to encourage restoration of function for work activities.
(HSA 2008)	[Irish Health and Safety Authority] (Vocational) rehabilitation is any method by which people with a condition resulting from sickness or injury which interferes with their ability to work can be returned to work. It is the process of restoration to good health of persons following injury or illness. In the context of this document, rehabilitation aims to restore the person to his/her optimum working capacity.
(ILO 2002)	[International Labour Organization] According to the C159 Vocational Rehabilitation and Employment (Disabled Persons) Convention, 1983: Vocational rehabilitation is a process which enables disabled persons to secure, retain and advance in suitable employment and thereby furthers their integration or reintegration into society. The ILO Convention includes two relevant requirements: • in planning and providing services for the vocational rehabilitation and employment of disabled persons, existing vocational guidance, vocational training, placement, employment and related services for workers generally should, wherever possible, be used with any necessary adaptations • vocational rehabilitation should be started as early as possible. For this purpose, health-care systems and other bodies responsible for medical and social rehabilitation should co-operate regularly with those responsible for vocational rehabilitation. *(The UK has not ratified C159)*
(Irving et al. 2004)	There is widespread recognition that the term 'vocational rehabilitation' is not readily understood by most people *(in 2004)*, and consequently it is adapted to more straightforward terms such as 'getting you back to work'. Ideas of what VR encompasses vary widely. At its core it is understood to be the process of getting people who have been sick or injured back to work or some meaningful activity. But some take a narrower definition and position VR as distinct from medical rehabilitation or as helping people back into a different job when they are unable to return to their original job. Others take a wider definition and see VR as covering initiatives to do with health and safety at work, prevention of injury or illness in the workplace, counselling and healthcare offered to staff as part of absence management. *What makes for good vocational rehabilitation:* Whilst there might be disagreements about what exactly VR comprises and its precise definition, there does seem to be some consistency of opinion about what makes for good VR. There is general agreement amongst the better informed that VR is a process often involving several different initiatives designed to help sick or injured people get back to work. In cases involving more acute illness/injury, VR can involve a whole range of interventions from cognitive behavioural therapy (CBT), provision of special equipment, training, identifying job opportunities, etc. Sometimes, quite simple interventions can have a disproportionate impact, for example, help with filling in job application forms, physiotherapy for back injuries, sorting out childcare arrangements and workplace adjustments.

TABLE 1: DEFINITIONS, DESCRIPTIONS AND CONCEPTS OF REHABILITATION

	Key elements of good VR include: • early intervention – it is generally accepted that the longer people stay off work sick or injured the more likely they are to lose contact with the world of work. A non-working self-image and lifestyle can take over, and often this is associated with the onset of mental health and/or financial problems and becoming acclimatised to the benefit system, potentially getting caught in the 'benefit trap'. The sooner people are offered appropriate support and assistance, the greater their chances are of avoiding a downward spiral and of retaining their existing employment or getting into other employment; • patient centric – it is acknowledged that it is crucial that VR interventions are relevant and appropriate for the individual's needs. This implies listening to and observing the person carefully to establish what they really want/need and would like to happen; Case management – especially with cases of more acute injury and illness, the patient is likely to have complex problems and need help on many different fronts, including housing modifications, transport, prosthetics and financial/ emotional counselling. Most insurers and providers agree that case managers have a key role in identifying appropriate and effective help, liaising with the various different agencies and facilitating interventions from the relevant parties. Inevitably, there are disagreements about what kind of case management works best, how hands on it should be, whether it should be face-to-face and so on. In short, more successful VR is likely to be initiated early, involve the patient in developing the solution, and involve a flexible, holistic, case management approach.
(Kendall & Thompson 1998)	**Hierarchy of occupational outcomes** There are a number of potential vocational rehabilitation outcomes, which can be placed in a hierarchy that can be pursued in sequence with each option being explored and exhausted before the next is considered. 1. Same job, same employer (SJSE). Worker returns to pre-injury job 2. Modified job, same employer (SJSE-Modified). Worker returns to similar or comparable job with pre-injury employer but with some restrictions or modifications 3. Different job, same employer (DJSE). Worker returns to pre-injury employer in an alternate job. Skills, aptitudes and experience are evaluated to determine if they are transferable to alternate work. Employer is encouraged to accommodate worker in a different position 4. Same job, different employer (SJDE). Pre-injury employer unable to accommodate, in any capacity. Alternatives in the same or related industry may be considered, making the most of the worker's skills in a similar or comparable job 5. Modified job, different employer (SJDE-Modified). Worker unable to return to work with pre-injury employer. Employment in a related industry may be considered with some restrictions or modified duties 6. Different job, different employer (DJDE). Worker is unable to return to employment in the same or related industry. Vocational exploration expanded to suitable opportunities in other areas where the worker's existing skills, aptitudes and interests will be used 7. Vocational and/or academic retraining. Existing skills are insufficient to restore the worker to suitable employment, the development of new occupational skills may be considered through on the job training, technical, vocational and/or academic programmes *(Adapted)*

TABLE 1: DEFINITIONS, DESCRIPTIONS AND CONCEPTS OF REHABILITATION

(Levack et al. 2006)	**Purposes and mechanisms of goal planning in rehabilitation** Goal planning is a fundamental component of contemporary rehabilitation practice and a prerequisite for inter-disciplinary teamwork. Interventions need to be goal oriented, and goal planning in rehabilitation should be integral to professional practice, guidelines and policy. The four major purposes of goal planning in rehabilitation are: (1) to improve patient outcomes, (2) to enhance patient autonomy, (3) to evaluate outcomes, and (4) built into contractual, legislative or professional requirements. The first of these purposes is associated with four distinct mechanisms: a) to influence patient motivation, b) to enhance the specificity of training effects, c) for secondary therapeutic effects, and d) to improve teamwork. The other three purposes require a flexible, open-ended approach.
(Lunt et al. 2005)	**HSE review of the risk prevention approach to occupational health: applying models to 21st century occupational health needs: health models information pack** [Health & Safety Executive] Definition of Occupational Health: A state of physical, mental and social well being at work, and not merely the absence of disease and disability, that is influenced by factors within and outside the work place. Occupational Health can be achieved by ensuring the work place is characterised by the principles underpinning Scottish Executive (2004) definition of Healthy Working Lives: A healthy working life is one that continuously provides working-age people with the opportunity, ability, support and encouragement to work in ways and in an environment which allows them to sustain and improve their health and wellbeing. It means that individuals are empowered and enabled to do as much as possible, for as long as possible, or as long as they want, in both their working and non-working lives.
(MBWDC 2000)	**Michigan Bureau of Workers' Disability Compensation (Report of The Task Force on Vocational Rehabilitation in Workers' Compensation):** Vocational rehabilitation is the coordinated and systematic process of professional services to enable and sustain the employment of an injured worker. The basic components of vocational rehabilitation services are vocational assessment, counselling, goal-setting, service planning, case management, service delivery, job placement and follow-up.
(Nocon & Baldwin 1998)	**Trends in rehabilitation policy: a review of the literature** Review of a range of ideas and definitions of rehabilitation - what it involves, who does it, and when it is carried out - and argued that the core objective is *restoration*. This might include restoration of function, capability, independence, or physical and mental health. Authors considered there was an emerging consensus that: • The primary objective of rehabilitation involves restoration (to the maximum degree possible) either of function (physical or mental activities) or of role (participation within the family, social network or work force). • Rehabilitation usually requires a combination of therapeutic and also social interventions that address the clinical problem *and* issues in the individual's physical and social environment. • Effective rehabilitation needs to be: responsive to users' needs and wishes; purposeful and goal-directed; involve a number of agencies and disciplines; and available when required. • Rehabilitation is often a function of services: it is not necessarily a separate service. *(Pre-2000 but included as key earlier review).*

TABLE 1: DEFINITIONS, DESCRIPTIONS AND CONCEPTS OF REHABILITATION

(Siegert & Taylor 2004)

Theoretical aspects of goal-setting and motivation in rehabilitation

The purpose of this article was to provide rehabilitation theorists and researchers with an introduction to some key theories of goals and motivation from the field of social cognition and to argue for increased dialogue between the two disciplines. The use of goals and goal-setting in rehabilitation is briefly surveyed and the somewhat ambivalent attitude toward the concept of motivation in the rehabilitation literature is highlighted. Summarises three major contributors to the study of goals and motivation from the field of social cognition. It is argued that there is a need for a greater emphasis upon theory development in rehabilitation research and that closer collaboration between researchers in rehabilitation and social psychology offers considerable promise. Goal setting is an important component of rehabilitation. It provides a framework for people and the associated rehabilitation professionals to work together to support the person back to their pre-injury lifestyle, or as close as possible. Rehabilitation can focus on short-term task oriented goals. Focusing on internal motivating factors and a range of goals may provide a greater level of personal satisfaction and motivation.

(Svensson et al. 2006)

Pride, empowerment, and return to work: on the significance of promoting positive social emotions among sickness absentees

Sickness absence is a great public health problem and there is a lack of knowledge concerning the hows and whys of success or failure in promoting return to work of sick-listed persons. Discussions of and research into social and psychological aspects of this problem area are in need of theoretical contextualisation. In this paper it is suggested that theories of social emotions may be useful, and that the concept of empowerment can be applied provided that it is reasonably well defined. The notions of pride/shame and empowerment are elucidated and discussed, and it is shown that they can be related in the context of research into emotional dimensions of sickness absentees' experiences of the rehabilitation process in a way that may help to guide empirical studies. A simple model of hypothetical relations between pride/shame, empowerment/disempowerment, work ability, health, and return to work is sketched:– Many people who are either off work or on long-term restricted duties suffer lowered self-esteem, sense of control and self determination. Social networks and family interaction are often lost, along with general participation in work life. Therefore being off work can cause a person to loose their sense of identity and place in society. If a person on sick leave evaluates themselves by the way they believe others see them, they may feel ashamed for being off work. The person may perceive or experience negative interactions with those around them. Negative feelings, such as shame, from social interactions are thought to be stronger and more readily felt than positive emotions, such as pride. When people feel shame they tend to withdraw into themselves, making rehabilitation more difficult. Rehabilitation in difficult circumstances pushes the injured person to extend themselves and may require sustained determination. In a situation where shame is the dominant emotion, the person is likely to feel disempowered. In contrast, pride can help people to feel psychologically empowered, and assists in rehabilitation. Interactions with rehabilitation and other health professionals that reduce hope and confidence and lower self-esteem are likely to be counterproductive to rehabilitation and return to work in the long term.

(TUC 2000)

(Vocational) rehabilitation is **any method** *[our emphasis]* by which people with a sickness or injury (that interferes with their ability to work to their normal or full capacity) can be returned to work. (*They stressed that no profession has a monopoly on rehabilitation and a multidisciplinary approach is almost always best*). This can involve medical or other treatment, vocational rehabilitation or retraining, adaptations to the work environment or working patterns. (*This definition is all-encompassing, but does not distinguish vocational rehabilitation from 'treatment'*).

(VRA 2007)

Vocational rehabilitation standards of practice

[Vocational Rehabilitation Association]

Vocational Rehabilitation is a process which enables persons with functional, psychological, developmental, cognitive and emotional impairments or health conditions to overcome barriers to accessing, maintaining or returning to employment or other useful occupation. (*The Vocational Rehabilitation Association, formerly the National Vocational Rehabilitation Association, is in the UK*).

TABLE 1: DEFINITIONS, DESCRIPTIONS AND CONCEPTS OF REHABILITATION

(Waddell & Burton 2004)	**Concepts of rehabilitation for the management of common health problems**

There is now broad agreement on the importance of rehabilitation and the need to improve occupational health and vocational rehabilitation in UK. However, there is considerable uncertainty about what 'rehabilitation' is, and about its (cost)-effectiveness, particularly for the common health problems that cause most long-term disability and incapacity. The aim of this paper is to develop a theoretical and conceptual basis for the rehabilitation of common health problems. The stereotype of disability is a severe medical condition with objective evidence of disease and permanent physical or mental impairment (e.g. blindness, severe or progressive neurological disease, or amputation). In fact, most sickness absence, long-term incapacity for work and premature retirement on medical grounds are now caused by less severe mental health, musculoskeletal and cardio-respiratory conditions. These 'common health problems' often consist primarily of symptoms with limited evidence of objective disease or impairment. Importantly, many of them are potentially remediable and long-term incapacity is not inevitable.

Rehabilitation was traditionally a separate, second-stage process, carried out after medical treatment had no more to offer yet recovery remained incomplete. The goal was then to overcome, adapt or compensate for permanent impairment. That approach remains valid for people with severe impairments. However, it is inappropriate for common health problems, where the obstacles to recovery are often psychosocial in nature rather than the severity of pathology or impairment. Here, rehabilitation should focus instead on identifying and overcoming health-related, personal/psychological and social/occupational obstacles to recovery and (return to) work.

This implies that rehabilitation can no longer be a separate, second stage intervention after 'treatment' is complete. Instead, to minimize the number of people going on to long-term incapacity, rehabilitation should be an integral part of good clinical and occupational management:

- Health care should provide timely and effective treatment, but that alone is not enough. Rehabilitation demands that clinical management should *both* relieve symptoms and restore function, and these go hand in hand. Work is not only the goal: work is generally therapeutic and an essential *part* of rehabilitation. Every health professional who treats patients with common health problems should be interested in and take responsibility for rehabilitation and occupational outcomes.

- Common health problems are not only matters for health care: they also require occupational management. Employers, unions and insurers must re-think workplace management of common health problems: addressing all of the health, personal and occupational dimensions of incapacity, identifying obstacles to return to work, and providing accommodations and support to overcome them.

- This should not obscure the importance of the individual's own role in the management of common health problems. Rehabilitation is an active process that depends on the participation, motivation and effort of the individual, *supported by* health care and the workplace.

Everyone – workers; employers, health professionals; government and society – has an interest in better outcomes for common health problems. Effective management depends on getting 'all players onside' and working together to that common goal. This is partly a matter of perceptions (by all the players). It depends on better communication. Even more, it requires a fundamental shift in the culture of how common health problems are perceived and managed, in health care, in the workplace, and in society.

TABLE 1: DEFINITIONS, DESCRIPTIONS AND CONCEPTS OF REHABILITATION

(WHO 2001)	**International classification of functioning, disability and health**
	[World Health Organization]
	The biopsychosocial model
	From a clinical perspective, symptoms and illness may *originate from* a health condition, but the development of chronic problems and incapacity often also depends on psychosocial factors. From the perspective of disabled people, restrictions of function are often imposed by the way society is organised for able-bodied living. There is now broad agreement that human illness and disability can only be understood and managed according to a biopsychosocial model that includes biological, psychological *and* social dimensions ((Engel 1977; Waddell et al. 2002)). 'Biopsychosocial' is a clumsy, technical term but it is difficult to find any adequate, alternative word. Put simply, this is an individual-centred model that considers the person, their health problem, *and* their social context:
	• *Biological* refers to the physical or mental health condition.
	• *Psychological* recognises that personal/psychological factors also influence functioning and the individual must take some measure of personal responsibility for his or her behaviour.
	• *Social* recognises the importance of the social context, pressures and constraints on behaviour and functioning.
	The *International Classification of Functioning, Disability and Health* (ICF) is based on the biopsychosocial model, and is now widely accepted as the framework for disability and rehabilitation (Davis et al. 1992; Post et al. 1999; Wade & de Jong 2000). ICF conceives functioning and disability as a dynamic interaction between the individual's health condition and contextual factors. This produces a classification in two parts, each with two components:
	Functioning and disability: (a) Body structures and functions (impairments); (b) Activities and participation (limitations and restrictions)
	Contextual factors: (a) Personal factors; (b) Environmental factors

[VR = vocational rehabilitation; RTW = return to work]

TABLE 1: ANNEX - CONTENT ANALYSIS AND EVIDENCE LINKING

Content	Key features	References
• Rehabilitation traditionally focuses on severe medical conditions and permanent impairments. However, vocational rehabilitation is equally important for people with common health problems.	[Key features: severe impairments; common health problems]	References: BSRM 2000, DWP 2004, Irving 2004, TUC 2000, Waddell & Burton 2004
• Rehabilitation for people with severe and permanent impairments is about overcoming, adapting or compensating for that impairment. However, in common health problems, psychosocial obstacles to recovery are often more important. Vocational rehabilitation for common health problems is more about identifying and addressing health-related, personal/psychological and social / occupational obstacles to (return to) work.	[Key features: biopsychosocial model and framework for disability and rehabilitation; physical and psychological factors; overcome barriers/obstacles]	References: BSRM 2000, 2003, VRA 2007, Waddell & Burton 2004. Additional references: Engel 1977, Waddell 2002, WHO 2001; Post et al. 1999; Wade & de Jong 2000
• Vocational rehabilitation is often seen as a separate intervention, carried out after medical treatment is complete. However, there is increasing recognition that the goals and principles of rehabilitation should be an integral part of all good clinical and workplace management.	[Key features: staging; rehabilitation principles]	References: DWP 2004, Waddell & Burton 2004
• Vocational rehabilitation is not a matter of health care alone. It commonly requires a combination of health care and workplace interventions, to address the health problem and work issues. In the last few years, there has been an important shift toward locating vocational rehabilitation in the workplace whenever possible (either entirely or in the latter stages).	[Key features: not solely healthcare; health and workplace interventions; including work and work-relevant tasks in rehabilitation; locating in workplace]	References: BSRM 2000, 2003, Hanson et al 2006, Nocon & Baldwin 1998, TUC 2000, Waddell & Burton 2004
• Vocational rehabilitation is goal directed and outcome focused. The core objective is restoration of capacity for work and translating that capacity into participation.	[Key features: goals; outcomes; focused; maximise and optimise capabilities; restore function while minimising risk to worker-others].	References: BSRM 2000, 2003, CARF 2007, ILO 2002, Levack et al 2006, Nocon & Baldwin 1998, Siegert & Taylor 2004, WHO 2001
• Vocational rehabilitation is a process of active change, facilitating the journey from sickness to (return to) work. It is often a function of health care and the workplace: it is not necessarily a separate programme or service.	[Key features: process; function of services]	References: BSRM 2000, 2003, Nocon & Baldwin 1998, VRA 2007, Waddell & Burton 2004.
• Provided a few, simple principles of vocational rehabilitation are followed, most people with common health problems should return to work uneventfully. The minority who are delayed returning to work may require a more structured programme, with several interventions in a range of settings (e.g. health care, workplace), delivered in sequence or in parallel.	[Key features: necessary, multifactorial, coordinated, structured steps, planned; case management]	References: BSRM 2000, 2003, CARF 2007, CMS(UK) 2008, Greenstreet Berman Ltd 2004, Hanson et al 2006, Irving 2004, MBWDC 2000, Nocon & Baldwin 1998
• The individual has an important role. Vocational rehabilitation is an active process that depends on the participation, motivation and effort of the individual, supported by the workplace and healthcare.	[Key features: individual responsibility; motivation]	References: BSRM 2003, CARF 2007, Irving 2004, Svenson et al 2006, Waddell & Burton 2004.
• Vocational rehabilitation requires 'all players onside' – the individual, the workplace and health professional(s) - working together to a common goal.	[Key features: all players onside, communication, common goal]	References: DWP 2004, ILO 2002, Irving 2004, MBWDC 2000, Waddell & Burton 2004

TABLE 2: 'WORK-RELATED' ISSUES

Table 2a: Definitions of accident, injury, and occupational disease

Authors	Key features *(Reviewers' comments in italic)*
TABLE 2a: DEFINITIONS OF ACCIDENT, INJURY, AND OCCUPATIONAL DISEASE	
Accident	
Concise Oxford Dictionary	Event without apparent cause, unexpected www.askoxford.com/dictionaries/?view=uk
Mirriam-Webster online dictionary	An unforeseen and unplanned event or circumstance. www.m-w.com/dictionary/accident
Dictionary.com	1. an undesirable or unfortunate happening that occurs unintentionally and usually results in harm, injury, damage, or loss; casualty; mishap: automobile accidents. 2. Law. such a happening resulting in injury that is in no way the fault of the injured person for which compensation or indemnity is legally sought. 3. any event that happens unexpectedly, without a deliberate plan or cause. 4. chance; fortune; luck: I was there by accident. 5. a fortuitous circumstance, quality, or characteristic: an accident of birth. 6. Philosophy. any entity or event contingent upon the existence of something else. — *Synonyms* 1. mischance, misfortune, misadventure; contingency; disaster. www.dictionary.reference.com/browse/accident
Oxford Concise Medical Dictionary	Traumatic incident involving any part of the body www.oxfordreference.com/pages/Subjects_and_Titles__2D_M01
Mirriam-Webster Medical Dictionary	1. an unfortunate event resulting from carelessness, unawareness, ignorance, or a combination of causes 2. an unexpected bodily event of medical importance especially when injurious e.g. a cerebrovascular *accident* 3. an unexpected happening causing loss or injury which is not due to any fault or misconduct on the part of the person injured but for which legal relief may be sought www.m-w.com/medical/accident
On-line medical dictionary	Literally, a befalling; an event that takes place without one's foresight or expectation; an undesigned, sudden, and unexpected event; chance; contingency; often, an undesigned and unforeseen occurrence of an afflictive or unfortunate character; a casualty; a mishap www.cancerweb.ncl.ac.uk/cgi-bin/omd? accident

TABLE 2a: DEFINITIONS OF ACCIDENT, INJURY, AND OCCUPATIONAL DISEASE

Source	Definition
HSE	any unplanned event that results in injury or ill-health to people, or damages equipment, property or materials but where there was a risk of harm. http://www.hse.gov.uk/costs/costs_of_injury/costs_of_injury.asp#section7
UK personal accident insurance	a sudden and unexpected event which happens after the 'Start date' (of the insurance policy) and results in 'Bodily injury'. http://www.nationwide.co.uk/insurance/personal_accident/accident_policy.htm#terms
Barron's dictionary of insurance terms	Unexpected, unforeseen event not under the control of the insured and resulting in a loss. The insured cannot purposefully cause the loss to happen; the loss must be due to pure chance according to the odds of the laws of probability. www.answers.com/topic/accident
The 'Lectric Law Library's Legal Lexicon	In chancery jurisprudence accident signifies such unforeseen events, misfortunes, losses, acts or omissions, as are not the result of any negligence or misconduct in the party. www.lectlaw.com/def/a145.htm
(Newman Taylor 2006)	An accident was defined in 1903 by case law as an event which is neither expected nor designed.
(ILO 1998)	[International Labour Organization] Sixteenth International Conference of Labour Statisticians: An occupational accident is an unexpected and unplanned occurrence, including acts of violence, arising out of or in connection with work which results in one or more workers incurring a personal injury, disease or death; as occupational accidents are to be considered travel, transport or road traffic accidents in which workers are injured and which arise out of or in the course of work, i.e. while engaged in an economic activity, or at work, or carrying on the business of the employer. *(Also used by Organisation for Economic Co-operation and development - OECD).* http://laborsta.ilo.org/applv8/data/c8e.html
UK Social Security Administration Act (1992)	An industrial accident is an accident whereby a person suffers personal injury [that] … arises out of and in the course of his employment

Injury

Source	Definition
Concise Oxford Dictionary	Wrongful action or treatment; harm, damage www.askoxford.com/dictionaries/?view=uk
Mirriam-Webster online dictionary	1 a: an act that damages or hurts: a 'wrong' b: violation of another's rights for which the law allows an action to recover damages 2: hurt, damage, or loss sustained www.m-w.com/dictionary/injury

TABLE 2a: DEFINITIONS OF ACCIDENT, INJURY, AND OCCUPATIONAL DISEASE

Wikipedia	Damage or harm caused to the structure or function of the body caused by an outside agent or force. www.en.wikipedia.org/wiki/Injury
American Heritage Dictionaries	1. Damage or harm done to or suffered by a person or thing: *escaped from the accident without injury* 2. A particular form of hurt, damage, or loss: *a leg injury.* 3. *Law.* Violation of the rights of another party for which legal redress is available. www.bartleby.com/61/63/I0146300.html
Dictionary.com	1. harm or damage that is done or sustained. 2. a particular form or instance of harm: an injury to one's shoulder; an injury to one's pride. 3. wrong or injustice done or suffered. 4. *Law.* any wrong or violation of the rights, property, reputation, etc., of another for which legal action to recover damages may be made. *Synonyms* 1. destruction, ruin, impairment, mischief. 1–3. injury, hurt, wound refer to impairments or wrongs. Injury, originally denoting a wrong done or suffered, is hence used for any kind of evil, impairment, or loss, caused or sustained: *physical injury: injury to one's reputation.* HURT suggests esp. physical injury, often bodily injury attended with pain: *a bad hurt from a fall.* A WOUND is usually a physical hurt caused by cutting, shooting, etc., or an emotional hurt: *a serious wound in the shoulder; to inflict a wound by betraying someone's trust.* www.dictionary.reference.com/browse/accident
Mirriam-Webster Medical Dictionary	hurt, damage, or loss sustained www.medical.merriam-webster.com/medical/injury
On-line medical dictionary	The damage or wound of trauma. *(The definition offered is tautological since 'Trauma' is defined as 'injury').* www.cancerweb.ncl.ac.uk/cgi-bin/omd?injury
Medline Plus	An injury (also called traumatic injury) is damage to your body. It is a general term that refers to harm caused by accidents, falls, blows, burns, weapons and more. www.nlm.nih.gov/medlineplus/injuries.html
UK personal accident insurance	'Bodily injury' means injury to your body (excluding sickness, disease or any naturally occurring condition or degenerative process) resulting from external violent and visible means. http://www.nationwide.co.uk/insurance/personal_accident/accident_policy.htm#terms
Personal Injury Information:	There are three basic categories of 'occupational injury': specific injuries sustained in a specific incident or 'accident'; 'repetitive injuries' are injuries or illnesses resulting from repetitive tasks; occupational diseases result from exposure to hazardous substances (?) at work. *(There is clearly some confusion between injury, disease and illness).* www.personal-injury-information.com/occupational_injury.html

TABLE 2a: DEFINITIONS OF ACCIDENT, INJURY, AND OCCUPATIONAL DISEASE

(ILO 1998)	Sixteenth International Conference of Labour Statisticians:
	An occupational injury is any personal injury, disease or death resulting from an occupational accident; an occupational injury is therefore distinct from an occupational disease, which is a disease contracted as a result of an exposure over a period of time to risk factors arising from work activity
	(There is clearly some circularity between the ILO definitions of occupational accident and occupational injury. There is also confusion between injury and disease. Note: the ILO definition of an 'occupational injury' seems somewhat confusing at first sight since it includes the term 'disease'. However, ILO does distinguish occupational disease from occupational injury. Disease occurs because of the work environment or conditions and is distinguished by exposure over time, whereas injury is the result of a specific incident). (Also used by the Organisation for Economic Co-operation and Development (OECD)).
	http://laborsta.ilo.org/applv8/data/c8e.html
UK Social Security Administration Act (1992)	*(Refers to personal injury but does not give any definition).*
(Haddon 1973)	Damage to the body produced by energy exchanges that have relatively sudden discernible effects
	(The concept of an energy exchange is useful, but has problems. The phrase 'damage to the body' may be interpreted as limited to tissue damage, which excludes psychological effects; and, the meaning of 'energy exchange' fails to capture intent since damage can occur from intentional causes such as surgery).

Occupational disease

Wikipedia	An occupational disease is any chronic ailment that occurs as a result of work or occupational activity. An occupational disease is typically identified when it is shown that it is more prevalent in a given body of workers than in the general population, or in other worker populations. Occupational hazards that are of a traumatic nature (such as falls by roofers) are not considered to be occupational diseases.
	www.en.wikipedia.org/wiki/Occupational_disease
Answers.com	A disease resulting from the conditions of a person's work, trade, or occupation.
	Illness contracted as the result of employment-related exposures and conditions.
	A disease that results from a particular employment, usually from the effects of long-term exposure to specific substances or from continuous or repetitive physical acts.
	The term 'occupational disease' refers to those illnesses caused by exposures at the workplace. They should be separated, conceptually, from injuries that may also occur at workplaces due to a variety of hazards.
	www.answers.com/occupational+disease?cat=health

TABLE 2a: DEFINITIONS OF ACCIDENT, INJURY, AND OCCUPATIONAL DISEASE

Source	Definition
Webster's Newworld Medical Dictionary	A disease due to a factor in a person's occupation. 1. Also called industrial disease. a disease caused by the conditions or hazards of a particular occupation. 2. a trait or tendency that develops among members of a particular profession: e.g. Cynicism was thought to be an occupational disease of reporters. http://eu.wiley.com/WileyCDA/WileyTitle/productCd-0764524615.html
Infoplease	Occupational disease: illness incurred because of the conditions or environment of employment. Unlike with accidents, some time usually elapses between exposure to the cause and development of symptoms. In some instances, symptoms may not become evident for 20 years or more. www.infoplease.com/ce6/sci/A0836318.html
(Cherry 1999)	An occupational disease may be defined simply as one that is caused, or made worse, by exposure *(to a hazard)* at work. *(No other definition includes aggravation.)* While epidemiological studies of populations can determine whether disease is attributable to a particular type or level of exposure, for an individual patient this is less clear.
(ILO 1998)	*Sixteenth International Conference of Labour Statisticians:* An occupational disease is a disease contracted as a result of an exposure over a period of time to risk factors arising from work activity. *(Also used by the Organisation for Economic Co-operation and Development (OECD)).* http://laborsta.ilo.org/applv8/data/c8e.html
Institut National de Recherché et de Securite	[French National Institute for Research and Safety] A disease is considered to be 'occupational' if it is the direct consequence of a worker's exposure to a physical, chemical or biological risk or if it is caused by the conditions in which the worker performs his or her occupation. Such a definition, whilst it sounds perfectly logical, is however much too vague for both lawyers and doctors. www.inrs.fr/safety/occupational_diseases.html
(Newman Taylor 2006)	**The prescription of disease** The 1897 Workmen's Compensation Act gave a duty on employers to compensate their employees for loss of earnings due to accidents arising out of and in the course of employment. a prescribed disease should be a) a recognised risk to workers in an occupation or exposed to a particular agent and b) that attribution of the disease to an occupation or agent should be based on the balance of probabilities, i.e. is more likely than not. IIAC Section 108(2) of the Contributions and Benefits Act 1992 requires that the disease: Ought to be treated, having regard to its causes and incidence and any other relevant considerations, as a risk of their occupations and not as a risk common to all persons; and

TABLE 2a: DEFINITIONS OF ACCIDENT, INJURY, AND OCCUPATIONAL DISEASE

	Is such that, in the absence of special circumstances, the attribution of particular cases to the nature of the employment can be established or presumed with reasonable certainty. In other words, a disease can only be prescribed if the risk to workers in a certain occupation is substantially greater than the risk to the general population, and the link between the disease and the occupation can be established in each individual case or presumed with reasonable certainty. In diseases which occur in the general population (e.g. chronic bronchitis and emphysema) there may be no difference in the pathology or clinical features to distinguish an occupational from a non-occupational cause. In these circumstances, in order to recommend prescription, IIAC looks for consistent evidence that the risk of developing the disease is more than doubled in a given occupation.
HSE	Self-reported work-related illness (SWI): conditions which respondents think have been caused or made worse by their current or past work http://www.hse.gov.uk/statistics/overall/hssh0506.pdf
Related concepts	
(HSC 1992)	**Risk, hazard and harm:** • A hazard is something with the potential to cause harm. • Risk is the likelihood that the harm from a particular hazard is realised. • Harm is a negative safety and health consequence (e.g. injury or ill health) (European Agency for Safety and Health at Work; Health and Safety Commission; Health and Safety Executive)
(Waddell & Aylward 2005)	*Disease* is objective, medically diagnosed, pathology. *Impairment* is significant, demonstrable, deviation or loss of body structure or function. *Symptoms* are bothersome bodily or mental sensations. *Illness* is the subjective feeling of being unwell. *Disability* is limitation of activities and restriction of participation. *Sickness* is a social status accorded to the ill person by society. *Incapacity* is inability to work because of sickness or disability.

Table 2b: Evidence on the impact of work-related, compensation and medicolegal factors

TABLE 2b: EVIDENCE ON THE IMPACT OF WORK-RELATED, COMPENSATION AND MEDICOLEGAL FACTORS[50]

Authors	Key features (Reviewers' comments in italic)
(AFOM/RACP 2001) Australian Report	**Compensable injuries and health outcomes** [Australian Faculty of Occupational Medicine + Royal Australian College of Physicians] *(A major Australian report based on a narrative literature review, interviews with stakeholders in the compensation process, and a multi-disciplinary seminar held in Sydney on 6 October 2000).* There is good evidence to suggest that people who are injured and claim compensation for that injury have poorer health outcomes (in the broadest sense - including functional capacity, return to work, return to prior activities, subjective perceptions of pain, depression, ability to function compared to the past, etc) than people who suffer similar injuries but are not involved in the compensation process. Although ***most people who have compensable injuries recover well,*** there is sufficient good quality evidence to show that a greater percentage of these people have poorer health outcomes than do those with similar but non-compensable injuries. There is significant agreement among practitioners in all relevant fields (medical, legal, insurance, government oversight bodies) to support the evidence and to suggest that a complex interaction of factors is responsible for this. However, research into the causes of poor health outcomes for these people has methodological problems and is inconclusive, but may include the following: Factors that are fully or partly implicated in the literature are: • The psychosocial environment of the injured person at the time of injury (for example, low job satisfaction, poor social networks, lack of purposeful use of time). This includes societal attitudes towards injury and compensation • The psychosocial environment of the injured person after the time of injury (for example, a workplace not prepared to adapt to a return to work program, family members unsupportive of rehabilitation programs) • The psychological vulnerability of the injured person (this will be affected by pain and by psychosocial factors) • The initial response to claimants by insurers (for example, acting as though claimants are automatically assumed to be fraudulent, thus pushing them into a defensive 'I'll show them I'm really sick' attitude) • The management of initial treatment (for example, in non-specific musculoskeletal injuries, not identifying psychosocial risk factors ['yellow flags'], not encouraging resumption of normal behaviours as far as possible, not encouraging return to work or normal activities, etc.) • The handling of case management by insurers (for example, not developing appropriate return to work programs nor monitoring these, not providing claimants with good information about the effects of long term sick leave, etc.) • The handling of case management by treating doctors, including specialists (for example, not reviewing treatment by service providers and continuing treatment which is not helping, providing unnecessary treatment, not giving early referral to pain management programs, not addressing psychological problems such as depression, etc.) • The number and type of medical examinations required by the insurers and by the claimant's lawyers. The effect of these appears to be twofold: to entrench illness behaviours and to prejudice the claimant further against the insurance company.)

50   This section of the evidence was extended back to 1990 as there was much more key material in the previous decade.

TABLE 2b: EVIDENCE ON THE IMPACT OF WORK-RELATED, COMPENSATION AND MEDICOLEGAL FACTORS[50]

- The length of time away from work. Unemployment is, in itself, a risk factor for poor health. There are multiple and interrelating effects of being away from work, including loss of sense of identity, loss of social networks, loss of economic control and independence, loss of social status, loss of financial security (such as loss of the family home), and so on. Long-term unemployment is notoriously hard to break. (Where unemployment is caused by injury, this is exacerbated by employer's reluctance to employ anyone with pre-existing injuries because of risk to workers' compensation premiums and the perceived risk of re-injury.)

Factors that have been identified through interviews or discussions with stakeholders but have not been formally tested are:

- The adversarial system of managing compensation cases, which encourages parties to take up fixed opposing positions and creates a climate where getting a result in the court case becomes the goal of both parties, rather than fully rehabilitating the injured person
- Encouragement from some plaintiffs' lawyers to remain inactive in order to ensure the highest possible settlement
- The length of time between injury and settlement. In one study, 29 months was the average time to settlement. While some legislation requires that the injury be 'stabilised' before settlement, stakeholders suggest that cases are often 'dragged out' unnecessarily, particularly by insurers' lawyers. Ordinary delays in the court system are also a problem
- The sense of powerlessness engendered by being caught up in 'the system'; having no control (except by dropping the claim) over when or how there will be a resolution, no control over decisions made about the claim, no control over number and content of medical examinations, etc.
- The type of compensation offered; systems with no or limited compensation for pain and suffering may produce better outcomes. (Why this is so has not been fully explored. Many of the points listed above may be relevant.)

The complexity of these lists makes it clear that there is no single, easily isolated cause of poorer health outcomes for compensable cases. Some of the factors that may affect outcomes have been identified by research, but it is very likely that it is a complex interaction of these factors that lead to poor health. Further research is needed to identify which of these factors, or the interaction of which factors, is most important in determining health outcomes.

It is generally agreed amongst representatives from the medical colleges that the quality of management of the most common types of compensable injuries (non-specific low back pain, 'whiplash' and other soft tissue injuries) should be improved. Research clearly indicates the importance of psychosocial factors in long-term disability and recent evidence suggests that appropriate early medical intervention that takes this into account can significantly reduce chronicity and long-term disability. Such intervention should ideally be a coordinated interdisciplinary effort (for example, medical, psychological and physiotherapy) to provide interventions that address as many levels of the case as possible.

(Bellamy 1997)	**Compensation neurosis: financial reward for illness as nocebo**
Narrative review	Results of medical treatment are notoriously poor in patients with pending litigation after personal injury or disability claims, and for those covered by workers' compensation programs. However, not all claimants exaggerate their injuries, many do recover despite their injuries and the results of treatment are not uniformly poor among such patients. Although some instances of overt malingering are documented by surveillance videos, most exaggerated illness behaviour in compensation situations takes place because of a combination of suggestion, somatisation, and rationalization. A distorted sense of justice, victim status, and entitlement may further the exaggerated sick role. Adversarial administrative and legal systems challenging the claimant to prove repeatedly he or she is permanently ill harden the conviction of illness and the individual's defence of the claim. Unfortunately, after advocating for one's injury before a sometimes doubting public for the several years required to

TABLE 2b: EVIDENCE ON THE IMPACT OF WORK-RELATED, COMPENSATION AND MEDICOLEGAL FACTORS[50]

	resolve such claims, care eliciting behaviour too often results in denial of disability status in the future, the claimant is compelled to guard against getting well and is left with no honourable way to recover from illness. Financial reward for illness thus functions as a powerful nocebo, a nonspecific force creating and exacerbating illness. Solutions require recognition that judging disability and work incapacity in others is an unscientific process and that adversarial systems rewarding permanent illness or injury, particularly self reported pain, are often permanently harmful. The remainder of the solution must be political. *(It is assumed throughout this review that clinical management and rehabilitation should follow standard lines).*
(Binder & Rohling 1996) Meta-analysis	**Money matters: the effects of financial incentives on recovery after closed-head injury** Included 18 studies and a total of 2353 subjects (673 receiving compensation and 1680 patients not receiving compensation). Patients with less severe head injuries were more likely to seek compensation. Patients receiving compensation were more likely to have late onset symptoms (which were considered to be less likely to have an organic aetiology). Financial incentives were associated with more symptoms and disability, including return to work *(though RTW data was not presented separately),* particularly in patients with less severe, mild head injuries: with a moderate mean effect size of 0.47 The reviewers estimated that if these financial effects were removed, the compensated group of patients would have 23% fewer problems. *(There is no suggestion in the review that these findings should alter standard clinical management or rehabilitation for compensated injuries).*
(Burton 1997) Narrative review	**Back injury and work loss: biomechanical and psychosocial influences** The basic 'injury/damage' model is based on the commonly held tenet that physically demanding work is detrimental to the back (i.e., it can cause injury leading to LBP and consequent disability). The sequence is considered to be one where exposure to mechanical overload, whether a single event or cumulative stress, results in some form of damage to spinal tissues and that further exposure leads to further damage and/or lack of recovery, which in turn leads to disabling consequences. On the face of it, this model would appear to be intuitively reasonable and valid. *(However, a selective exploration of the literature challenged this basic premise and led to the conclusion that describing non-specific LBP as a work-related 'injury' is unhelpful).* Workers commonly believe their LBP is attributable to work, but these beliefs are not necessarily well-founded. When looking at worker-rated job demands and back injury rates, purportedly high risk jobs can have quite diverse demands; not all jobs with high 'injury' rates require the same physical abilities, and not all jobs with high physical demands result in high symptom reports. Many epidemiological studies show an association between heavy work (physical stress) and LBP but that must be viewed against a high prevalence in the (non-working) population, there are methodological problems to this evidence, and the findings are not entirely consistent. The physical demands of modern work have diminished, while incapacity attributed to LBP has increased. The biomechanical basis of 'work injury' is also under question. Biomechanics/ergonomic factors/physical stressors do appear to be related to the first onset of low back pain, but not to persistent/recurrent problems or to disability: chronicity and long-term incapacity are related much more strongly to psychosocial factors. Recent studies show that disc degeneration is influenced only modestly by work history. Objective signs of the overload damage to the discs and vertebral bodies from exposure to mechanical stress predicted by *in vitro* studies and models remain elusive *in vivo.* Of course, structures other than vertebrae and discs (*i.e,* muscles and ligaments) may become damaged, but for the most part there are no objective means for detecting such damage.

TABLE 2b: EVIDENCE ON THE IMPACT OF WORK-RELATED, COMPENSATION AND MEDICOLEGAL FACTORS[50]

	The question of when and how to return workers with LBP to their job has attracted considerable attention. Intuitively, it seems a sensible presumption that too early a return to the same task would increase the risk of symptom recurrence (or do further damage), and a recent literature review concluded that programs involving a return to modified work (e.g., reduction of physical stress through biomechanical modifications or transfer to less demanding tasks) can be successful. However, such programmes often include other elements such as organisational policies, early reporting and prompt active treatment, rendering it difficult to ascribe 'success' just to modified tasks. The use of work restrictions does not necessarily correlate with reduced symptoms after returning to work. Thus, the traditional secondary prevention strategies of rest and return to restricted work duties are seemingly suboptimal. More promising in this respect are programs that take account of the psychosocial influences surrounding disability. Work organizational issues are clearly important, but so also is the behaviour of clinicians. The balance of the available evidence suggests that clinicians generally should adopt a proactive approach to rehabilitation: the majority of workers can be encouraged to return to normal rather than restricted duties (within sensible limits and with appropriate advice) at the earliest opportunity. They should also be given psychosocial advice with the focus on the secondary prevention of persistent disability rather than short-term pain relief. (*These recommended principles of clinical management and vocational rehabilitation are comparable to modern best practice for LBP (Table 3). This review also emphasises the importance of beliefs irrespective of whether they are correct*).
(Burton et al. 2008) Report	**Management of upper limb disorders and the biopsychosocial model** Upper limb disorders are experienced by most people, predominantly during working age: in that sense they can be considered to be common health problems. There is considerable uncertainty over classification and diagnosis for upper limb disorders; the inconsistent terminology impacts on studies of their epidemiology, treatment, and management. Upper limb disorders are commonly experienced irrespective of work and can lead to difficulty undertaking everyday tasks; this applies to specific diagnoses as well as non-specific complaints. Work has a limited overall role in the primary causation of ULDs, yet the symptoms are frequently work-relevant (some work tasks will be difficult for people experiencing upper limb symptoms, and may sometimes provoke symptoms that may otherwise not materialise). Management of cases shows more promise than attempts at primary prevention.
(Butler et al. 1996) Narrative review	**Increasing claims for soft tissue injuries in workers compensation: cost shifting and moral hazard** During the 1980s, the distribution of workers compensation claims showed a 30% shift towards soft tissue injuries such as sprains, strains and low back claims. There are three possible explanations for this trend: 1) safety incentives induced by the workers compensation system or the Occupational Safety and Health Administration (OSHA) may have reduced other injury claims; 2) the movement away from heavy manufacturing and the 1980 construction recession may have changed the underlying risks of workplace injuries; or 3) there has been a moral hazard behaviour on the part of workers and health care providers. Using claim data from the US National Council on Compensation Insurance from 1980–89 and a new estimation framework, the authors concluded that the moral hazard response (*rather than any biological difference*) explained most of the increase in the proportion of soft tissue injury claims during the 1980s. (*This implies that these compensable soft tissue injuries are no different biologically and that clinical management and vocational rehabilitation remain unchanged*).
(DeGood & Kiernan 1996) Single study	**Perception of fault in patients with chronic pain** (*Single study but included as a key piece of evidence*.) The beliefs and expectancies of chronic pain patients have been shown to be critical cognitive facilitators or impediments to the recovery process. In the present study patients presenting to an outpatient pain centre were classified according to their response to the question 'Who do you think is at fault for your pain?': 'employer', 'other' (primarily 'doctors' and 'other drivers'), or 'no one'. The resulting 3 groups of patients did not differ in type or duration of pain, current pain intensity or activity limitation (*i.e. these patients' pain was the same*). Patients who attributed fault to their employers and to a lesser extent to 'others', reported greater concurrent mood.

TABLE 2b: EVIDENCE ON THE IMPACT OF WORK-RELATED, COMPENSATION AND MEDICOLEGAL FACTORS[50]

distress and behavioural disturbance, as well as poorer response to past treatments, and lesser expectations of future benefits, relative to the no-fault patients. The authors concluded that attribution of blame may be an under-recognized cognitive correlate of pain behaviour, mood disturbance, and poor response to treatment. (*This study demonstrates the importance of addressing beliefs about causation and 'fault'. The authors do not suggest any other change in clinical management and rehabilitation of chronic pain*).

(Dembe 2001) Narrative & conceptual review	**The social consequences of occupational injuries and illnesses** There is extensive evidence on the social consequences of illness, but most studies of occupational injuries and illnesses focus on the duration of work disability and direct economic costs. This review considers a wider range of social consequences of work-related injuries and illnesses, including injured workers' psychological and behavioural responses, vocational function, stress, vocational function, rehabilitation and return to work. It also considers their family and community relationships, and the impact on workers' families, coworkers, and community: Such social consequences are complex, inter-related and mutually dependent. Understanding the social consequences of workplace injuries and illnesses is essential in order to appreciate the full impact of workplace accidents, minimize their repercussions, and plan appropriate rehabilitation measures.
(Dersh et al. 2004) Narrative review	**The management of secondary gain and loss in medicolegal settings: strengths and weaknesses** Individuals with chronic illness and disability are among the most difficult patients to treat. The health-care provider is faced with an array of physical, psychological, and social factors, requiring adoption of a biopsychosocial approach to treatment. This approach necessitates consideration of the benefits for the patient of remaining ill and disabled. These benefits have been termed the 'secondary gains' of illness, and they may serve to perpetuate disability and illness behaviour. This paper focuses on secondary gain and loss issues in patients with chronic, non-progressive illness associated with chronic disability, who are evaluated and treated in medicolegal settings. In working with this population of patients, the health-care provider is faced not only with the usual secondary gains of illness (e.g., escape from family responsibilities), but must also deal with the myriad of secondary gain issues unique to medicolegal settings (e.g., seeking financial compensation). Consequently, identifying and managing secondary gain issues can be quite challenging. Freud first proposed the concept of secondary gain, which he described as interpersonal or social advantage attained by the patient as a consequence of . . . illness. In more recent years, the term secondary gain has developed increasing use and has generally referred to the financial rewards associated with disability. In turn, the presence of potential financial rewards is often equated with conscious malingering. This suspicion can interfere with the doctor-patient relationship. Secondary gain issues are then often used as an excuse for treatment failures. However, there is limited or conflicting evidence for may of these interpretations. Most patients, even in a medicolegal context, are not malingerers. The psychosocial factors influencing illness behaviour and disability are complex. Internal and external 'secondary gains' include: In general, secondary losses of chronic illness and disability outweigh secondary gains. Other family members may also have tertiary gains and losses. Awareness of all these gains and losses may help to understand patients' behaviour and entry into the sick role.

TABLE 2b: EVIDENCE ON THE IMPACT OF WORK-RELATED, COMPENSATION AND MEDICOLEGAL FACTORS[50]

(Dersh et al. 2004) Narrative review	**The management of secondary gain and loss in medicolegal settings: strengths and weaknesses**
	The main conclusion of this review is that conscious and unconscious secondary gain issues can be identified and managed appropriately. The authors found their model of managing secondary gain to be a good complement to the functional restoration rehabilitation model, which focuses on increasing function rather than ameliorating symptoms, with the assumption that subjective illness and disability will change only when there is an improvement in functional level. The large majority of their chronically disabled, workers' compensation pain patients demonstrated good long-term outcomes in terms of work return and retention, case closure, decreased health utilization, and decreased pain. Their most significant lesson was the importance of both a skilled disability case manager and a skilled psychologist or psychiatrist collaborating in the effectively management of secondary gain issues, preferably in the context of an interdisciplinary team approach to treatment.
(Fishbain et al. 1995) Systematic review	**Secondary gain concept: a review of the scientific evidence**
	Included 24 studies of 'secondary gain' and 14 'reinforcement' studies. The original concept of secondary gain came from psychoanalysis (*see van Egmond 2003*.) Sociologically, secondary gain has been extended to include interpersonal or social advantage, and is incorporated into the concept of the 'sick role' – when illness has been legitimised by medical sanction, the sick role relieves the person of the usual demands and obligations and takes priority over other social roles. Based upon a review of the psychiatric literature, the authors considered there were problems surrounding the concept and diagnosis of secondary gain. Only five studies could be found in the pain literature that dealt directly or indirectly with the issue of disability benefits influencing disability and treatment outcome in (chronic) pain. Four of these five studies showed that disability benefits reinforced disability perception, though there were major methodological problems. The reinforcement studies showed that positive or negative reinforcement could modify pain behaviour. Discusses the methodological problems and conflicting findings in the compensation literature and concludes that workers compensation chronic pain patients appear to have a worse prognosis than non-compensation chronic pain patients. This literature, however, does not provide evidence that the worse prognosis is directly related to financial secondary gain. *(This part of the review was not systematic but was a very limited and selective narrative review of 5 papers; c.f. Rohling 1995 about the same time (Table 2b). The main concern of this review was abuse of the term 'secondary gain'. The implicit conclusions are that these issues are often over-stated and should not interfere with clinical management).*
(Fordyce 1995) IASP Report	**Back pain in the workplace (PIW): management of disability in non-specific conditions**
	[International Association for the Study of Pain]
	PIW addressed prolonged disability *(in a workers compensation setting)* from non-specific low back pain (LBP), which was distinguished from specific spinal pathologies that remained a matter for medical management and standard social support. The fundamental theoretical basis of PIW was that LBP should be re-conceptualised as activity intolerance, which depended not only on physical impairment but also on psychosocial factors. The original, radical and controversial proposal of PIW was to apply this concept to social policy. PIW proposed fundamental conceptual changes:
	• Re-conceptualise chronic non-specific LBP as a problem of activity intolerance, not a 'medical' problem.
	• Non-specific LBP considered a temporary and not a permanent disability.
	• Complaints of pain, per se, are not adequate to define a medically based pain problem.
	• Psychological factors are critical to a worker's activity intolerance (inability to work). Disability status should not continue beyond the limits set forth - - without comprehensive evaluation.
	• Medical management on a time-contingent rather than a pain-contingent basis.
	• Emphasise work-site based interventions to minimise and limit disability.
	• Provide comprehensive re-evaluation in cases where function is not restored and return to work is not achieved, including social and vocational assessment components.

TABLE 2b: EVIDENCE ON THE IMPACT OF WORK-RELATED, COMPENSATION AND MEDICOLEGAL FACTORS[50]

(This review focused on entitlement, compensation arrangements, incentives and behavioural modification, but a fundamental part of the proposed solution was to link compensation to vocational rehabilitation. Proposals for clinical management and vocational rehabilitation were almost identical to current guidelines for non-specific LBP (Table 3)). (See Waddell 2004 (Table 2b) for a detailed analysis and critique of this report).

(Gatchel et al. 2002)

Narrative review

Secondary loss and pain-related disability: theoretical overview and treatment implications

In the area of occupational pain disability, issues of secondary gain have traditionally been viewed as major barriers to recovery in patients with workers' compensation injuries. Disability behaviours were thought to be perpetuated by the perceived financial, vocational, and emotional rewards that might arise from the psychosocial context of 'being sick' for an extended period of time. Reviews the evidence against this being 'conscious' and 'malingering'. In fact, a much larger barrier to effective treatment of pain patients may be the extensive personal losses that can arise as secondary features of chronic pain. Secondary loss issues are extremely important to consider in any rehabilitation program in order to ensure the most comprehensive and compassionate treatment of these patients. Reviews psychological concepts of loss and in particular of loss of employment.

This has important implications for treatment and rehabilitation. The patient with chronic pain is an individual who has sustained, at the very least, a significant primary loss (of good health and normal physical functioning), and consequent secondary losses that are determined by the psychosocial contexts of the illness. Recommends early intervention of appropriate interdisciplinary treatment, including social support and group therapy, in order to help circumvent the downward spiral of loss, psychological distress and depression, and diminished coping. Such rehabilitation programs may include:

- Treating depression when necessary.
- Implementing other effective medication and psychological techniques to manage pain and disability.
- When appropriate, offering grief counselling, and adaptive readjustment to perceived losses, as well as addressing family dysfunction when necessary.
- Providing group therapy and social support in dealing with losses.
- Addressing physical dysfunctions through physical/occupational therapies and accommodations.
- Helping patients to apply for appropriate entitlements to help offset financial and physical losses.

These secondary gain issues need not be major barriers to recovery, and may actually do a major disservice to patients who may erroneously be labelled as unmotivated and resistant to treatment. In fact, a much larger barrier to effective treatment of chronic pain. An early intervention of appropriate interdisciplinary treatment will help to circumvent the downward spiral of loss, psychological distress, and diminished coping. Once such issues are identified, they may be addressed within the context of interdisciplinary rehabilitation programs, which may include, when appropriate:

- Treating depression
- Implementing other effective medication and psychological techniques to manage pain and disability.
- Offering grief counselling, and adaptive readjustment to perceived losses
- Addressing family dysfunction.
- Providing group therapy and social support in dealing with losses.
- Addressing physical dysfunctions through physical/occupational therapies and accommodations.

(These recommendations for rehabilitation follow typical approaches as in Table 3).

TABLE 2b: EVIDENCE ON THE IMPACT OF WORK-RELATED, COMPENSATION AND MEDICOLEGAL FACTORS[50]

(Guthrie & Jansz 2006)
 	
Narrative review
	Women's experience in the workers compensation system
	
	Introduction: Gender differences are a question of major importance within workers' compensation given the increased role of women in the workforce over the past several decades. This article reviews literature relating to women's experiences following work injury.
	
	Methods: An Australian study is used as background to exploring the broad issue of the question of gender equity in workers' compensation. In doing so it takes account of historical, legal and medical issues.
	
	Results: Literature reviews in the fields of occupational health and safety issues, workplace injuries and diseases, and workers' compensation show that women's experiences may be affected by a range of gender specific issues, including:
	
	  • Gender-segregation in work
	
	  • Differing forms of injury and disease for men and women
	
	  • Lower pay for women and lower bargaining power
	
	  • Poor return to work rates for women in part-time and casual work circumstances.
	
	Conclusion: The Australian experience suggests that as a consequence of the combination of lesser industrial bargaining power, lower wages and differing forms of injury and disease women often receive less than men in compensation payments, struggle to obtain equity in the dispute resolution process and experience greater difficulties in returning to work following injury or disease. *(Rehabilitation should take account of these gender issues. However, otherwise appears to assume that clinical management and vocational rehabilitation should follow standard lines.*

(Hadler et al. 2007) Editorial	**Back pain in the workplace** The primary purpose of (US) workers compensation insurance is to indemnify medical costs and lost wages when a worker has experienced a work-related personal injury, generally defined as an injury that arose out of and in the course of employment. The back 'injury' construct holds that physical demands that render the pain less tolerable are the proximate cause of the back pain and hence the agent of 'injury'. This is a damaging misconception for the medical and workers' compensation systems. From the outset, the notion of 'injury' was contentious. Back pain frequently affects adults of working age who are generally otherwise well and who experienced no unusual, let alone traumatic, precipitant. Back pain is common both in and out of the workplace: whatever the biomechanical precipitants, they cannot be shown to be specific to the workplace. Multiple cohort studies in the contemporary workplace can discern little if any influence of a vast array of task demands on the incidence of disabling backache. Disc 'rupture' is a flawed pathogenetic theory and compensable back 'injury' an iatrogenic sophism. The causes of non-specific back pain continue to elude scientific inquiry. 'Degenerative changes' increase in prevalence with each passing decade until they are ubiquitous but have almost nothing to do with life activities. The age of onset and the degree of degenerative change are largely genetically determined; the contributions of environmental influences *(including work)* are barely discernable. Age-appropriate spines, however hoary, do not bear witness to a life of damaging trauma, nor do they offer anatomical clues as to the cause of backache. They mark longevity, not decrepitude. Therefore, 'wear and tear' and 'injury' are no longer tenable pathogenetic inferences. Furthermore, the incidence of back 'injury' has proved refractory to successive waves of ergonomic advice and devices, of clinical and rehabilitative inventiveness, and of regulatory and legal machinations in the United States and across the resource-advantaged world. Fortunately, modern science has probed for and discerned associations with disabling backache that supersede the 'injury' paradigm. The result is an entirely different conception of backache. Like the 'common cold', backache is an intermittent and remittent predicament of life. Extensive and compelling science supports the premise that inability to cope with backache, chronicity and long-term disability have much more to do with psychosocial factors than with the physical demands of tasks at work.

TABLE 2b: EVIDENCE ON THE IMPACT OF WORK-RELATED, COMPENSATION AND MEDICOLEGAL FACTORS[50]

	Does it matter that back 'injury' is often a surrogate complaint? After all, the backache can be disabling nonetheless — not because of what is lifted, but rather the context in which it is lifted. Such a surrogate might be countenanced if launching a workers' compensation claim benefited the worker who is hurting, but too often that outcome proves elusive. Resources are expended in attempts to 'fix' the 'injured' spine; in demanding the worker prove that the 'injury' is disabling; in attempting to teach the disabled worker that the 'injury' is not disabling; and in blaming the worker for not returning to (often unsatisfactory) work. In the aggregate, great sums of money are spent on an exercise that misses the forest for the trees. More important, these expenditures miss the central issue and capture the worker in escalating iatrogenicity. *(Main argument is that the 'injury model' is unfounded and unhelpful and should not distort clinical management and rehabilitation of LBP. Hadler argues, here and elsewhere, for major reform of the US workers compensation system).*
(Hirsch 1997) Narrative review	**Incentive effects of workers compensation** *(Written by an economist.)* Moral hazard typically refers to a situation where insurance coverage affects the actions of insured parties or, in the case of workers' compensation, the probability and extent of injury and illness claims. Economic theory and evidence indicate that workers, employers, and healthcare personnel respond to the incentives built into state workers' compensation systems. Although empirical studies cannot provide precise estimates of the quantitative effects resulting from specific policy changes, research is useful in evaluating the qualitative effects of alternative policies. Studies show that workers' compensation claims are higher the more generous the level of benefits, the shorter the waiting period, and the more readily available is information on benefits to workers. States that decreasing real benefit levels and lengthening the waiting period required before workers are compensated for lost earnings can constrain future growth in workers' compensation costs, while continuing to provide partial compensation for workers with the most serious injuries. The most difficult problem facing policymakers is to design and implement reforms that take into account what are often the incompatible incentives of workers, employers, and medical care providers. *(Provides an economic analysis of how financial incentives affect claimant behaviour, but no evidence on the magnitude of this effect).*
(IIAC 2007a) Position statement	**Back and neck pain – position paper 18** [Industrial Injuries Advisory Council] The Industrial Injuries Advisory Council has identified significant barriers to prescription, including problems with diagnosis. Back and neck pain are symptoms, and not diseases. However, injuries to the back and neck, occurring as a result of an identifiable accident, continue to be covered under the accident provisions of the Industrial Injuries Disablement Benefit (IIDB) Scheme. Reform of the IIDB Scheme is currently being considered, including the possibility of a greater focus on vocational rehabilitation and support. Research suggests back pain may be one disorder where rehabilitation could be used effectively to enable people to remain in work. This position paper also highlights several preventative measures to combat back and neck pain. Given this inherent limitation, the Council decided not to pursue a full literature review. It has concluded that further consideration of prescription is currently ruled out because the diagnosis rests on a self-report of LBP or neck pain with no robust and effective process for independent corroboration. However, workers injured as a result of acute trauma to the spine will continue to be compensated by the Scheme's accident provisions. The Council notes that several other European countries have scheduled back and neck disorders for prescription – a common focus being on the outcomes of degenerative disc disease or disc prolapse on the one hand and the exposures of heavy lifting and whole body vibration on the other.

TABLE 2b: EVIDENCE ON THE IMPACT OF WORK-RELATED, COMPENSATION AND MEDICOLEGAL FACTORS[50]

	Currently, consultations are underway about the future structure of the IIDB Scheme, including the potential to deploy resources to aid vocational rehabilitation. Back pain is a condition that might be targeted under such a configuration. Research evidence suggests that the longer a person is off work with low back pain the greater the likelihood of long-term health-related unemployment. Many authorities believe that more intensive and earlier efforts at rehabilitation are required in sub-chronic cases (e.g. those with 6 to 12 weeks of sickness absence) to avoid this outcome. The challenge of corroborating diagnosis would be no less great in such cases, but would be less important in the context of functional rehabilitation, as would the distinction between symptoms caused by work, as compared with symptoms aggravated by work. Arguably, such a use of funds could be beneficial to employers and employees alike and cost-effective from the taxpayer's perspective.
(IUA/ABI 2007) Guidance	**The 2007 Rehabilitation Code** [International Underwriting Association + Association of British Insurers] The Rehabilitation Code provides an approved framework for injury claims within which claimant representatives and compensators can work together. Whilst the Code is voluntary, the court Pre-action Protocol provides that its use should be considered for all types of personal injury claims. The objective is to ensure that injured people receive the rehabilitation treatment they need to restore quality of life and earning capacity as soon as possible and for as long as the parties believe it is appropriate. Some key features: • 1 the claimant is put at the centre of the process • 2 the claimant's lawyer and the compensator work on a collaborative basis to address the claimant's needs, from first early notification of the claim and through early exchange of information • 3 the need for rehabilitation is addressed as a priority and sometimes before agreement on liability: fixed time-frames support the Code's framework • 4 rehabilitation needs are assessed by those who have the appropriate qualification, skills and experience The new 2007 Code simplifies the original version, first published in 1999, at the same time as underlining the important principles. It has the support of all the important stakeholders in the claims process including the ABI, IUA, APIL, FOIL, MASS, the Civil Justice Council and major insurers. (*A consensus statement demonstrating desire by UK stakeholders in the litigation industry to set a code supportive of early rehabilitation for injured parties*).
(Leavitt 1992) Single study	**Physical exertion factor in compensable work injuries: a hidden flaw in previous research** (*Single study but included as a key piece of evidence*). Argues that the literature on the negative impact of compensation is biased, that the evidence is much less conclusive than commonly assumed, and that there are a number of conflicting studies. This study compared patients injured at work vs. patients injured away from work. The two groups were quite similar in age, education, and previous back surgery, though they differed in gender and racial make-up. They showed very similar duration of pain and pain intensity. Injury at work was clearly linked to prolonged disability time. Employed people injured away from work but displaying equivalent levels of pain intensity and presumably similar severity back injuries, had shorter periods of disability. The level of physical exertion in the job also significantly affected disability time. Multivariate analysis showed that injury at work appeared to operate both independent of the level of exertion, as well as in interaction with it, to extend the period of disability. Also pointed out that workers compensation patients are more often male, with lower levels of education, heavier and less skilled manual jobs, who are more likely to be injured at work, have less free choice over their treatment and their work, are more likely to experience delays caused by third-party involvement, and require clearance for return to work from employer / supervisor. (*Main conclusion was that the impact of work injury and compensation on return to work is less than commonly assumed, and that physical demands of work are more important. Vocational rehabilitation should take account of work demands*).

TABLE 2b: EVIDENCE ON THE IMPACT OF WORK-RELATED, COMPENSATION AND MEDICOLEGAL FACTORS[50]

(Loeser et al. 1995) Literature synthesis	**Incentive effects of workers' compensation benefits** Included 24 studies that directly addressed the relationship of benefits to claims incidence and duration within the workers compensation system. The best available evidence shows that an increase of 10% in workers compensation benefits is associated with a 1-11% increase in the frequency of claims and a 2-11% increase in the duration of claims. *(Provides strong evidence that the level of compensation benefits influences claims, but the magnitude of this effect is much less than commonly believed).*
(Lunt et al. 2005) Review	**HSE review of the risk prevention approach to occupational health** [Health & Safety Executive/Health & Safety Laboratory] Britain has a world-class record for safety at work and HSE is widely respected for playing a major role in achieving this. However, HSE has not been as successful in achieving the same record for health issues. One contribution to this difference is thought to be a reliance on a philosophy of regulation that is grounded in the prevention of the realization of risks. While this has proved successful for safety problems and for traditional health issues such as chemicals and noise, it has not been successful for health issues such as musculoskeletal disorders (MSD), work-related stress, depression and anxiety, that predominate in the working age population. These are likely to require a different approach. Other approaches and models, derived from, for example, occupational medicine, psychology, economics, horizon scanning, legal and public health domains, may offer equally or more successful ways of thinking about and tackling the problems. This is likely to be particularly the case for rehabilitation, which cannot easily be embraced by the risk prevention model. Moreover, there is a view that, since not all illness can be prevented, intervention strategies that rely solely on prevention will not succeed. Encouraging people to cope with less than perfect health may be a more useful way of framing the issue. The review aims to provide HSE and its partners with a flexible decision-making framework for handling more effectively the spectrum of health issues arising in the 21st Century workplace. *(A critical review of the strengths and limitations of risk assessment for return to work, particularly relevant when there is any question of the health condition being caused by work. Remainder of this review describes the current HSE approach to risk assessment, other government initiatives, future scanning of occupational health needs, and various models of individual and organizational health, health behaviour, disability, and intervention, and how they might apply to occupational health.).*
(Melhorn & Hegmann 2008) Book chapter	**Methods of determining work-relatedness** [American Medical Association] In general, a disease or injury is considered occupational if: 1. The medical findings of disease or injury are compatible with the effects of a hazard to which the worker has been exposed; 2. The worker has had sufficient exposure to have caused the disease or injury; and 3. The balance of the evidence supports the disease or injury being occupational rather than non-occupational. Assessment of whether these criteria are met is in 6 parts (adapted from NIOSH): 1. Evidence of disease – clinical history and examination, diagnostic tests. 2. Epidemiological data – does it support a relationship to work? 3. Objective evidence that the occupational exposure (frequency, intensity, duration) could cause the disease 4. Other relevant factors about causation, e.g. individual risk factors 5. Validity of the evidence, e.g. confounding or conflicting factors 6. Evaluation and conclusions: Does the above evidence support an occupational cause for the disease? This approach can be applied to a particular disease, to an individual case or to a group of workers.

TABLE 2b: EVIDENCE ON THE IMPACT OF WORK-RELATED, COMPENSATION AND MEDICOLEGAL FACTORS[50]

(Merrill 1997) Narrative review	**Worker's compensation, litigation and employment factors in return to work** Focused particularly on outcome studies of multidisciplinary treatment programmes including physical modalities and exercises, education, psychological counselling, job simulation activities and vocational counselling for work low-back injuries. Concludes that considerable evidence has accumulated suggesting that psychological and social factors interact with physical findings in injury, affecting recovery and rate of return to work. The evidence is inconclusive regarding the effect of workers compensation upon return to work, but shows that litigation has a notable negative influence and that length of pre-morbid employment, duration of sickness absence, and availability of a job following injury all impact on employment prognosis following rehabilitation. It is not clear whether the effect of litigation and adversarial proceedings is direct or whether it is related to different employment patterns and increased duration of time off work. *(Concludes that the impact of compensation is less than commonly assumed and that litigation has a greater effect).*
(O'Donnell 2000) Narrative review	**Will Australian workers' compensation insurance management get better soon?** The major aim of workers' compensation legislation is to provide support, rehabilitation, and re-employment for injured workers. Employers have stated their concern that an unacceptably wide definition of occupational injury was leading to increased claims for injuries of gradual onset, where the cause of the injury was unclear and perhaps not work-related. Trade unions were concerned about slow processing of claims, high levels of disputed claims, and the necessity for workers to be provided with more information about the system in order to gain more effective rehabilitation and return to work. Concern was also expressed about the continuing problem of workers ending up unemployed because of disputed claims. To use an adversarial method to estimate the level of permanent disability inhibits rehabilitation and is also illogical and costly in a supposedly no-fault system. Argues for the need to give rehabilitation professionals greater opportunities to take a more pro-active role. To maximise their effectiveness, however, rehabilitation professionals require a broader perspective on their service provision. They must interact clearly, practically and objectively with all parties in the economic and industrial context which drives workers' compensation, in order to achieve effective rehabilitation and work return, in the interests of their clients and the public. The development and provision of a holistic, evidence-based rehabilitation service and widespread dissemination of information about outcomes is crucial to ensure that rehabilitation services do not simply add to current costs. Workplace rehabilitation coordinators and rehabilitation professionals who can demonstrate effective assistance with client problems which relate to all the services under the workers' compensation act are likely to be most effective at achieving rehabilitation and re-employment. Widespread dissemination of comparable, reliable information about outcomes of health, rehabilitation, dispute resolution and employment services is necessary for assessment of their competitive performance in promoting health, employment and productivity. *(Most of this paper is about the organization of Australian Workers Compensation schemes. However, it also provides a strong argument that workers compensation systems should focus on (vocational) rehabilitation which follows typical approaches as in Table 3).*
(Rohling et al. 1995) Meta-analysis	**Money matters: the association between financial compensation and the experience and treatment of chronic pain** Included 32 studies (72% of low back pain) with 3802 patients receiving compensation and 3849 non-compensated controls. *(Most of these studies were representative and cross-sectional.)* Compensated patients were more likely to have low back pain, to be male, younger and have lower levels of education. Patients receiving compensation reported more pain: effect size 0.60 p<.0002 while adjustment for physical severity made no significant difference to this figure. However, compensation status only accounted for 6% of the variance of pain intensity. Patients receiving compensation had poorer results of physical, psychological and surgical treatment (effect sizes generally .50-.60). Such an effect size could mean that if this effect was removed, the compensated group might have 24% fewer days off work. The authors stress that these data do not suggest that compensated patients cannot benefit from surgery or any other form of treatment. They stated: In fact, it is our experience that compensated patients do indeed benefit from a variety of treatments. *(An implicit similar conclusion would apply to vocational rehabilitation).*

TABLE 2b: EVIDENCE ON THE IMPACT OF WORK-RELATED, COMPENSATION AND MEDICOLEGAL FACTORS[50]

(Smith et al. 2006) Analysis of US national data	**Blurring the distinctions between on and off the job injuries: similarities and differences in circumstances** The new, revised National Health Interview Survey (NHIS) collects population-based data on the cause, location, and work relatedness of all medically attended injuries. National US estimates of non-fatal work and non-work injuries were compared by cause and place/location for working age adults (18–64 years). Overall 28.6% of injuries to working age adults were work related (37.5% among employed people). The causes and locations of many work and non-work injuries were similar, supporting the premise that injuries often share common characteristics irrespective of where they occur. Falls, overexertion, and struck/caught by were leading causes for work and non-work injuries. Motor vehicle injuries were less likely to be work-related (3.4% at work v 19.5% non-work) and overexertion injuries more likely to be work related (27.1% v 13.8%). Work and non-work injuries share many similarities regardless of where they occur. Moreover, place is not a good indicator of work-relatedness as 3.5% of home injuries, 9.9% of street/highway injuries, and 66% of injuries in public buildings occurred while working. While certain injuries are unique to the workplace, many causes were similar to non-work injuries: falls were the first or second leading cause of work and non-work injuries and three of the top four causes were the same. The main conclusion of this review is that work and non-work injuries are more similar than different. This suggests opportunities to broaden injury prevention programmes that are commonly limited to one or other setting; comprehensive programmes are likely to be more effective and cost-saving. *(And exactly the same arguments and conclusions would apply to vocational rehabilitation principles and interventions for work- and non-work-related injuries).*

(Teasell & Bombardier 2001)
 	
Systematic review
	Employment-related factors in chronic pain and chronic pain disability
	
	Work disability is a multifactorial problem. Social scientists suggest that non-clinical factors, including personal, psychosocial and work-related factors, can influence (the development of) disability. The aim of this review was to investigate employment related factors associated with the development of chronic pain disability. It concluded that they include:
	
	  • Lack of availability of modified work (moderate evidence)
	  • Lack of work autonomy (moderate evidence)
	  • Low job satisfaction (limited evidence)
	  • Type of work (limited evidence)
	  • Job history (limited evidence)
	  • Public sector vs. private sector (limited evidence)
	  • Lower socioeconomic status (limited evidence)
	  • Number of years employed with firm (contradictory evidence).

TABLE 2b: EVIDENCE ON THE IMPACT OF WORK-RELATED, COMPENSATION AND MEDICOLEGAL FACTORS[50]

(van Egmond 2003) Narrative review	**The multiple meanings of secondary gain** The advantages of an illness experienced by the patient and that hinder recovery are generally termed 'gain'. Freud made the original distinction between 'primary gain', in which (neurotic) illness is the result of unconscious psychological mechanisms, and 'secondary gain', where there is a preconscious holding on to the illness because of supposed or real advantages. However, Freud himself changed the definition of secondary gain several times during his career, and since that time it has become widely used outwith psychoanalysis. In psychoanalysis, the focus is on internal psychological mechanisms. Outwith psychoanalysis, there is often greater emphasis on inter-personal or social aspects, though there is often confusion about whether the gain is perceived (i.e. subjective) or 'real' (i.e. external), and whether the process is conscious or unconscious. In practice, the concept and term 'secondary gain' is often used but with different meanings. For instance, it can be used to describe an unconscious mechanism with an intrapsychological reward for holding on to a neurotic symptom complex, or to describe a conscious attempt to obtain an external reward irrespective of any psychiatric disorder. All variants between these two extremes are also possible. *(Main conclusion seems to be that 'secondary gain' is often used with very different meanings, which can cause confusion).*
(Waddell et al. 2002) Monograph	**Back pain, incapacity for work and social security benefits** *(Section on Workers compensation pp 61-71)* The injury event can have a lasting impact on perceptions about work and health. Many studies show that there is little difference in the physical findings of patients receiving compensation. They do consistently report more pain, though the difference is quite small – about 6%. Several studies show that injuries that occur at work lead to slightly but significantly longer work loss than comparable non-work injuries. There is considerable evidence that the level of financial benefits influences claims rates and duration, though the effect is quite modest. There is conflicting evidence on the effect of lump-sum settlements. The balance of the evidence suggests that the structure of the benefits system and the availability and ease or difficulty of getting benefits (i.e. the control mechanisms: eligibility criteria, the definition and assessment of incapacity, and the claims, adjudication and appeals procedures) have more impact than the actual financial level of benefits (i.e. the financial self-risk to the individual) on the number of claims and the number and duration of benefits paid. Nevertheless, compensation is only one, and probably one of the less powerful, factors in the decision to stop work and to return to work. Workers compensation patients respond less well to pain management and rehabilitation, though many do benefit. To put this all in context, 75–90% of compensation patients do respond well to health care and rehabilitation, and do recover and return to work rapidly. It is only a small proportion who go on to long-term incapacity. Claimants who appeal disallowance of benefits have particularly poor outcomes and few return to work. *(Main conclusion is that there is a lot of evidence that workers compensation benefits can influence claims behaviour, but the magnitude of this effect is modest. There is no suggestion this should influence clinical management or vocational rehabilitation).*
(Waddell 2004) Monograph	**Compensation for chronic pain** *(The conceptual, legislative and legal debate about compensation for chronic pain in the Workers Compensation Boards of Canada 1994-2003).* Addressed the problem of compensation for chronic pain which persists longer than expected after physical injury in the absence of organic findings to explain the reported severity of pain and disability. Referred back to the debate that surrounded Back Pain in the Workplace (Fordyce 1995). The Workers Compensation Boards of Canada are the only agencies that have tried to implement these proposals, which led to prolonged legislative and legal debate. Most of the review addressed the medical evidence on disability evaluation, the incorporation of psychosocial issues and evidence, implementing this in legislation and the resulting legal debate. However, a key part of the proposals was the provision of vocational rehabilitation, which was almost identical to current principles and guidelines for vocational rehabilitation for non-specific musculoskeletal conditions (Table 3).

TABLE 2b: EVIDENCE ON THE IMPACT OF WORK-RELATED, COMPENSATION AND MEDICOLEGAL FACTORS[50]

(Wise 2001)	**Does workers' compensation influence recovery rates?** [Report prepared for the Workers' Compensation and Rehabilitation Commission of Western Australia]
Narrative review	A comparative analysis of published findings indicates that patients who sustain injuries that are compensated under a workers' compensation system, can experience longer recovery periods than patients with similar injuries not covered by any form of compensation. This conclusion was reached in the majority of studies included in this critical review and was irrespective of geographical location of the research, injury type or bodily location of the injury. Australian and international statistics revealed patients with compensable work-related injuries received a greater number of medical and rehabilitation services and had higher costs associated with their medical care than their non-compensable peers. It is suggested that various 'system' factors may influence this: • The medical profession: insufficient understanding of the workers' compensation system and contextual issues related to the workplace and work-related injuries; poor and/or unwilling communication with the employer and other key stakeholders; negative stereotyping of workers compensation cases'; unlimited numbers of treatments. • Specific workers compensation legislation and systems – though there is little published evidence. • Employers not providing suitable alternative duties. • Provision (or lack of) multidisciplinary vocational rehabilitation. • Legal representation The role of psychological issues in creating barriers to physical and functional recovery and return to work.

TABLE 3: REVIEWS AND REPORTS ON MUSCULOSKELETAL DISORDERS

Table 3: Musculoskeletal disorders

TABLE 3: MUSCULOSKELETAL DISORDERS	
Authors	**Key features** *(Reviewers' comments in italic)*
(Adams & Sim 2005) Narrative review	**Rehabilitation approaches in fibromyalgia** An overview of the evidence for the principal approaches taken to the rehabilitation of patients with fibromyalgia. Owing to factors such as methodological shortcomings of existing studies, and the lack of evidence on individual modalities, it is difficult to draw definitive conclusions as to which is the most appropriate rehabilitation approach in fibromyalgia. However, there is growing evidence for the role of exercise training, and clear indications that if appropriately prescribed, this can be undertaken without adverse effects. Similarly, psychologically-based interventions such as cognitive-behavioural therapy have received some support from the literature. Evidence for other interventions is more equivocal. Overall, it appears that a combination of interventions, in a multimodal approach (e.g., exercises combined with education and psychologically-based interventions) is the most promising means of managing patients with fibromyalgia. *(Most of the studies used physiological and physical outcomes rather than occupational outcomes (work capacity)).*
(Abenhaim et al. 2000) Task force report	**Role of activity in the therapeutic management of back pain** The authors introduce a conceptual framework for the relation between back pain and occupational activity. Pain is the initiator of a series of psychological and occupational manifestations that are linked together in the biopsychosocial model. Workers with back pain may or may not experience activity limitations or restriction in employment participation. Occupational activity may be regular, reduced (activity disrupted), or interrupted (completely incapable of performing any occupational activity). In all three categories, the relation between health care, the workplace environment, and the patient is iterative (pain providing a feedback mechanism in response to medical or occupational interventions); workers with back pain have two courses of action – seek medical attention to reduce their pain, or attempt to modify their activity in the workplace, to accommodate the pain. *(Other options include complementary therapies, self-treatment, self-certification or simply coping).* The Task Force recommended that rest beyond the first few days of back pain (or nerve root pain) was contraindicated. Activity was considered appropriate for back pain at all stages. Work, as tolerated (perhaps with temporary modification), was considered appropriate for back pain at all stages. The importance of establishing return to regular occupational activities as soon as possible was emphasised as a therapeutic goal – this being a reflection of the necessity of minimising the duration of work absence to avoid compromising the probability of work-return.
(ARMA 2004) Consensus	**Standards of care** [UK Arthritis and Musculoskeletal Alliance] *(Derived from working groups and consultation. The Standards are intended to inform health care policy makers, and cover back pain, osteoarthritis and inflammatory arthritis. Although focused on care services, the Standards do include work issues).* The high economic impact of back pain, osteoarthritis and inflammatory arthritis is acknowledged in respect of sickness absence and disability as well as health care. The following Standards in respect of work are set down: • Back pain: People with back pain should be encouraged and supported to remain in work or education wherever possible – vocational rehabilitation should be available to support people in staying in existing employment or finding new employment. • Osteoarthritis: People with joint pain or osteoarthritis should be encouraged to remain in work or education wherever possible. Vocational rehabilitation should be available to support people staying in existing employment or finding new employment. • Inflammatory arthritis: People should be supported to remain in or return to employment and/or education, through access to information and services such as occupational therapy, occupational support and rehabilitation services. *(A statement of what is needed more than evidence of effectiveness).*

TABLE 3: MUSCULOSKELETAL DISORDERS

(Developed by expert working group with access to the evidence. The Standards are intended to inform health care policy makers in respect of regional musculoskeletal pain). The Standards take a biopsychosocial perspective and are given for: Promoting musculoskeletal health; Information on self-management and prevention; Information on services, treatments, and providers; Access to diagnosis; Assessment of needs; Individualised care plans; Pain relief; Support to remain in, or return to, work, education, or the home environment; Involvement of people with regional musculoskeletal pain in; Multidisciplinary teams, Self-management. The Standards state most regional musculoskeletal pain can and should be managed in the community. Notes role of psychosocial factors (identified by the 'flags' system) as obstacles to recovery: management requires adequate information (to remain active, to continue at work or in education wherever possible and maintain other normal activities), pain control (adequate to allow reactivation), biopsychosocial assessment and intervention in or near the workplace (for improved early management). *(A statement of what is more needed than evidence of effectiveness).*

(Athanasou 2005) Narrative review	**Return to work following whiplash and back injury: a review and evaluation**

The purpose was to review the reported return-to-work rates following whiplash and back-injury. The return-to-work rates for the 71 relevant studies that were reviewed varied from 29% to 100% with a median of 67%. The results suggest considerable residual return-to-work potential for persons with whiplash and back injury. Return-to-work rates were substantially higher for motor vehicle (96%) compared to work-related (71%) studies and also considerably higher for whiplash (95%) compared to back injuries (65%). It is suggested that these indices may form potential benchmarks for personal injury claims outcomes. Results often range from either no return to a very high return rate, with an approximate average of 68% following multimodal treatment procedures. *(No specific information on interventions, but illustrates variability in return to work rates across different types of injury).*

(Backman 2006) Narrative review	**Psychosocial aspects in the management of arthritis pain**

Summarizes psychosocial factors associated with arthritis pain and highlight recent evidence for psychosocial approaches to managing arthritis pain (considered in a generic sense). By definition, psychosocial factors refer to two dimensions of experience: the psychological (cognitive, affective) and social (interacting with others, engaging in life activities). Psychosocial approaches to managing arthritis pain include educational programs, coping skills training, and cognitive behavioural therapy. As a group of interventions, the focus is the provision of information necessary to understand the rationale for the approach selected, and techniques to enhance self efficacy, manage stress, decrease helplessness and catastrophising, and perhaps most importantly, develop and practice specific skills, applied to the person's unique life situation. Psychosocial approaches enhance medical regimes of care. There is evidence that psychosocial interventions improve coping and self efficacy, reduce psychological distress, and reduce pain, at least in the short term. While there is a body of literature examining psychosocial approaches, the volume addressing any one specific approach or research question (condition) is not large enough to draw confident conclusions. Truly interdisciplinary collaborations may advance the understanding between physiological and psychological processes, and advance the rather sparse evidence for efficacy of biopsychosocial approaches. Cost-effectiveness has yet to be adequately assessed.

TABLE 3: MUSCULOSKELETAL DISORDERS

| (Baldwin & Butler 2006) Narrative review with | **Upper extremity disorders in the workplace: costs and outcomes beyond the first return to work**

Noted that majority of workers compensation claims in Quebec for work-related upper extremity disorders are resolved quickly and the worker returns to work, although a small but significant proportion experience unusually lengthy spells of work absence. A small fraction of injured workers with the longest spells of work absence have extremely low probabilities of returning to work. These imply large productivity losses for employers. Mean workers compensation claim costs in the US are between $5000 and $8000, but this is not a good measure due to the highly skewed nature of the duration distribution for upper extremity claims. The total cost burden of work-related upper extremity disorders is large because of the relatively high incidence of the conditions. Estimates of the costs of work-related upper extremity disorders derived from administrative data are certain to underestimate the true costs on society, however, because many cases go unreported, and because indemnity benefits may not cover periods of prolonged or recurrent spells of work absence. Some evidence suggests that recurring spells of work absence may increase the disability burden further. Approximately one-third of workers with upper extremity disorders are at risk of prolonged employment instability following their injury. *(The results of this study have two important implications for vocational rehabilitation approaches – may be a need to target work-maintenance and sustainability, in addition to RTW).* |
|---|---|
| (Bevan et al. 2007) Report | **Fit for work? Musculoskeletal disorders and labour market participation**

[The Work Foundation]

Reports on a review of the recent academic and practitioner research on the relationship between musculoskeletal disorders and labour market participation, and conducted 15 interviews with acknowledged experts in this field. Focus on back pain, work-related upper limb disorders – two groups of conditions which are usually characterised by non-specific and short episodes of pain and incapacity – and rheumatoid arthritis and ankylosing spondylitis, two specific conditions that are often progressive and increasingly incapacitating. Authors consider the evidence supports a biopsychosocial approach, and identified five principles which GPs, employers, employees and the government should focus on if the working lives of workers with MSDs are to be improved:

- early intervention is essential;
- focus on capacity not incapacity;
- imaginative job design is the key to rehabilitation *(transitional work arrangements)*;
- think beyond the physical symptoms
- assess the direct and indirect costs of musculoskeletal disorders *(authors suggest that changes to the NICE Statutory Instrument would allow them to take appropriate account of the benefits of full and active labour market participation).*

Authors reported finding no shortage of clinical, epidemiological, psychological and economic evidence on the nature, extent and consequences of the musculoskeletal disorder problem in the UK. However, there still seems to be a lack of coherence or 'joined-up' thinking and action which focuses on the musculoskeletal disorder patient as worker. While the number of advocates of the biopsychosocial model as it applies to all musculoskeletal disorders is growing, the authors noted that some of those who can have most impact on fulfilling the labour market participation of workers with musculoskeletal disorders have yet to embrace its principles as fully as they might. |

TABLE 3: MUSCULOSKELETAL DISORDERS

(Bongers et al. 2006) Narrative review	**Epidemiology of work-related neck and upper limb problems: (2) effective interventions from a bio-behavioural perspective** There are few controlled trials of individual or organisational interventions for work-related neck and upper limb symptoms. This precludes any conclusions on effectiveness of bio-behavioural interventions for reduction of neck and upper limb problems and return to work after symptoms. From the low back pain intervention research there is evidence that interventions should be targeted at both the worker and the organisation and that interventions will only be successful when all the players are involved.
(Boocock et al. 2007) Systematic review	**Interventions for prevention and management of neck/upper extremity musculoskeletal conditions** Review of non-clinical intervention programmes for neck/upper extremity musculoskeletal conditions: 31 studies included, covering mechanical exposure interventions; production systems/organisational culture; modifier interventions – directed variously at people without pain, with pain, or with chronic pain. Heterogeneity of subjects and outcome measures, and limited information on the interventions (*predominantly ergonomics, quasi-ergonomics, and exercise*). No one single-dimensional or multidimensional strategy for intervention was considered effective across occupational settings. Limited evidence that work environment/workstation adjustments (mouse/keyboard design) can improve neck/upper extremity musculoskeletal conditions in display screen workers, but insufficient evidence for equipment interventions among manufacturing workers. Evidence to support the benefits of production systems/organisational culture interventions is lacking. Until better evidence is available, interventions for the prevention and management of neck/upper extremity musculoskeletal conditions should continue to use multifactorial approaches. (*Health outcomes defined as symptoms (questionnaire or examination) – no vocational outcomes*).
(Breen et al. 2007) Narrative review	**Early pain management for musculoskeletal disorders** The aim was to establish the usefulness of early pain management techniques in helping people, within the first 2 weeks of the onset of symptoms of a musculoskeletal disorder, to stay at work or get back to work. Evidence-based care pathways are offered for employees, employers and health professionals and start within the first week of onset. The evidence was variable in quality across MSDs, with ULDs in need of greatest development. Latest evidence and current thinking supports the use of biopsychosocial assessment and intervention in close proximity to work for improved early management of MSDs. The employee and employer have the main roles, with musculoskeletal practitioners being the preferred healthcare providers. Psychosocial influences are significant predictors of outcome for non-specific MSDs, together with high level of initial pain. Combinations of physical load factors potentially implicated in tenosynovitis or peritenonitis of wrist or forearm, but imprecise measurement of exposure makes the association undependable. <u>Back pain</u>: Consistent messages that for work-related problems, early intervention should be a collaborative approach that includes the employer, worker empowerment, and biopsychosocial rehabilitation. Interventions for acute non-specific back pain: information and reassurance; stay active, adequate pain control; manual therapy if not improving; temporary modified work if needed. <u>Neck pain</u>: Current thinking (albeit in a climate of largely inconclusive evidence) supports a very similar approach to that for back pain. <u>Shoulder pain</u>: Some support for combined interventions including active exercises, stretching, and hot and cold. Tentative evidence for ultrasound for calcific tendonitis. <u>Upper limb disorders</u>: Current thinking focuses more on work modifications and physical and mental reconditioning than on treatment. But, treatment may be of value for resistant problems: rotator cuff tendonitis (local steroid injection); epicondylitis (topical NSAID); carpal tunnel syndrome (individual exercise/keyboard adaptations).

TABLE 3: MUSCULOSKELETAL DISORDERS

	Generic care pathway:- Stage 1 – within 1 week: Discussion, assessment and action planning with employer → activity modification considered → involvement of health professional (if concerned). Stage 2 – if not recovered in 2 weeks: Reassessment and revised action plan → monitor and amend staged recovery plan, together with employer with focus on activity and function (as distinct from pain alone). Employee pathway: Stage 1 – within 1 week: Advice – MSDs common, self-limiting and may have nothing to do with work or injury; control the pain, stay at work (even if some pain); stay active, perhaps with modified activities → tell employer about problem and discuss effect of work activities → if worried, consider seeing health professional (active physical treatment) + keep in touch with work → Stage 2 – if not recovered in 2 weeks: Do not be discouraged; use pain control and (if necessary) + modified activities at work and/or seek other treatment; plans with employer for workplace accommodation; if the plan not helping recovery, need to identify with employer and healthcare professional what needs to be done.
(Brox et al. 2007) Systematic review	**Systematic review of back schools, brief education, and fear-avoidance training for chronic low back pain** Assesses the effectiveness of back schools, brief education, and fear-avoidance training for chronic low back pain. Assessment of effectiveness was based on pain, disability, and sick leave. Conflicting evidence for back schools compared with waiting list, placebo, usual care, and exercises, and a cognitive behavioural back school. Seven trials, six of high quality, evaluated brief education in the clinical setting: strong evidence of effectiveness of brief education on sick leave and short-term disability compared with usual care; conflicting or limited evidence for back book or Internet discussion (*clinical not occupational outcomes*), compared with no intervention, massage, yoga, or exercises. Moderate evidence that there is no difference between rehabilitation including fear-avoidance training and spinal fusion. Consistent recommendations are given for brief education (examination, information, reassurance, advice to stay active) in the clinical setting, and back schools may be considered in the occupational setting.
(BSRM 2004) Report	**Musculoskeletal rehabilitation** [British Society of Rehabilitation Medicine] Musculoskeletal disorders are common, and half of all disability in the UK can be attributed to their presence. Relatively little attention is focussed on common MSD such as osteoarthritis and their consequences. Instead, there is a tendency to regard the resultant disability as an inevitable consequence of ageing for which little can be done. Services for those with MSD conditions are poorly planned. Services for those with MSD remain too focused within secondary care and have not kept pace with improvements in community-based rehabilitation. Multidisciplinary teamwork is a cardinal feature of the management of complex Musculoskeletal disability. These teams may embrace specialist nurses and therapists but need both psychological and medical support. Commissioners of services and local providers should meet to review the overall provision of services for those with a musculoskeletal disorder and how they can be provided most cost-effectively. (*Focus was on service provision rather than vocational rehabilitation*).

TABLE 3: MUSCULOSKELETAL DISORDERS

(Burton & Waddell 2002) Narrative	**Educational and informational approaches** Reviews written educational material for back pain, and provides empirical evidence about the information and advice that should be given to patients with back pain. The evidence indicates that carefully selected, suitably presented information and advice about back pain in line with current management guidelines (conducive with biopsychosocial principles) can have a positive effect on beliefs and on clinical outcomes. Demonstrating that educational materials have an influence on return to work is more problematic: because many primary care patients do well and return to work, manageable trials may have insufficient statistical power to test any effect on work loss or subsequent health care. Furthermore, a booklet in isolation is unlikely to have much impact on work absence and having a real impact requires complete management strategies that get all the players on one side – there is some evidence that this is the case. Arguably, the very low per-person cost of written information may render it a worthwhile use of resources.
(Burton et al. 2008) Evidence synthesis	**Management of upper limb disorders and the biopsychosocial model** Work has a limited overall role in the primary causation of upper limb disorders, yet the symptoms are frequently work-relevant (some work tasks will be difficult for people experiencing upper limb symptoms, and may sometimes provoke symptoms that may otherwise not materialize). Management of cases shows more promise than attempts at primary prevention. Neither medical treatment nor ergonomic workplace interventions alone offer an optimal solution; rather, multimodal interventions show considerable promise, particularly for vocational outcomes. Some specific diagnoses may require specific biomedical treatments, but the components of supplementary interventions directed at securing sustained return to work seem to be shared with regional pain disorders. Early return to work, or work retention, is an important goal for most cases and may be facilitated, where necessary, by transitional work arrangements. The emergent evidence indicates that successful management strategies require all the players to be onside and acting in a coordinated fashion, in order to overcome obstacles to recovery and return to work. • Early return to work is important – it contributes to the recovery process and will usually do no harm; facilitating work retention and return to work requires support from workplace and healthcare • All players onside is fundamental – sharing goals, beliefs and a commitment to coordinated action. • Promote self-management – give evidence-based information and advice – adopt a can-do approach, focusing on recovery rather than what's happened. • Intervene using stepped care approach – treatment only if required (beware detrimental labels and over-medicalisation); encourage and support early activity; avoid prolonged rest; focus on participation, including work. • Encourage early return to work – stay in touch with absent worker; use case management principles; focus on what worker can do rather than what they can't; provide transitional work arrangements (only if required, and time-limited). • Endeavour to make work comfortable and accommodating – assess and control significant risks; ensure physical demands are within normal capabilities, but don't rely on ergonomics alone; accommodating cases shows more promise than prevention. • Overcome obstacles – principles of rehabilitation should be applied early: focus on tackling biopsychosocial obstacles to participation – all players communicating openly and acting together, avoiding blame and conflict.

TABLE 3: MUSCULOSKELETAL DISORDERS

(Carter & Birrell 2000; Waddell & Burton 2000) Guideline	**UK Occupational Health Guidelines: - Management of the worker having difficulty returning to normal occupational duties at 4-12 weeks:** [Faculty of Occupational Medicine] • There is strong evidence that the longer a worker is off work with LBP, the lower their chances of ever returning to work. Once a worker is off work for 4-12 weeks they have a 10-40% risk (depending on the setting) of still being off work at one year; after 1-2 years absence it is unlikely they will return • to any form of work in the foreseeable future, irrespective of further treatment. • Various treatments for chronic LBP may produce some clinical improvement, but there is strong evidence that most clinical interventions are quite ineffective at returning people to work once they have been off work for a protracted period with LBP. • There is moderate evidence that for the patient who is having difficulty returning to normal activities at 4-12 weeks, changing the focus from purely symptomatic treatment to a 'back school' type of rehabilitation programme can produce faster return to work, less chronic disability and less sickness absence. There is no clear evidence on the optimum content or intensity of such packages, but there is generally consistent evidence on certain basic elements. There is moderate evidence that such interventions are more effective in an occupational setting than in a health care setting. • From an organisational perspective, there is moderate evidence that the temporary provision of lighter or modified duties facilitates return to work and reduces time off work. (Conversely, there is some suggestion that clinical advice to return only to restricted duties may act as a barrier to return to normal work, particularly if no lighter or modified duties are available.) • There is moderate evidence that a combination of optimum clinical management, a rehabilitation programme, and organisational interventions designed to assist the worker with LBP return to work, is more effective than single elements alone.
(Cole et al. 2006) Narrative review	**Integrative interventions for MSDs: nature, evidence, challenges & directions** Review focused on neck and upper extremity, with the aim of exemplifying 'integrative' interventions, rather than being an exhaustive review. They describe 'integrative' workplace interventions to include both biomechanical and psychosocial aspects, aiming at achieving both primary and secondary prevention, and/or consisting of multiple components versus only a single component. Authors noted that currently there are mixed messages on workplace intervention effectiveness due to a variety of reasons, including a lack of participation in research by workplaces. They argued that there are many opportunities to expand the range of 'integrative interventions'. They find an integrated approach to both biological and psychosocial Interventions to be appealing, since it allows the targeting of two main categories of risks, to better prevent and manage musculoskeletal disorders in the workplace. They pointed out that given there are multiple causes for workplace injury, illness and disability, then preventing these problems requires multiple solutions, operating in synergy. Also, that effort to reduce workplace injury, illness and disability should build on combined strategies for primary and secondary prevention. They highlighted the use of multiple component interventions such as combining proactive case management from insurers with workplace ergonomic interventions to facilitate faster return to work. *(Although vocational outcomes were a primary interest, there was limited data specifically in respect of return to work).*

TABLE 3: MUSCULOSKELETAL DISORDERS

(COST B13 Working Group 2004) Guideline	**European guidelines for management of low back pain** [European Commission Research Directorate General] The guidelines were based on systematic evidence reviews in three areas: management of acute low back pain, management of chronic low back pain, and prevention in low back pain. • The clinical guidelines for acute LBP considered there was evidence that advice to stay active led to less sick leave and less disability. There was consensus that advice to stay at work or return to work if possible is important. Longer duration of work absenteeism is associated with poor recovery (lower chance of ever returning to work). An appendix on back pain at work, which included information and recommendations taken from various occupational health guidelines, echoed these points. • The clinical guidelines for chronic LBP noted that after an initial episode of LBP, 44-78% people have relapses of pain and 26-37% experience relapses of work absence. In workers having difficulty returning to normal occupational duties at 4-12 weeks, the longer a worker is off work with LBP the lower the chances of ever returning to work. Intensive physical training ('work hardening') programs with a cognitive-behavioural component are more effective than usual care in reducing work absenteeism. • The guidelines for prevention in low back pain suggest that the general nature and course of commonly experienced LBP means that there is limited scope for preventing its incidence (first-time onset). Primary causative mechanisms remain largely undetermined: risk factor modification will not necessarily achieve prevention. Nevertheless, there is evidence suggesting that prevention of various consequences of LBP (e.g. recurrence, care seeking, disability, and workloss) is feasible. Overall, there is limited robust evidence for numerous aspects of prevention in LBP; for interventions where there is acceptable evidence, the effect sizes are rather modest. For workers with or without back pain the following statements are made: (1) physical exercise is recommended in the prevention of LBP, for prevention of recurrence of LBP, and for prevention of recurrence of sick leave due to LBP; (2) temporary modified work and ergonomic workplace adaptations can be recommended to facilitate earlier return to work for workers sick listed due to LBP; (3) there is insufficient consistent evidence to recommend recommended physical ergonomics interventions alone for prevention in LBP; (4) there is insufficient consistent evidence to recommend stand-alone work organisational interventions; (5) multidimensional interventions at the workplace can be recommended in principle.
(Crawford & Laiou 2005) Review + survey	**Effective management of upper limb disorders by general practitioners and trainee occupational physicians** [UK Health & Safety Executive Research Report] Study to identify best practice in the clinical management of work related upper limb disorders by reviewing the literature and contacting relevant institutions and associations; to determine the nature of teaching on this subject in the training of Occupational Physicians and GPs The literature review identified that there is evidence for the efficacy of conservative treatments in the management of carpal tunnel syndrome (the use of steroids and steroid injection, range of motion exercises), epicondylitis (topical nonsteroidal anti-inflammatory agents and steroid injection), rotator cuff tendonitis and bicipital tendonitis (nonsteroidal anti-inflammatory agents and steroid injection), impingement syndrome (home exercise programmes and manual therapy) and tension neck (workplace intervention). There was no evidence to support the use of conservative treatments for tenosynovitis, tendonitis, de Quervain's disease, cervical spondylosis or diffuse non-specific upper limb disorders. The evidence reviewed was not always found to be high quality and there are serious methodological issues with much of the research reviewed. *(Focus was clinical rather than occupational outcomes. See entry in Table 6a for delivery information).*

TABLE 3: MUSCULOSKELETAL DISORDERS

(Crawford & Laiou 2007) Quasi-systematic review	**Conservative treatment of work-related upper limb disorders** Summarises the evidence base for conservative clinical management of ULDs including specific and non-specific conditions (articles published 1993-2004; variable quality). Much of the evidence for the efficacy of various conservative treatments for the management of ULDs is generally limited and of low quality – positive statements given with caution: Carpal tunnel syndrome: +ve for local steroid injection, exercise, stretching: no evidence for non-specific anti-inflammatory drugs (NSAID) and workplace intervention strategies. Epicondylitis: +ve for short term symptomatic relief from local steroid injections, acupuncture, topical NSAIDs; longer-term relief from 'physiotherapy'. Rotator cuff syndrome and bicipital tendonitis: +ve for local steroid injection, NSAIDs, although evidence unclear. (Straps/braces not included in review). Shoulder capsulitis: +ve for local steroid injection: no evidence for other conservative approaches. Impingement syndrome: +ve for exercise and NSAIDs, but evidence low quality. Tension neck syndrome: +ve for ergonomic interventions to reduce discomfort; physical training does not have an impact. Tenosynovitis, tendonitis, de Quervain's disease, or diffuse non-specific ULDs: no evidence to support or refute conservative treatment. General management of work-related MSDs: few papers found with inconclusive findings. Pain management programmes: +ve for cognitive behavioural programmes (especially early) for occupational outcomes: +ve for hypnosis with biofeedback for RSI pain, but low quality. *(The included papers are notable for largely omitting occupational outcomes, thus preventing appraisal of the impact of these conservative treatments on return to work).*
(de Buck et al. 2002) Systematic review	**Vocational rehabilitation in patients with chronic rheumatic diseases: a systematic literature review** Subjects were work disabled or on sick leave with a chronic rheumatic disease (considered generically) at the start of the vocational rehabilitation programme. Methodological considerations reduced the selection to 6 articles. 5 of 6 vocational rehabilitation programmes consisted of multidisciplinary intervention and 15% to 69% of the patients successfully returned to work. Although 5 of the 6 studies showed marked positive effects on work status, proof of the benefit is limited, mainly because of methodological shortcomings (none were controlled studies). The components of the studies showing an effect were: • Assistance in placement in suitable employment (including skills retraining) • Physical restoration; training; work adjustments and behavioural instruction; support services (transport etc) • Counselling, guidance, placement services, physical/mental restoration, training/education, transportation • Skills training, capability assessment, signposting opportunities, counselling, work trials, adaptations, social support • Structured group meetings – didactic, peer interaction, exercise, job search, social support, community services Although increased attention is being paid to preventing disability and promoting return to work for people with rheumatic conditions, knowledge regarding the effectiveness of vocational rehabilitation programs is insufficient.

TABLE 3: MUSCULOSKELETAL DISORDERS

(de Vries et al. 2006) Cochrane review	**Interventions for treating chronic ankle instability** Objective was to compare different treatments, both conservative and surgical, for chronic lateral ankle instability. In view of the low quality methodology of almost all the studies, this review does not provide sufficient evidence to support any specific surgical or conservative intervention for chronic ankle instability. However, after surgical reconstruction, early functional rehabilitation (supervised programme starting following initial immobilisation and then remobilisation for 6 weeks) was shown to be superior to six weeks immobilisation regarding time to return to work and sports.
(Dunstan & Covic 2006) Narrative review	**Compensable work disability management: A literature review of biopsychosocial perspectives** For work-related musculoskeletal injury, empirical findings support the following management based on a biopsychosocial framework and time. Acute stage: control of pain ('bio'); reassurance about the benign nature and prognosis of the condition ('psycho'); and encouragement and support to remain active and to stay at work or RTW as early as possible ('social'). Furthermore, avoid over-investigation, medicalisation and contributing to iatrogenic disability. Sub-acute stage (4+ weeks): medical review to exclude serious pathology; screen for psychosocial risk factors for long-term disability (yellow flags); multidisciplinary, biopsychosocial rehabilitation addressing psychosocial issues and linked to the workplace. Chronic stage: All workers still off work should receive specialist, multidisciplinary rehabilitation to address expected limitations in physical, social and occupational functioning. Although interventions for chronic pain-related disability, such as medical care (the relief of symptoms), functional restoration (the re-establishing of physical performance) and pain management (improving quality of life by addressing beliefs and behaviour), can deliver varying improvements in physical and psychological functioning, only multidisciplinary biopsychosocial rehabilitation shows positive effects on work resumption.
(Durand et al. 2007) Descriptive review	**Workplace interventions for workers with musculoskeletal disabilities: a descriptive review of content** This review identifies the different objectives pursued through workplace interventions carried out in the context of a rehabilitation program, and to describe the activities involved. There is great heterogeneity in the content of interventions offered in the workplace to workers with musculoskeletal disabilities. The objectives of workplace interventions may range from gathering information in order to reproduce work demands in a clinical setting, to gradually exposing workers to the demands of the real work environment, or permanently reducing the demands of the work situation. A descriptive analysis of the literature also brings to light the diversity of actions carried out, human resources used, and workplace environments involved, while highlighting the few documented process outcome evaluations that have been done of workplace interventions. *(Review is about content of interventions not effectiveness).*
(Elders et al. 2000) Systematic review	**Return to work after sickness absence due to back disorders – a systematic review on intervention strategies** Twelve articles with quantitative information on the effect of ergonomic interventions on return to work were included. In eight studies, introduction of a back-school programme was the preferred intervention, combining exercise and functional conditioning, and training in working methods and lifting techniques. In seven out of eight back-school studies, return to work was significantly better in the intervention group. Intervention after 60 days, in the subacute phase of back pain, showed the most promising results. In these studies the preventable fraction varied between 11% and 70%, largely depending on the stage and phase of back disorders and the time of follow-up. The success of intervention also depended on the profile of the referents when left untampered. In all studies compliance during the intervention was fairly good, but there was a lack of information on sustainability of the intervention during the follow-up and on recurrence of back complaints and consequent sickness absence.

TABLE 3: MUSCULOSKELETAL DISORDERS

(EASHAW 2007)	**Work-related musculoskeletal disorders: back to work report**
Report	[European Agency for Safety and Health at Work]

This report aimed to evaluate the effectiveness of interventions in the workplace, and to provide an overview of policy initiatives regarding the retention, reintegration, and rehabilitation of workers with MSDs. The publication search that was carried out for this report covered scientific literature concerning work-related interventions aimed at the rehabilitation, reintegration and retention of workers with MSDs. These included interventions such as work modifications, exercise therapy, behavioural treatment, psychosocial interventions and multidisciplinary treatment. The main findings with respect to particular body parts were:

Back pain

• there is clear evidence that it is important for patients to stay active and return to ordinary activities as early as possible;

• a combination of optimal clinical management, a rehabilitation programme and workplace interventions is more effective than single elements alone;

• taking a multidisciplinary approach offers the most promising results, but the cost effectiveness of these treatments needs to be examined;

• temporarily modified work is an effective return-to-work intervention, if it is embedded in good occupational management;

• some evidence supports the effectiveness of exercise therapy, back schools, and behavioural treatment;

• lumbar supports such as back belts and corsets appear to be ineffective in secondary prevention.

Upper limb pain

• a multidisciplinary approach involving a cognitive-behavioural component might be the most effective type of intervention;

• there is limited evidence on the effectiveness of some technical or mechanical interventions and exercise therapy;

• in the scientific literature, sufficient evidence is not available for the effectiveness of psychosocial interventions.

Lower limb pain

• no information on work-related intervention strategies has been found;

• the results of studies concerning lower limb treatment in general indicate that exercise programmes might be effective for hip and knee problems.

In spite of the lack of strong scientific evidence, anecdotally many of these workplace interventions are reported as being effective. The evaluation of workplace interventions should probably adopt different criteria on which to base its evidence. These criteria are currently lacking, but policymakers and employers should not be discouraged from carrying out preventive action simply because there is no 100% proof that it will work. Moreover, secondary and tertiary prevention should go hand in hand with primary prevention in order to prevent the recurrence of MSD episodes.

Most of the Member States' policies focus on integrating into the workforce people with disabilities who are not currently employed, rather than retaining, reintegrating and rehabilitating workers who have developed MSDs at work. There should be an increased awareness regarding the needs of this target group. |

TABLE 3: MUSCULOSKELETAL DISORDERS

A number of countries have policies that cover the reintegration and rehabilitation of workers after illness or accident. Variations between the countries are large, with advantages and disadvantages:

- Emphasis on early recognition of problems and avoidance of long-term incapacity for work, including returning people with MSDs to work as quickly as possible. [Reintegration and rehabilitation are often offered only to workers who have suffered occupational accidents or have recognised occupational diseases. Providing help only to the severely disabled tends to exclude individuals with less severe MSDs, many of whom could return to work after being given a little help or offered simple adjustments to their jobs].

- Provision of comprehensive care including medical, occupational and social rehabilitation. Multidisciplinary approach — enhanced collaboration between the treating physician, the occupational physician and the insurance fund's medical advisor. This would facilitate better case management and earlier return to work among workers with MSDs. [The Bismarckian social health insurance system (the 'dual system') that exists in many member States strictly separates work and social insurance, which is not compatible with offering integrated counselling and help to workers with health problems].

- The introduction of financial incentives for employers, such as funding for work adaptations and improving workplace conditions or an obligation to pay employees a wage during their sickness, stimulates the employer to provide occupational rehabilitation in order to facilitate the employee's early return to work. [In countries with adversarial legal systems, employers may be reluctant to reintegrate an employee for fear of aggravating a musculoskeletal condition. Similarly, employees may be reluctant to return to work in case it reduces any compensation for personal injury.

(EFILWC 2007)

Report

Managing musculoskeletal disorders

[European Foundation for the Improvement of Living and Working Conditions]

This report was compiled on the basis of individual national reports submitted by the European Working Conditions Observatory correspondents. The importance of return-to-work policies increases as the workforce is ageing and quality of work and promotion of health at work strategies are put in place. Opportunities for early retirement due to incapacity are limited in the case of musculoskeletal disorders (MSD), and absenteeism is a major symptom. Different countries take differing routes in respect of return to work policies. Overall, three approaches may be identified. A first approach emphasises intervention on the employer side. This strategy may be advanced by providing employers with support in consultancy and job redesign to ease the return to work of affected workers. Alternatively, legislation may underline the employer's responsibility in setting up a recovery plan under the supervision and with the support of social security institution and/or national guidelines. Intervention on the employee side represents a second approach. This method may be addressed by categorising affected workers as disabled, thus offering them: rehabilitation training and clinical treatment, training and placement support, or reserve shares at workplaces. The third approach is to address the needs of the social partners in an integrated way: taking an integrated approach addressing the roles of – and challenges for – various stakeholders, including workplaces, employer and employee organisations, the healthcare system and the managing municipal authorities, as well as researchers from a broad array of disciplines. It is stated that return to-work policies do not aim to reduce sick leave but rather ease employability. Although the impact of return-to-work policies is positive in most countries, the effect seems to be more relevant from a social security approach in terms of work absence days and permanent incapacity to work rather than in terms of self-reported work-related MSDs. Therefore, the impact on mild MSDs seems rather uncertain. Further evidence is needed in order to better assess the impact of these policies.

TABLE 3: MUSCULOSKELETAL DISORDERS

(Faber et al. 2006) Systematic review	**Treatment of impingement syndrome: a systematic review of the effects on functional limitations and return to work** Nineteen articles were included. For functional limitations, there is strong evidence that extracorporeal shock-wave therapy is not effective, moderate evidence that exercise combined with manual therapy is more effective than exercise alone, that ultrasound is not effective, and that open and arthroscopic acromioplasty are equally effective on the long term. For all other interventions there is only limited evidence. Functional limitations not often used as an outcome measure. Duration of sick leave was seldom included as an outcome measure. *(Concerned 'treatments' rather than rehabilitation, but helps to make the point that treatment alone is insufficient. No data on occupational outcomes).*
(Feldman 2004) Narrative review	**The prevention of occupational low back pain disability: evidence-based reviews point in a new direction** Review of the findings of recent (at that time) extensive evidence-based reviews of the literature on occupational low back pain disability. There is strong evidence that variables other than biomedical or biomechanical have impact on occupational low back pain disability. A shift toward conceptualizing and treating occupational low back pain disability according to its duration post-injury provides a promising new direction. Increasing evidence points to the subacute stage post-injury (4-12 weeks) as a critical period in preventing disability. In limited studies to date, interventions implemented in the subacute stage that address maladaptive cognitions and behaviour, and focus on return to work have demonstrated reductions in lost work time and disability. Collaborative approaches that combine the proactive efforts of the physician, rehabilitation professionals, and the workplace hold the most promise for future prevention of occupational low back pain disability.
(Feuerstein & Harrington 2006) Conference consensus	**Secondary prevention of work-related upper extremity disorders: recommendations from the Annapolis conference** Narrative summary of recommendations from a 2005 conference aimed at preventing disability due to work-related upper limb disorders. The intent of the meeting was to review 'state of the art' evidence in epidemiology and intervention research in order to develop suggestions regarding next steps in intervention research and application. Consensus conclusions included the following: (1) new conceptual models are required with a broad biobehavioral perspective (2) the workplace is dynamic with continuously changing characteristics of fluctuating demands, tasks, work areas, and postures (3) effective interventions seem to need an interdisciplinary approach (4) the ergonomics field needs to expand in order to adapt to the changing workplace (5) non-occupational health practitioners are neither prepared nor knowledgeable about ergonomics and other risk factors in the workplace (6) programmes with both management and worker participation are likely to be best (7) insurance systems fail to account for all relevant costs appropriate to an injury, and this prevents focus on secondary prevention. *(More a collection of promising ideas than data on effectiveness – supports concepts of disability prevention requiring all players onside).*
(Franche et al. 2005b) Systematic review	**Workplace-based return-to-work interventions: a systematic review of the quantitative literature** Reviews return-to-work interventions provided at the workplace to workers disabled with musculoskeletal or other pain-related conditions. 10 studies included (out of >4000 identified). Strong evidence that work disability duration is significantly reduced by work accommodation offers and contact between healthcare provider and workplace. Moderate evidence that work disability is reduced by interventions which include early contact with worker by workplace, ergonomic work site visits, and presence of a return-to-work coordinator. For these 5 intervention components, there was moderate evidence that they reduce costs associated with work disability duration. There was limited evidence on the sustainability of these effects. Overall, the evidence base shows workplace-based interventions can reduce work disability duration and associated costs.

TABLE 3: MUSCULOSKELETAL DISORDERS

(Gobelet et al. 2007b) Narrative review	**Work in inflammatory and degenerative joint diseases** Focuses on work disability and sick leave and their cost; also discusses the value of vocational rehabilitation programmes in rheumatic conditions such as rheumatoid arthritis, ankylosing spondylitis, hip and knee osteoarthritis. Authors make the general point that vocational rehabilitation should not be regarded as bolt-on activity after drug treatment but an integral part of effective management. Publications dealing with return to work are relatively common in rheumatoid arthritis, less common in ankylosing spondylitis and relatively rare in osteoarthritis. Data suggest that after conservative treatment around a third of patients with osteoarthritis return to work, 5% may change jobs and 20% may retire. The authors felt vocational rehabilitation would probably have much to offer these patients, but recognised their age range might mean a proportion retire rather than take sick leave. Also, it may be that patients are a valued and experienced part of the workforce who are helped to stay at work (even with increasing pain and diminishing mobility). The authors indicate that vocational rehabilitation programmes should aim to facilitate job retention (stay at work) or; failing that, to improve the ability to return to work. The process must be started within the health arena and it has to be recognised that slow or poor practice in the health service can jeopardise the patient's work potential. (*Although inflammatory joint disease is excluded from the present review, the information on degenerative conditions is relevant*).
(Grant et al. 2004) Systematic review	**Evaluation of interventions for rotator cuff pathology: a systematic review** The best available evidence from our review of conservative treatment options for rotator cuff disease (grades A and B) lends support for electrotherapy, steroid injections, exercise therapy, and acupuncture. With respect to return-to-work outcomes, generally it was noted that individuals undergoing less invasive treatment procedures, those with less severe cuff damage, and workers in sedentary positions returned to their previous jobs sooner and more frequently. In addition, individuals receiving workers' compensation generally took longer to return to their previous duties. The one study that included outcomes for patients receiving workers' compensation found that significantly fewer claimants reported good to excellent outcomes as compared with those in the non-claimant group.
(Green et al. 2003) Cochrane review	**Physiotherapy interventions for shoulder pain** Twenty six trials met the inclusion criteria. Methodological quality was variable and trial populations were generally small (median sample size = 48, range 14 to 180). Exercise was demonstrated to be effective in terms of short term recovery in rotator cuff disease (RR 7.74), and longer term benefit with respect to function (RR 2.45). Combining mobilisation with exercise resulted in additional benefit when compared to exercise alone for rotator cuff disease. Laser therapy was demonstrated to be more effective than placebo (RR 3.71 (1.89, 7.28)) for adhesive capsulitis but not for rotator cuff tendinitis. Both ultrasound and pulsed electromagnetic field therapy resulted in improvement compared to placebo in pain in calcific tendinitis (RR 1.81 and 1.9 respectively). There is no evidence of the effect of ultrasound in shoulder pain (mixed diagnosis), adhesive capsulitis or rotator cuff tendinitis. When compared to exercises, ultrasound is of no additional benefit over and above exercise alone. There is some evidence that for rotator cuff disease, corticosteroid injections are superior to physiotherapy and no evidence that physiotherapy alone is of benefit for adhesive capsulitis. (*Included studies focused on clinical (eg pain) and functional (eg range of movement) outcomes, so no information on return to work*).

TABLE 3: MUSCULOSKELETAL DISORDERS

(Gross et al. 2006) Practice guide	**Disability management of injured workers: a best practice guide for physical therapists** Collaborative venture between four stakeholder groups in the physical therapy profession. Representatives from education, regulation, practice and a payer organization came together to develop a resource guide intended to support physical therapists in the treatment of injured workers (musculoskeletal disorders). Combination of literature review and professional consensus. Model for the physical therapist disability management of injured workers. Physical therapists need to collaborate with an extended return-to-work team and make the right connection at the right time. • Maximizing the Worker-Physical Therapist Connection: understand the worker; introduce concept of early return to work; formulate return to work plan. • Maximizing the Case Manager-Physical Therapist Connection: establish contact with injured worker's case manager; for workers not progressing as expected, make the connection; work collaboratively to solve return to work problems. • Maximizing the Workplace-Physical Therapist Connection: directly contact the workplace; clarify job demands with employer; plan for return to work. • Maximizing the Physician-Physical Therapist Connection: contact the physician; discuss return to work plan with physician. • Maximizing the Health Care Provider-Physical Therapist Connection: create collaborative approach. *(Strong focus on the (physical) therapist being proactive in the communication and collaboration between the players).*
(Guzmán et al. 2001) Systematic review	**Multidisciplinary rehabilitation for chronic low back pain: systematic review** Multidisciplinary biopsychosocial rehabilitation varied in setting (inpatient or outpatient) and the time and intensity of the three components (physical, psychological, and social or occupational). !0 trials reviewed. Subjects had disabling back pain for > 3 months. Programmes fell into two main categories: daily intensive programmes with more than 100 hours of therapy and once or twice weekly programmes with less than 30 hours of therapy. There was contradictory evidence regarding vocational outcomes of intensive multidisciplinary biopsychosocial rehabilitation, although intensive multidisciplinary biopsychosocial rehabilitation with functional restoration improved function and pain. Less intensive multidisciplinary biopsychosocial rehabilitation did not show improvements in pain, function or vocational outcomes compared with non-multidisciplinary outpatient rehabilitation or usual care.
(Hagberg 2005) Narrative review	**Clinical assessment, prognosis and return to work with reference to work related neck and upper limb disorders** 65 relevant articles were identified (published between 1980 and 2002) that addressed assessment, prognosis and RTW for neck and upper limb problems. Many of these were found to be review articles and the author noted a paucity of randomised studies of prognosis and return to work with reference to neck and upper limb disorders. Treatment that focuses on keeping the patient active and maintains contact with the workplace is recommended. Non-specific neck and upper arm pain and discomfort may be decreased but not eliminated in the majority of cases. Rehabilitation is best started early and should provide workplace accommodation, and if this is not available RTW may not be indicated.

TABLE 3: MUSCULOSKELETAL DISORDERS

(Hanson et al. 2006) Narrative review	**The costs and benefits of active case management and rehabilitation for musculoskeletal disorders** Project aimed to review evidence on the costs and benefits of active case management and rehabilitation programmes for musculoskeletal disorder; to identify potential incentives, and obstacles to, the adoption of these programmes; and, to describe a model programme based on the evidence and assess its acceptability to stakeholders There is strong evidence that rehabilitation programmes using a cognitive-behavioural orientation and an activity focus are effective, and cost-effective at reducing pain and increasing productive activity in both the sub-acute and the chronic groups. There is also strong evidence that the use of these interventions at the sub-acute stage can prevent the development of long-term problems and reduce time off work. Furthermore, there is good evidence that this is highly cost-effective, especially when the intervention is selectively delivered to individuals screened as having a high risk for a poor outcome. The key components of good quality rehabilitation service delivery were outlined. An evidence-based delivery model was outlined (with high acceptability to UK providers, although there was acknowledgement that applicability to small employers was uncertain) using the following key features: create the right culture; manage workers with musculoskeletal disorder; manage the return to work process; and, monitor and review the programme effectiveness. (*See also Table 6c*)
(Harris & Susman 2002) Guideline summary	**Managing musculoskeletal complaints with rehabilitation therapy: summary of the Philadelphia Panel evidence-based clinical practice guidelines on musculoskeletal rehabilitation interventions** [Philadelphia Panel] The Philadelphia Panel has published evidence-based guidelines for selected rehabilitation interventions in the management of low back, knee, neck, and shoulder pain. This article provides a summary and overview. (*Although the outcomes of interest to the panel included return to work, it was not possible to extract specific data concerning interventions specific to occupational outcomes*).
(Hayden et al. 2005) Cochrane review	**Exercise therapy for non-specific low back pain** Evaluates the effectiveness of exercise therapy in adult non-specific acute, subacute and chronic low back pain. Looked at randomized, controlled trials evaluating exercise therapy and measuring pain, function, return to work or absenteeism, and global improvement outcomes. Exercise therapy is effective in chronic back pain (for pain and function) relative to comparisons at all follow-up periods. Some evidence suggests effectiveness of a graded-activity exercise program in subacute low back pain in occupational settings (for pain), although the evidence for other types of exercise therapy in other populations is inconsistent. In acute low back pain, exercise therapy and other programs were equally effective (for pain). In subacute low back pain populations, some evidence suggests that a graded activity program improves absenteeism outcomes, although evidence for other types of exercise is unclear.
(Henrotin et al. 2006) Systematic review	**Information and low back pain management: a systematic review** To determine whether information is an effective preventive action and/or therapy for low back pain and which type of information is most effective. There is strong evidence that a booklet increases knowledge and moderate evidence that physician-related cues increase the confidence in a booklet and adherence to exercises. There is limited evidence that a biopsychosocial booklet is more efficient than a biomedical booklet to shift patient's beliefs about physical activity, pain, and consequences of low back trouble. There is strong evidence that booklets are not efficient on absenteeism. There is no evidence that e-mail discussion or video programs alone are effective to reduce low back pain, disability, and healthcare costs. Information based on a biopsychosocial model is recommended in primary care to shift patient beliefs on low back pain. Nevertheless, information delivery alone is not sufficient to prevent absenteeism and reduce healthcare costs. (*The studies concerned investigated information as an isolated intervention rather than part of a vocational rehabilitation intervention*).

TABLE 3: MUSCULOSKELETAL DISORDERS

(Hestbaek et al. 2003) Systematic review	**Low back pain: what is the long-term course? A review of studies of general patient populations** It is often claimed that up to 90% of low back pain episodes resolve spontaneously within 1 month. However, the literature in this area is confusing due to considerable variations regarding the exact definitions of low back pain as well as recovery. Therefore, the claim – attractive as it might be to some – may not reflect reality. Thirty-six articles were reviewed. The proportion of patients who still experienced pain after 12 months was 62% on average, the percentage who experienced relapses of pain was 60%, and the percentage who had relapses of work absence was 33%. The mean reported prevalence of low back pain in cases with previous episodes was 56% (range 14–93%), which compared with 22% for those without a prior history of low back pain. The risk of low back pain was consistently about twice as high for those with a history of low back pain. The overall picture is that LBP does not resolve itself when ignored. (*This suggests that vocational rehabilitation needs to consider sustained return to work and stay at work issues against a background of labile symptoms and sickness absence*).
(Heymans et al. 2004) Cochrane review	**Back schools for non-specific low-back pain** Nineteen RCTs (3584 patients) were included in this updated review. Overall, the methodological quality was low, with only six trials considered to be high quality. There is moderate evidence suggesting that back schools, in an occupational setting, reduce pain, and improve function and return-to-work status, in the short and intermediate-term, compared to exercises, manipulation, myofascial therapy, advice, placebo or waiting list controls, for patients with chronic and recurrent LBP.
(Hlobil et al. 2005) Systematic review	**Effectiveness of a return-to-work intervention for subacute low-back pain** Best-evidence synthesis of the effectiveness of return-to-work intervention for subacute low-back pain on work absenteeism, pain severity, and functional status: comparison was with 'usual care'. Five of nine studies were methodologically high-quality. Strong evidence was found for the effectiveness of return to work intervention on the return-to-work rate after 6 months and for the effectiveness of return-to-work intervention on the reduction of days of absence from work ≥ 12 months. It can be concluded that return-to-work interventions are equal or more effective regarding absence from work due to subacute low-back pain than usual care. All the studies used a return-to-work intervention that was designed for use in clinical practice. Although some of the studies did not show statistically significant differences, all showed an effect from the intervention that was at least equal to or greater than usual care – importantly none reported a potential harm to the workers. The optimal return-to-work intervention for subacute low back pain is probably a mixture of exercise, education, behavioural treatment and ergonomic measures, but it is not clear which (or which combination) is most effective.
(Hoffman et al. 2007) Meta-analysis	**Meta-analysis of psychological interventions for chronic low back pain** The purpose of this meta-analysis of randomized controlled trials was to evaluate the efficacy of psychological interventions for adults with chronic low back pain. Outcomes included pain, healthcare variables, physical functioning, and employment/disability compensation status. Positive effects of psychological interventions, contrasted with various control groups, were noted for pain intensity, pain-related interference, health-related quality of life, and depression. Cognitive-behavioural and self-regulatory treatments were specifically found to be efficacious. Multidisciplinary approaches that included a psychological component, when compared with active control conditions, were also noted to have positive short-term effects on pain interference and positive long-term effects on return to work. The results demonstrated positive effects of psychological interventions for chronic low back pain.

TABLE 3: MUSCULOSKELETAL DISORDERS

(Hogelund 2001) Narrative review	**Work incapacity and reintegration: a literature review** Reviewed literature from 4 main research disciplines (clinical studies; economics; public policy; social studies) in order to develop a model of work incapacity and reintegration. Taken alone, none of the research disciplines seems able to offer a convincing explanation of why some incapacitated workers return to work whereas others do not. Each of the 4 theoretical disciplines seems able to contribute to an explanation, and several variables are of importance. The proposed model comprises: Input: Person characteristics – medical condition, psychological condition, life style, socio-demographics. Work characteristics – work conditions, job demands, environment, employment background Processes: Disincentives for work resumption – employee related; employer related Interventions for work resumption – assessment of work incapacity; medical treatment; vocational training/education; work accommodations; employment services Outcomes: employment/benefit status *(Whilst the review did not consider the content or effectiveness of interventions, it follows that successful intervention will require integrated elements to deal with the various issues related to all the players).*
(HSE 2002) Report	**Initiative evaluation report: back in work** [Health & Safety Executive] A report evaluating the results of 19 projects (>300 businesses and 2700 employees) set up jointly between the Department of Health and the HSE to develop innovative ideas to tackle back pain in the workplace. The projects encouraged stakeholders to work in partnership with others, particularly small and medium sized enterprises, to determine what approaches for the prevention, treatment and rehabilitation of back pain actually work. The results show that a proactive partnership approach to managing back pain is effective. The key lessons that came out of the initiative were: • early treatment should be sought for back pain • most back pain is not due to a serious condition • simple back pain should be treated with basic pain killers and mobilisation • it is important to keep active both to prevent and to treat back pain • getting back to work quickly helps prevent chronic back pain • adopt the correct posture while working • all workplace equipment should be adjustable • take breaks from repetitive or prolonged tasks or postures • avoid manual handling and use lifting equipment where possible • clear information should be provided to employees about back care • health and safety policies should be implemented to cover all aspects of day-to-day work and should be reviewed regularly. *(Regrettably, this Contract Research Report is no longer available – thus, the precise contents of the projects remain a mystery. The key points have been taken from an HSE press release).*

TABLE 3: MUSCULOSKELETAL DISORDERS

(Huisstede et al. 2006) Systematic review	**Incidence and prevalence of upper-extremity musculoskeletal disorders. a systematic appraisal of the literature** A systematic appraisal of the worldwide incidence and prevalence rates of upper extremity disorders (UED) available in scientific literature. Studies that recruited at least 500 people, collected data by using questionnaires, interviews and/or physical examinations, and reported incidence or prevalence rates of the whole upper-extremity including neck, were included. No studies were found with regard to the incidence of UEDs and 13 studies that reported prevalence rates of UEDs were included. The point prevalence ranged from 1.6–53%; the 12-months prevalence ranged from 2.3–41%. One study reported on the lifetime prevalence (29%). We did not find evidence of a clear increasing or decreasing pattern over time. In general, higher prevalence rates of UEDs were found in women then in men and the estimates of self-reported complaints were higher than those acquired by using (in addition) physical examinations. The case definitions for UEDs used in the studies, differed enormously, which impacted on the prevalence rates.
(IASP 2005) Professional curriculum	**Work rehabilitation** [International Association for the Study of Pain] *(This chapter form the IASP Core Curriculum for professional education relates primarily to competencies for work rehabilitation of musculoskeletal disorders, with much of the supporting evidence coming from the back pain field: it is implicit that the principles apply to other regional musculoskeletal pain and possibly to pain in general).* Key areas of knowledge for the clinician include the importance of psychosocial factors, the applicability of the stepped care approach, the detrimental effects of long periods of work absence, equating work-related symptoms with work-related injury is counterproductive, a comprehensive rehabilitation programme includes general exercise, cognitive therapy, and vocational elements (ie interventions that address both the clinical problem and issues in the individual's physical and social environment), even those who have been absent from work for prolonged periods can be rehabilitated. Individuals who do not return to work within a few weeks require intensive multidisciplinary approaches (including active exercise, attention to distorted beliefs about pain, enhancement of positive coping strategies, and promotion of self-management – delivered as near to the workplace as possible – modified work arrangements can facilitate early return, but that alone is insufficient.
(IIAC 2007a) Position statement	**Back and neck pain – position paper 18** [Industrial Injuries Advisory Council] The Industrial Injuries Advisory Council has identified significant barriers to the prescription of back and neck pain, including problems with diagnosis. However, injuries to the back and neck, occurring as a result of an identifiable accident, continue to be covered under the accident provisions. Research suggests back pain may be one disorder where rehabilitation could be used effectively to enable people to remain in work. This position paper also highlights several preventative measures to combat back and neck pain. Given this inherent limitation, the Council decided not to pursue a full literature review. It has concluded that further consideration of prescription is currently ruled out because the diagnosis rests on a self-report of LBP or neck pain with no robust and effective process for independent corroboration. The Council notes that several other European countries have scheduled back and neck disorders for prescription – a common focus being on the outcomes of degenerative disc disease or disc prolapse on the one hand and the exposures of heavy lifting and whole body vibration on the other. The possibility of a greater focus on vocational rehabilitation and support is being considered; back pain is a condition that might be targeted. Research evidence suggests that the longer a person is off work with low back pain the greater the likelihood of long-term health-related unemployment. Many authorities believe that more intensive and earlier efforts at rehabilitation are required in sub-chronic cases (e.g. those with 6 to 12 weeks of sickness absence) to avoid this outcome. The challenge of corroborating diagnosis would be no less great in such cases, but would be less important in the context of functional rehabilitation, as would the distinction between symptoms caused by work, as compared with symptoms aggravated by work. Arguably, such a use of funds could be beneficial to employers and employees alike and cost-effective from the taxpayer's perspective.

TABLE 3: MUSCULOSKELETAL DISORDERS

(Karjalainen et al. 2000) Cochrane review	**Multidisciplinary biopsychosocial rehabilitation for sub-acute low back pain (Cochrane review)** Working age patients suffering from subacute low back pain (more than 4 weeks but less than 3 months). The rehabilitation program was required to be multidisciplinary, i.e.; it had to consist of a physician's consultation plus either a psychological, social or vocational intervention, or a combination of these. The only two included studies were considered to be methodologically low quality randomized controlled trials. The level of scientific evidence for the effectiveness of multidisciplinary rehabilitation was moderate on subacute low back pain showing that multidisciplinary rehabilitation which includes workplace visit or more comprehensive occupational health care intervention helps patients to return to work faster, makes sick leaves less and alleviates subjective disability.
(Karjalainen et al. 2003a) Cochrane review	**Biopsychosocial rehabilitation for upper limb repetitive strain injuries (RSI) (Cochrane review)** The rehabilitation program was required to be multidisciplinary, i.e.; it had to consist of a physician's consultation plus either a psychological, social or vocational intervention, or a combination of these. Only two included studies found, both low quality. Little scientific evidence for effectiveness of biopsychosocial rehabilitation for RSI. One small trial suggested hypnosis supplementary to comprehensive treatment can decrease pain intensity for acute RSI at 6-weeks. Need for high quality trials. *(Occupational outcomes not assessed in either study).*
(Karjalainen et al. 2003b) Cochrane review	**Multidisciplinary biopsychosocial rehabilitation for neck and shoulder pain (Cochrane review)** Trials had to assess the effectiveness of biopsychosocial rehabilitation for patients suffering from neck and shoulder pain among working age adults. The rehabilitation program was required to be multidisciplinary, i.e.; it had to consist of a physician's consultation plus either a psychological, social or vocational intervention, or a combination of these. Only two studies were included: 1 low quality randomised trial and 1 low quality controlled trial. Limited scientific evidence for effectiveness of multidisciplinary biopsychosocial rehabilitation for neck and shoulder pain, compared with other commonly used intervention: no benefits were seen for absence-related outcomes. Using a clinical psychologist as a supervisor for the multidisciplinary team is more cost-effective than the psychologist giving behavioural treatment individually to the patients.
(Karjalainen et al. 2003c) Cochrane review	**Multidisciplinary rehabilitation for fibromyalgia and musculoskeletal pain (Cochrane review)** The rehabilitation program was required to be multidisciplinary; that is, it had to consist of a physician's consultation, plus a psychological, social or vocational intervention, or a combination of both. Only seven (low quality) studies were included: 4 randomised trials on fibromyalgia suggested no quantifiable benefit; 3 randomised trials on widespread musculoskeletal pain showed that, based on limited evidence, no evidence of efficacy was observed. Behavioural treatment and stress management appear to be important components. Education combined with physical training showed some positive effects in the long term. Only one study focused on occupational outcomes: the effects were 'neutral'. Overall, little scientific evidence for effectiveness of multidisciplinary rehabilitation for these conditions.
(Kay et al. 2005) Cochrane review	**Exercises for mechanical neck disorders** The evidence summarised in this systematic review indicates that there is a role for exercises in the treatment of acute and chronic mechanical neck disorder and neck disorder plus headache. Exercise for neck disorders with radicular findings is not assessed. The relative benefit of each type of exercise needs extensive research. Phase II trials would help identify the most effective treatment characteristics and dosages. *(No conclusions are drawn for occupational outcomes).*

TABLE 3: MUSCULOSKELETAL DISORDERS

(Kool et al. 2004) Meta-analysis	**Exercise reduces sick leave in patients with non-acute non-specific low back pain: a meta-analysis** The results of the qualitative and quantitative analysis are consistent. Treatments using exercise alone or as a part of a multidisciplinary treatment reduce sick leave in patients with non-specific non-acute LBP. The effects are greater in more severely disabled patients and tend to decline with increasing follow-up duration. There is strong evidence that sick days are reduced during the first year after treatment especially in severely disabled patients with >90 sick days per year under usual care in the control group. There is no evidence in this review for the assumption that early intervention is more effective. The reduction in the number of sick days is greater in patients who had more sick leave. It remains unclear whether the number of patients receiving a disability allowance is reduced, and there is insufficient research comparing the effectiveness of different treatments.
(Kunkel & Miller 2002) Narrative review	**Return to work after foot and ankle injury** Workplace foot and ankle injuries (including fractures) are common. Return to work is critical, but because several parties are involved in the process, the potential for substandard care is high. The speediest possible return to the workplace is usually best for all concerned, the injured worker, the employer and the physician. The treatment team within the workers' compensation system assists in the facilitation and coordination of the medical care and assists in bringing the patient back to work. The team includes the nurse case manager, the insurer, and physical and occupational therapists. Appropriate use of work hardening programs or functional capacity evaluations can be valuable in the return-to-work effort. Brief but frequent communication between the physician and the workers compensation case manager is seen as important. The outcome for rehabilitation and return to work in cases of occupational foot and ankle injury depends on communication and cooperation among the employee, the employer, the insurance company, the physical therapist, and the case manager.
(Kupper et al. 2004) Narrative review	**The challenge of managing upper limb disorders – how can health professionals become more effective?** Combination of literature review and interview/questionnaire survey. The review examined the current available literature for evidence concerning the effectiveness of various management options for people suffering from upper limb disorders. Effective management should result in reduced pain and discomfort and increased function. In terms of work, effective management should aim to achieve early return to work and prevent reoccurrence and long-term sick leave. Focus was those management and treatment techniques that may be used by occupational health nurses and physiotherapists. Authors found that there was not enough quality research (e.g. randomised controlled trials and systematic reviews) that studied the effectiveness of treatments and management approaches to enable them to determine what best practice should comprise. Generally physiotherapists and OH nurses were aware of psychosocial issues and favoured keeping the ULD sufferer active and in employment rather than taking sick leave. There was a limited amount of evidence to suggest that this overall approach is favourable. Numerous recommendations were made, with a strong theme of inter-professional communication and communication between healthcare and the workplace: written information and advice for all the players was advocated.
(Linton 2002) Descriptive review	**Cognitive behavioural therapy in the prevention of musculoskeletal pain: description of a program** Description of a cognitive behavioural programme that converges on the secondary prevention of disability, and summary of results from 3 randomised controlled trials. This six-session, manual-directed, group treatment by specially trained therapists focuses on psychological risk factors ('yellow flags'). Identified in the programme. The trials showed the intervention helps prevent the development of long-term disability (reduced sick leave days). A particular advantage of the programme may be that it key on psychological risk factors identified individually and provides a method for dealing with them, and provides an alternative to merely providing larger doses of traditional treatment to a persistent problem.

TABLE 3: MUSCULOSKELETAL DISORDERS

(Loisel et al. 2001) Narrative review	**Disability prevention: new paradigm for management of occupational back pain** The causes of disability are not only due to the patient's personal characteristics (physical and psychosocial), but also stem from the patient's environment in the disability problem – the workplace, the compensation system and even the healthcare delivery system. In addition, successful intervention studies have used an approach to disability prevention through patient reassurance and interventions linked to the workplace, instead of using a medical model of back pain treatment. It is evident that the present disease treatment paradigm should be replaced by a disability prevention paradigm for patients with subacute or chronic back pain to avoid unnecessary evolution towards prolonged disability. A disability prevention management model is proposed to encourage clinicians, employers, unions and insurers to work within the perspective of the disability paradigm. Adopting this paradigm does not mean that efforts to better understand and relieve back pain should be abandoned. Rather, it means that more efforts should be made, through appropriate and timely disability management, to find a fit between the worker experiencing back pain and the workplace to make work suitable to those with back pain as well as to others.
(Loisel et al. 2003) Descriptive review	**From evidence to community practice in work rehabilitation: the Quebec experience** The causes of prolonged disability due to low back pain are multiply determined. This review describes three phases of the process of transfer of evidence from rehabilitation research to community practice in the province of Quebec (Canada). (A) Based on literature review and expert knowledge, the Sherbrooke model was developed and assessed through a population-based, randomized clinical trial. Results at 1-year follow-up showed quicker return to regular work and improvement of quality of life; the 6-year follow-up showed the cost-effectiveness of the method. (B) Based on the Sherbrooke model experience and recent evidence, a new program addressing the disability paradigm was developed and implemented in the province of Quebec (also offered to workers with other musculoskeletal disorders). Results at 1- and 3-year follow-ups showed that only 24% of workers were not working owing to their musculoskeletal disorder. (C) To implement the program at a provincial level, a network for management, research and education in work rehabilitation was developed. An external assessment is presently planned to evaluate return to work and economic outcomes and quality of implementation of the program in various settings. • The Sherbrooke Model involves three steps for cases at risk of disability at the 4th week of absence: (1) Occupational intervention (worker visits occupational health department; participatory ergonomics intervention → (2) Clinical intervention at 8-12 weeks absence (worker sees back pain specialist and attends back school) → (3) Early rehabilitation at 13-26 weeks absence (functional rehabilitation therapy and therapeutic return to work). Return to work is possible at any time and stops any further interventions (apart from possible ongoing work modifications). • The new disability management programme has 2 main steps starting with the: (1) Work disability diagnosis, set in primary care (general practitioner and occupational therapist engage in identifying psychosocial disability predictors and recommend a plan to worker: immediate return to work may be possible); (2) Therapeutic return to work, set in the workplace (tailored to worker's needs dependent on step 1; progressive return to regular work or permanently modified work; workplace becomes a rehabilitation setting; intervention requires all stakeholders to make efforts to attain a common return to work goal. The programme has a multidisciplinary team (general practitioner with special interest; occupational therapist; physical educator; ergonomist; back pain specialist; team coordinator) which meets regularly. *(Not strictly a review, rather a description of what one influential group has done to construct and implement what is very much a programme, requiring trained and committed team members, and successful rehabilitation requires employer engagement - see also data from other sources in Tables 6 and 7).*

TABLE 3: MUSCULOSKELETAL DISORDERS

(Loisel et al. 2005) Narrative review + expert opinion	**Prevention of work disability due to musculoskeletal disorders: the challenge of implementing the evidence** The process of returning disabled workers to work presents numerous challenges, and there has been little uptake of the evidence (which may not yet be practical for immediate use). The problem is complex and subject to multiple legal, administrative, social, political, and cultural challenges. A literature review and collection of experts' opinion is presented, on the current evidence for work disability prevention, and barriers to evidence implementation. The current evidence regarding work disability prevention shows that some clinical interventions (advice to return to modified work and graded activity programs) and some non-clinical interventions (at a service and policy/community level but not at a practice level) are effective in reducing work disability. Implementation of evidence in work disability is a major challenge because intervention recommendations are often imprecise and not yet practical for immediate use, many barriers exist, and many stakeholders are involved. Future studies should involve all relevant stakeholders and aim at developing new strategies that are effective, efficient, and have a potential for successful implementation.
(Mahalik et al. 2006) Narrative review	**A review of employability and worksite interventions for persons with rheumatoid arthritis and osteoarthritis** The current review paper built upon past reviews of the worksite intervention literature and determined that there continues to be a rather small albeit growing base of research studies. Ranging from psychoeducational, behavioural, and psychological worksite interventions for the general population or persons with musculoskeletal disorders, the reviewed studies demonstrate varying degrees of effectiveness (primarily due to methodological limitations). Psycho-educational interventions were generally found to be less effective without behavioural components, there is also a need to incorporate a cognitive-behavioural approach to worksite interventions to enhance effectiveness. In addition to the use of combined psycho-educational and behavioural interventions within a cognitive-behavioural approach, the reviewed literature reveals that focusing on psychological variables may enhance job-seeking ability, and the use of vocational rehabilitation interventions is effective in minimizing job loss for persons with arthritis.
(MacEachen et al. 2006) Systematic review	**Systematic review of the qualitative literature on return to work after injury** Review was undertaken in order to better understand the dimensions, processes, and practices of return to work. Because return to work often includes early return before full recovery while a person is undergoing rehabilitation treatment, physical recovery is embedded in complicated ways with workplace processes and practices and social organization. These process-oriented dimensions of return to work are well described in the qualitative literature. Focus was on musculoskeletal and pain-related injuries – evidence synthesis using the meta-ethnographic approach. Found that return to work extends beyond concerns about managing physical function to the complexities related to beliefs, roles, and perceptions of many players. Good will and trust are overarching conditions that are central to successful return-to-work arrangements. In addition, there are often social and communication barriers to return to work, and intermediary players have the potential to play a key role in facilitating this process. Key mechanisms of workplace practice, process, and environment can affect the success of return to work.
(Martimo et al. 2007) Cochrane review	**Manual material handling advice and assistive devices for preventing and treating back pain in workers** Reviews the effectiveness of manual materials handling advice and training and the provision of assistive devices in preventing and treating back pain and back-related disability. Six randomised controlled trials and five cohort studies were evaluated. All studies focused on prevention of back pain (with some including back-related disability). There is limited to moderate evidence that manual materials handling advice and training with or without assistive devices do not prevent back pain, back pain-related disability or reduce sick leave when compared to no intervention or alternative interventions. *(Although the ergonomic interventions studied here are not effective for prevention of LBP, this review does not enable assessment of their value if integrated into a return-to-work intervention).*

TABLE 3: MUSCULOSKELETAL DISORDERS

(Meijer et al. 2005) Systematic review	**Evaluation of effective return-to-work treatment programs for sick-listed patients with non-specific musculoskeletal complaints: a systematic review** Eighteen high quality studies reporting on 22 treatment programmes. Overall, the findings were inconsistent: only 7 programmes resulted in faster return to work, though none had negative findings. What appeared to be essential to the success of treatment programs was knowledge, psychological, physical and work conditioning, possibly supplemented with relaxation exercises. However, most of the study populations (64%) were limited to low back pain patients – four studies did include patients with a wide variety of musculoskeletal disorders but did not itemize the treatment effects on return to work by sub-population. No studies were found that examined the effect of treatment programs on return to work by itemized region of the musculoskeletal system, such as non-specific upper extremity musculoskeletal complaints.
(Mueller et al. 2003) Narrative review	**What have physicians learned about returning chronically disabled back patients to work?** Proper timing for adequate interventions ('window of opportunity') is important for returning back pain patients to work before they are chronically disabled. The medical system takes some responsibility in the so-called medicalisation of the reported complaint of back pain. There needs to be a shift of focus the interaction between patient and physician from pain and spinal pathology toward restoration of function and ability to perform the duties of daily life, including work. For physician and physiotherapist, a time-contingent approach for functional restoration is more effective than a pain-contingent approach. A multidimensional or biopsychosocial view and an honest partnership between physician and patient helps to reveal and address obstacles for return to work. A local network of general practitioners, physiotherapists, and surgeons with a similar approach and therapeutic language helps to better guide the patient. Different messages from the health care system will lead to insecurities on the patient's side and may prolong the pain problem. Functional restoration programs are effective in restoring function and reducing pain in chronically disabled patients. There is yet insufficient data on whether these programs are cost-effective. *(See also Table 7b).*
(Nash et al. 2004) Systematic review	**Resting injured limbs delays recovery: a systematic review** The authors noted that rest is commonly used as primary treatment, rather than just palliation, for injured limbs. They identified 49 eligible randomised controlled trials of immobilisation for soft tissue injuries and fractures of both upper and lower limbs (total of 3,366 subjects), in order to seek evidence of benefit or harm from immobilisation or mobilisation of acute limb injury in adults. The outcomes considered by the reviewers included pain, swelling, cost, range of motion, days lost from work, and complications from treatment. The reviewers noted that all the studies concluded there was either no difference between rest and early mobilisation, or there was a benefit from early mobilisation over rest. The reported benefits included: earlier return to work; decreased pain, swelling, and stiffness; and, a greater preserved range of joint motion. Furthermore, early mobilisation caused no increased complications, deformity or residual symptoms. The reviewers concluded there is strong evidence that early mobilisation decreases pain, swelling and stiffness, especially in the short-term, without longer-term cosmetic or radiological deformity. They also found there is moderate evidence to conclude patients usually (but not always) prefer early mobilisation, and return to work sooner. The final conclusion was that we should not assume any benefit from resting or immobilising acute upper or lower limb injuries in adults, and that therefore rest appears to be an overused treatment.

TABLE 3: MUSCULOSKELETAL DISORDERS

(NHMRC 2004) Guideline	**Evidence-based management of acute musculoskeletal pain** [National Health and Medical Research Council] Australian evidence-based clinical guidelines for management of a variety of painful musculoskeletal conditions. Conditions covered comprise: acute low back pain, acute thoracic pain, acute neck pain, acute shoulder pain, acute knee pain. (*Occupational issues and return to work were not the focus of this guidance, but the recommendations regarding activity are of relevance to work*). For low back pain, advice to stay active reduces sick leave compared to bed rest (as well as having small benefits for pain and function). For thoracic pain, it is, in general, important to resume normal activities as soon as possible. For neck pain, encouraging the resumption of normal activities and movement of the neck is more effective than a collar and rest. For shoulder pain, although pain may make it difficult to carry out usual activities, it is important to resume normal activities as soon as possible. For knee pain, maintenance of normal activity has beneficial effect on patellofemoral pain compared to no treatment or use of orthoses. (*Limited occupational outcomes*).
(Nordin et al. 2006) Narrative review	**Nonspecific low back pain: surgical versus nonsurgical treatment** Expert opinion review of evidence-based treatments for patients seeking care for lower-back pain and patients who have been diagnosed with nonspecific lower-back pain. Based on selected systematic reviews and national and international guidelines for the treatment of lower-back pain, with some additional randomized controlled trials. In acute nonspecific lower-back pain (0–4 weeks duration of pain) there is moderate to strong evidence that self-care with over-the-counter medication and maintaining activity as tolerated or treatment with a limited number of sessions of manipulative therapy is effective for pain relief. In subacute nonspecific lower-back pain (4-12 weeks duration of pain) there is weak to moderate evidence that a graded activity program including exercises and cognitive behavioural treatment in combination (especially at the workplace) is more efficient than usual care with regard to return to work. There is strong evidence that these programs reduce work absenteeism. In cases of chronic nonspecific lower-back pain (> 12 weeks duration of pain) a variety of treatments are available with limited and similar efficacy on pain and disability reduction. A structured approach seems to have the best results where the healthcare providers treat the patients as a team and provide a clear and common message. Patient adherence to treatments remains a complex problem, but it may not be deviance but a reasoned behaviour based on their beliefs and experiences – treatments tailored to patients' needs will enhance adherence.
(Ostelo et al. 2005) Cochrane review	**Behavioural treatment for chronic low-back pain** Combined respondent-cognitive therapy (a type of behavioural therapy) and progressive relaxation therapy are more effective than waiting list control on short-term pain relief. However, it is unknown whether these results sustain in the long term. No significant differences could be detected between behavioural treatment and exercise therapy. There is limited evidence (1 trial, 98 people) that a graded activity program in an industrial setting is more effective than usual care for early return to work and reduced long-term sick leave.
(Pengel et al. 2002) Systematic review	**Systematic review of conservative interventions for subacute low back pain** Reviews the effect of conservative interventions on clinically relevant outcome measures for patients with subacute low back pain (pain, disability and return to work). For a strict duration of low back pain (six weeks to three months), some evidence was found for the efficacy of advice (alongside routine care) for return to work. When a broader view is taken of the duration of subacute low back pain (seven days to six months), other treatments (e.g. manipulation, exercise, TENS) and coordination of primary healthcare may reduce disability.

TABLE 3: MUSCULOSKELETAL DISORDERS

(Poiraudeau et al. 2007) Systematic review	**Functional restoration programs for low back pain: a systematic review** The term 'functional restoration' has been associated with a full-day multidisciplinary program lasting from 3 to 6 weeks. Consensus exists on proposing multidisciplinary programs for patients with disabling chronic LBP. Functional restoration programs should probably be reserved for this population. Results from most published controlled studies on the efficacy of functional restoration programs are positive regarding the return-to-work rate. Maintaining job status with the pre-injury employer is often best accomplished by the provision of suitable modified duties. Finally, results of functional restoration programs in terms of return-to-work rate probably depend strongly on the social security system of the country where the program was developed.
(Pransky et al. 2002) Narrative review	**Stress and work-related upper extremity disorders: implications for prevention and management** Stress and work-related upper limb disorders are linked. Although evidence is incomplete, it is suggestive that individual and workplace interventions (targeted at stress reduction) delivered in primary care or workplace may be helpful. Examples studied included: numerous outcomes including stress, upper limb symptoms, and work outcomes; numerous (combined) interventions including stress reduction techniques, cognitive behavioural therapy, physical rehabilitation, pain management. Tabulated examples indicated that effects of 'ergonomics-only' interventions were inconsistent. Further research warranted. *(Preliminary evidence that combining ergonomics and stress management/rehabilitation interventions may be effective).*
(Rainville et al. 2005) Narrative review	**The physician as disability adviser for patients with musculoskeletal complaints** Review of the literature about the performance of physicians as mediators of temporary and permanent disability for patients with chronic musculoskeletal complaints. While caring for patients with musculoskeletal injuries, physicians are often asked to recommend appropriate levels of activity and work, which have significant consequences for patients' general health, employment, and financial well-being. Physician recommendations limiting activity and work after injury are highly variable, often reflecting their own pain attitudes and beliefs. Patients' desires strongly predict disability recommendations (i.e. physicians often acquiesce to patients' requests). Other influences include jurisdiction, employer, insurer, and medical system factors. Physician recommendations for work and activity have important health and financial implications. Systemic, multidimensional approaches are necessary to improve performance.
(Schonstein et al. 2003) Cochrane review	**Work conditioning, work hardening and functional restoration for workers with back and neck pain** To determine the effect on time lost from work of physical conditioning programs for workers with back and neck pain. Based on cost considerations, authors nominated a mean saving of 10 sick days per year, or a number needed to treat to return 1 person to work of 10, as the smallest treatment effects that would be clinically worthwhile. 19 trials, none of which studied the effectiveness of interventions on workers with neck pain. Most included men and women. Five trials included subjects who were off work, 4 included subjects either not working or on suitable duties, and 9 included subjects working and not working. Physical conditioning programs were defined as those interventions that are work- or function-related physical rehabilitation programs specifically designed to restore an individual's systemic, neurologic, musculoskeletal, or cardiopulmonary function. These trials provide evidence that physical conditioning programs that included a cognitive-behavioural approach could produce a clinically worthwhile reduction in the number of sick days taken at 12 months (average of 45 days; 95% confidence interval 3–88) when compared to general practitioner care or advice for workers with chronic back pain. There was little evidence that specific exercise programs that did not include a cognitive- behavioural component had any effect on time lost from work.

TABLE 3: MUSCULOSKELETAL DISORDERS

(Seferiadis et al. 2004) Systematic review	**A review of treatment interventions in whiplash-associated disorders** The methodological quality of 26 randomised controlled trials of common treatments for whiplash associated disorder (WAD) was analyzed; the trials were rated as low quality. However, a best evidence synthesis indicated that some treatments may have beneficial effects for occupational outcomes: early physical activity reduces pain, increases cervical range of motion and reduces sick leave in patients with acute WAD; cognitive behavioural therapy combined with Physical therapy reduces pain and sick leave in patients with chronic WAD.
(Selander et al. 2002) Quasi-systematic review	**Return to work following vocational rehabilitation for neck, back and shoulder problems: risk factors reviewed** Musculoskeletal problems were defined as neck, back and shoulder problems. Authors considered that high-quality studies now support the hypothesis that multidisciplinary treatment is more effective than single-mode treatment regarding return to work. Education may be more effective than work training. Inconsistent evidence for value of early vocational rehabilitation. Involvement of client/patient in vocational rehabilitation seen as important. A vocational rehabilitation counsellor to guide client through system may be helpful, but depends on competences. A great number of demographic, psychological, social, medical, rehabilitation-related, workplace-related and benefit-system-related factors are associated with return to work. The different types of risk factor are associated in many ways. People with greater chances of job return after vocational rehabilitation are younger, native, highly educated, have a steady job and high income, are married and have stable social networks, are self-confident, happy with life, not depressed, have low level of disease severity and no pain, high work seniority, long working history and an employer that cares and wishes them back to the work place. Unfortunately, people with the above profile are seldom found among the long-term sick. *(Focus of the review was largely on 'obstacles': no programme details given in discussion of 'effective' rehabilitation).*
(Shaw et al. 2001) Narrative review	**Early prognosis for low back disability: intervention strategies for health care providers** Purpose was to synthesize findings from available studies of prognostic factors for disability related to occupational low back pain in a clinically-relevant framework. Significant prognostic factors included low workplace support, personal stress, shorter job tenure, prior episodes, heavier occupations with no modified duty, delayed reporting, severity of pain and functional impact, radicular findings and extreme symptom report. Physicians can decrease occupational low back pain disability by using standardized questionnaires, improving communication with patients and employers, specifying return to work accommodations, and employing behavioural approaches to pain and disability management. *(Does not include effectiveness data, but illustrates that using prognostic data can highlight the necessary components of an occupational rehabilitation intervention).*
(Shaw et al. 2002) Conceptual review	**Secondary prevention and the workplace** Conceptually, 'secondary prevention interventions in the workplace' may focus on early detection and treatment of mild/moderate symptoms, and on accommodating temporary functional limitations to aid recovery and reduce likelihood of recurrence. Review examines several interventions aimed at physical work environment, modified duty, educational and exercise approaches, case management, and programmes for supervisors. Integrating care and facilitating communication among workers, health-care providers and the workplace emerge as salient features. As a whole the evidence shows that there is considerable potential to reduce disability and longer-term problems associated with work-related musculoskeletal pain. Efforts to reduce ergonomic risk factors, to enhance education and fitness, and to influence case managers and supervisors provide opportunities for effective secondary prevention. Integrating care and facilitating communication among workers, health care providers and the workplace emerge as particularly salient. *(A carefully conducted and argued review displaying the potential for modern joined-up management, though robust scientific evidence limited).*

TABLE 3: MUSCULOSKELETAL DISORDERS

(Shaw et al. 2006) Review of reviews	**Reducing sickness absence from work due to low back pain: how well do intervention strategies match modifiable risk factors?** From 17 review articles (2000–2005), disability risk factors and interventions were cross-tabulated to assess levels of relative concordance. Potentially modifiable risk factors included 23 variables describing 3 workplace and 3 personal domains. Three intervention clusters that were most highly supported by risk factor evidence were: workplace technical and organizational interventions, graded activity exposure, and cognitive restructuring of pain beliefs. Experimental interventions within each of these areas have continued to evolve, with many studies showing meaningful reductions in lost work time. Effective interventions included 25 strategies that were personal (physical or behavioural), engineering, or administrative in nature. There was a strong risk factor concordance for workplace technical and organizational interventions, graded activity exposure, and cognitive restructuring of pain beliefs. There was less risk factor concordance for exercise, back education, and RTW coordination. Few interventions focused on relieving emotional distress or improving job dissatisfaction, two well-supported risk factors. One area of potential controversy is whether risk factors for LBP disability must be altered to achieve successful outcomes. If risk factors are indeed causal mechanisms in the development of chronic pain and disability, then reduction of these factors should lead to improved health and work outcomes. If, on the other hand, these variables are merely risk markers and are confounded by other causal factors, then interventions may appear to be successful without a commensurate reduction in risk factors.
(Shaw et al. 2007) Systematic review	**A literature review describing the role of return-to-work coordinators in trial programs and interventions designed to prevent workplace disability** Return-to-work (RTW) coordination has been suggested as an effective strategy for preventing workplace disability, but the scope of these services is not well described. The objective of this review was to describe the activities of RTW coordinators in published trials to provide a basis for establishing necessary competencies. The interest was RTW coordinators providing direct, on-site workplace liaison to reduce work absences associated with physical health ailments. 40 articles (22 studies) met criteria for inclusion. All but two studies (of traumatic brain injury) focused on musculoskeletal conditions or work injuries. Twenty-nine RTW coordinator activities were identified, but there was variation in the training background, workplace activities, and contextual setting of RTW coordinators. Based on reported RTW coordinator activities, six preliminary competency domains were identified: (1) ergonomic and workplace assessment; (2) clinical interviewing; (3) social problem solving; (4) workplace mediation; (5) knowledge of business and legal aspects; and (6) knowledge of medical conditions. The principal activities of RTW coordination involve workplace assessment, planning for transitional duty, and facilitating communication and agreement among stakeholders. It was concluded that successful RTW coordination may depend more on competencies in ergonomic job accommodation, communication, and conflict resolution than on medical training.
(Sinclair & Hogg-Johnson 2002) Narrative review	**Early rehabilitation: the Ontario experience** A province-wide early active intervention for MSDs (community clinic program based on a sports medicine model) did not have expected benefits. The key ingredient missing from the clinics was any meaningful tie to the workplace, or even a legitimisation of clinics' role in helping to negotiate modified work. Concept of early intervention is variable both temporally and with regard to type of care provided. Appropriately matching interventions with stage in recovery is an approach that may prove more effective. *(More a constructive critique of the intervention program than a review. Points out that timing and intervention need to be put in context).*

TABLE 3: MUSCULOSKELETAL DISORDERS

(Smidt et al. 2005) Systematic review	**Effectiveness of exercise therapy: a best-evidence summary of systematic reviews** The goal of this review was to summarise the available evidence on the effectiveness of exercise therapy for patients with disorders of the musculoskeletal, nervous, respiratory, and cardiovascular systems. Reviews were selected by two reviewers that included at least one RCT investigating the effectiveness of exercise therapy, used clinically relevant outcome measures, and were written in English, German or Dutch. Then 13 independent and blinded reviewers were asked to participate in review selection, quality assessment, and data extraction. The authors reported that 104 systematic reviews were selected, of which 45 were considered to be 'reasonable or good quality'. 26 studies concerned musculoskeletal disorders (back, neck, shoulder or knee pain; 'repetitive strain injury'; hip or knee osteoarthritis; ankylosing spondylitis; rheumatoid arthritis). (The remainder concerned cardio-circulatory-respiratory conditions). The reviewers concluded that exercise therapy is effective for patients with knee osteoarthritis, sub-acute (6 to 12 weeks) and chronic (≥12 weeks) low back pain. Furthermore, there are indications that exercise therapy is effective for patients with ankylosing spondylitis and hip osteoarthritis. However, they found there is currently insufficient evidence to support or refute the effectiveness of exercise therapy for patients with neck pain, shoulder pain, repetitive strain injury, and rheumatoid arthritis. They also concluded that exercise therapy is not effective for patients with acute low back pain. (No data on occupational outcomes (though doubtless some of the original reviews included RTW)).
(Staal et al. 2003) Systematic review	**Occupational health guidelines for the management of low back pain: an international comparison** There was general agreement across all the international guidelines on numerous issues fundamental to occupational health management of back pain. The assessment recommendations consisted of diagnostic triage, screening for 'red flags' and neurological problems, and the identification of potential psychosocial and workplace barriers for recovery. The guidelines also agreed on advice that low back pain is a self limiting condition and, importantly, that remaining at work or an early (graduated) return to work, if necessary with modified duties, should be encouraged and supported.
(Staal et al. 2005) Narrative review	**Physical exercise interventions to improve disability and return to work in low back pain: current insights and opportunities for improvement** Acknowledges the body of literature indicating that physical exercise might be effective to stimulate return to work and improve function in workers who are absent from work due to low back pain. However, in cases of occupational low back pain, it is often a physical incident or activity that is blamed for the precipitation of back pain or sciatica and held responsible for damaging spinal structures. Physical exercises are not associated with an increased risk for recurrences. The effects of interventions may vary depending on content-related factors (i.e., type of exercises, dosage, frequency, skills of the healthcare providers, etc.) and contextual factors (i.e., treatment setting, compensation system, etc.). Treatment confidence and patients' expectations also significantly influence outcomes of physical exercise interventions. Timing is also important; interventions targeting return to work, applied during the acute phase of work absenteeism, compete with a high rate of spontaneous recovery and may therefore be inefficient. Authors consider staying active and increasing the level of physical activity are safe, despite increased loading of spine structures.

TABLE 3: MUSCULOSKELETAL DISORDERS

(Sullivan et al. 2005) Narrative review	**Integrating psychosocial and behavioural interventions to achieve optimal rehabilitation outcomes** Selective review of scientific literature on psychosocial and behavioural interventions and work disability. Most prior interventions focused on psychosocial risk factors that exist primarily within the individual (e.g., pain catastrophising, beliefs, expectancies). Successful disability prevention *(translates into earlier return to work)* will require methods to assess and target psychosocial risk factors 'outside' of the individual (e.g., interpersonal conflict in the workplace, job stress, etc.) using cost-effective, multipronged approaches. Cognitive behavioural approaches have dominated intervention research on psychosocial risk factors for work disability. The term cognitive-behavioural does not refer to a specific intervention, but rather to a class of intervention strategies that might include self-instruction, relaxation, developing coping strategies, increasing assertiveness, minimizing negative or self-defeating thoughts, changing maladaptive beliefs about pain, and goal setting. Intervening with cognitive behavioural principles is not confined to psychologists: increasing front-line rehabilitation professionals' ability to detect and intervene on psychosocial risk factors can facilitate early implementation of risk factor targeted interventions, whilst integrating the same principles into community/public health programmes or the workplace can be effective. Challenges to effective secondary prevention of work disability include developing competencies to enable a range of providers to deliver interventions, standardization of psychosocial interventions, and maximizing adherence to intervention protocols.
(Talmage & Melhorn 2005) Physician guidance	**Working with common musculoskeletal problems** [American Medical Association] *(Guidance book for primary care physicians and care providers to assist in the navigation of return to work issues, supported by science and consensus – the approach involves consideration of risk, capacity and tolerance at the individual level).*
(Haralson 2005)	Common lower extremity problems: Lower extremity injuries are a common cause of the loss of the ability to work. With proper job accommodations (e.g. redesign to reduce the need for locomotion) people with lower extremity problems can return to work relatively quickly (with general health benefit) and there seems little reason to keep workers with most lower extremity problems off work for extended periods.
(Melhorn 2005)	Common upper extremity problems: Returning an individual with an upper extremity problem to work requires a balance between the demands of the job and the capability of the patient. Temporary workplace advice on accommodations and tolerance should focus on an early return to work and improve the outcome for work-related injuries, and advance the patients' quality of life.
(Sherrer 2005)	Common rheumatological disorders: Rheumatological disorders are varied, but they uniformly have a negative impact on work. Emerging data suggest that the majority of patients can continue to work with certain parameters, and will need aggressive control of disease activity and pain, along with appropriate workplace adaptations. *(Entries related to cardio-respiratory conditions are in Table 5.*

TABLE 3: MUSCULOSKELETAL DISORDERS

(Tveito et al. 2004) Systematic review	**Low back pain interventions at the workplace: a systematic literature review** The aim of this review was to assess if controlled workplace interventions have a positive effect on low back pain, and which interventions are most effective. Four outcome classes: sick leave, costs, future episodes, pain. • Educational interventions (mostly back schools/lifting training): No evidence of effect on sick leave; no evidence of any effect on costs. • Exercise: Limited evidence for a positive effect from exercise on sick leave; limited evidence that exercise has a positive effect on costs. • Multidisciplinary interventions: There is limited evidence of no effect on sick leave; no evidence for effect on costs or new episodes; limited evidence for effect on pain. • Treatment interventions (at workplace): There is moderate evidence of a positive effect on sick leave; no evidence of effect on costs; limited evidence of reduction in new episodes. *(The main positive finding at that time was that exercise and treatment interventions at the workplace can reduce sick leave. More recent reviews provide more positive evidence and conclusions).*
(van Geen et al. 2007) Systematic review	**The long-term effect of multidisciplinary back training: a systematic review** To determine the long-term effect of multidisciplinary back training on the work participation of patients with nonspecific chronic low back pain. Ten studies met the inclusion criteria. All 5 high-quality studies found a positive effect on at least one of the 4 outcome measures used. The various studies used different elements in their multidisciplinary training programs. Based on our criteria, effectiveness was found for the outcome measures of work participation and quality of life. The interventions ranged from 4 elements (physical, educational, psychological, and social) to 2 elements (physical and educational or psychological). The duration and intensity of the treatments ranged from 2 hours to 35 hours a week. The intensity of the intervention seems to have no substantial influence on the effectiveness of the intervention. In the long-term, multidisciplinary back training has a positive effect on work participation in patients with nonspecific chronic low back pain.
(van Tulder et al. 2002) Narrative review	**Low back pain** Low back pain is a major burden to society. Many people will experience an episode of low back pain during their life. Some people develop chronic low back pain, which can be very disabling. Low back pain is associated with high direct and indirect costs. Recent epidemiological data suggest that there is a need to revise our views regarding the course of low back pain. Low back pain is not simply either acute or chronic but fluctuates over time with frequent recurrences or exacerbations. Also, low back pain may frequently be part of a widespread pain problem instead of being isolated, regional pain. Although epidemiological studies have identified many individual, psychosocial and occupational risk factors for the onset of low back pain, their independent prognostic value is usually low. Similarly, a number of factors have now been identified that may increase the risk of chronic disability but no single factor seems to have a strong impact. Consequently, it is still unclear what the most efficient strategy is for primary and secondary prevention. In general, multi-modal preventative approaches seem better able to reflect the clinical reality than single-modal interventions.

TABLE 3: MUSCULOSKELETAL DISORDERS

(Varekamp et al. 2006) Narrative review	**How can we help employees with chronic diseases to stay at work? A review of interventions aimed at job retention and based on an empowerment perspective** Vocational rehabilitation used to focus on (re)entering the labour market. Recently more attention is paid to interventions aimed at job retention. Some of these use an empowerment perspective. Nine studies were detected. The aims of the intervention programs were to improve psychosocial skills or implement work accommodations. There is some evidence that vocational rehabilitation interventions that pay attention to training in requesting work accommodations and feelings of self-confidence or self efficacy in dealing with work-related problems are effective. There is no evidence for greater effectiveness of group programs compared to individual programs. Attention has to be paid to feasibility aspects such as recruitment of participants and cooperation between medical professionals, occupational physicians, and vocational rehabilitation experts. Medical specialists and nursing specialists should pay more attention to work. Although many studies claim effectiveness, evidence for this was often weak due to short follow-up and the lack of control groups.
(Verbeek 2001) Discussion paper	**Vocational rehabilitation of workers with back pain** Discussion concerns the concepts and practices currently in use in occupational health for the rehabilitation of workers with back pain. No conclusive evidence exists for an etiologic model for nonspecific back pain. A difference between acute and chronic back pain is backed up by evidence from the literature. Apart from having the patient stay active and return to ordinary activities as early as possible, there are no significant forms of intervention for acute back pain that effectively decrease the time off work. For chronic back pain multidisciplinary treatment in an occupational setting is effective in enhancing return to work. Clinical practice guidelines consist of diagnostic triage, the assessment of 'red flags' for medical emergencies, and guidance in the appropriate application of diagnostic facilities. Occupational health guidelines concentrate on gradual return to work, psychosocial issues, and multidisciplinary rehabilitation facilities.
(Verhagen et al. 2006) Cochrane review	**Ergonomic and physiotherapeutic interventions for treating work-related complaints of the arm, neck or shoulder in adults** Conservative interventions such as physiotherapy and ergonomic adjustments (such as keyboard adjustments or ergonomic advice) are frequently offered as treatments for most work-related complaints of the arm, neck or shoulder. This review aimed to determine their effectiveness. 21 studies (mostly with low methodological quality) were included, evaluating 25 interventions. The authors concluded there is limited evidence for the effectiveness of keyboards with an alternative force-displacement of the keys or an alternative geometry, and limited evidence for the effectiveness of exercises compared to massage; breaks during computer work compared to no breaks; massage as an add-on treatment to manual therapy; and manual therapy as an add-on treatment to exercises. *(Only 4 of the trials used occupational outcomes – thus any differences between clinical and occupational outcomes cannot reliably be assessed).*

TABLE 3: MUSCULOSKELETAL DISORDERS

(Verhagen et al. 2007) Systematic review	**Exercise proves effective in a systematic review of work-related complaints of the arm, neck, or shoulder** The Netherlands has achieved consensus about the term 'complaints of the arm, neck, and/or shoulder' (CANS), which can be either work related or not work related. Work-related CANS can be divided into specific conditions such as carpal tunnel syndrome, which has relatively clear diagnostic criteria and pathology, or nonspecific conditions such as tension neck syndrome, which is primarily defined by the location of complaints and whose pathophysiology is less clearly defined or relatively unknown. Data from randomised studies of frequently performed interventions in work-related upper extremity musculoskeletal disorders: pain was the outcome measure for most, though some included return to work/sick leave. Findings: Exercises: There is limited evidence that exercises are more effective compared to massage. There is conflicting evidence concerning the efficacy of exercises over treatment or as add-on treatment, and no differences between various kinds of exercises can be found yet. Behavioural therapy *(the term used by the authors, but actually refers mostly to relaxation therapy):* There is conflicting evidence about the effectiveness of behavioural therapy when compared to no treatment or waiting list controls. Ergonomics: There is conflicting evidence concerning the effectiveness of ergonomic programs over no treatment, although there is limited evidence that breaks during computer work are effective. There is limited evidence for the effectiveness of some keyboards in people with carpal tunnel syndrome compared to placebo but conflicting evidence compared to other keyboards. Group therapy vs individual therapy: There is conflicting evidence concerning the effectiveness of individual vs. group therapy. Massage: There is limited evidence for the effectiveness of massage as add-on treatment to manual therapy. Manual therapy: There is limited evidence for the effectiveness of manual therapy as add-on treatment to exercises. Energized splint: There is one low-quality study comparing an "energized splint" with placebo, but no data are available *(The effectiveness of the treatments in respect of occupational outcomes cannot be disentangled from pain outcomes).*
(Walker-Bone & Cooper 2005) Narrative review	**Hard work never hurt anyone: or did it? A review of occupational associations of soft tissue musculoskeletal disorders of the neck and upper limb** Focus was occupational associations with neck and upper limb musculoskeletal disorders. Considered separately neck disorders, shoulder disorders, epicondylitis, non-specific forearm pain, and carpal tunnel syndrome. • Neck disorders: High background prevalence of neck pain among adults in developed countries (point prevalence up to 34%); contributes to sickness absence and demands on medical services. Neck pain and neck disorders are associated with mechanical and psychosocial workplace factors (with complex interactions) – preventive strategies are not convincing. • Shoulder disorders: High background prevalence of shoulder pain (point prevalence up to 26%). Symptoms/disorders are associated with overhead work and possibly repetitive work: occupational psychosocial factors are also implicated (this holds true even when the outcome studied is a specific diagnosis). • Epicondylitis: Strenuous manual tasks seem to be associated with epicondylitis, but unclear if mechanical factors initiate the disorder or aggravate a tendency among predisposed people: emerging evidence suggesting association with psychosocial factors. • Non-specific forearm pain: Rare among working age adults (point prevalence 0.5%). Significantly associated with psychological distress but not with any mechanical exposures. • Carpal tunnel syndrome: Aetiology controversial due to problem of case definition. Overall, workplace factors may be contributory (force, repetition, and vibration). Neck and upper limb pain is a common problem among working age adults and contributes to sick leave. Workplace factors such as prolonged abnormal posture and repetition contribute to these conditions. Psychosocial influences show the aetiology is complex, and both types of factor may be important, though there is insufficient evidence to determine the relative contribution.

TABLE 3: MUSCULOSKELETAL DISORDERS

(Waddell & Burton 2004) Evidence synthesis	**Concepts of rehabilitation for the management of common health problems** [Report commissioned by UK Department for Work and Pensions] *(The review covered the range of common health problems but only information related to musculoskeletal disorders is noted here)* • Low back pain: Advice to stay active and continue ordinary activities (including work) as normally as possible despite pain leads to faster return to work, fewer recurrences and less work loss over the following year than more passive approaches. Most workers with back pain are able to continue working or to return to work within a few days or weeks, even if they still have some residual or recurrent symptoms. • Other musculoskeletal disorders: There seems to be common strands to the different musculoskeletal symptoms/disorders. The themes were broadly consistent with back pain (where there is a much higher quantity of evidence) and there was nothing contrary to the evidence on back pain. • Modified work: Helpful for assisting return to work for back pain and other musculoskeletal disorders. Modified work should be a temporary measure to accommodate reduced capacity; it facilitates early return to normal duties, assuming the risks are suitably assessed and controlled – assignment to permanent modified work can be harmful.
(Waddell & Watson 2004) Narrative review	**Rehabilitation** Review of rehabilitation interventions for low back pain, analysed within a biopsychosocial framework to test the hypothesis that effective rehabilitation interventions should have all three biological, psychological and social elements to address all of the potential obstacles to recovery. Virtually all the interventions included some form of exercise or physical activity element to address the biological problem and restore physical function. However, it seems clear from this review and the evidence on exercise and functional restoration programmes that this physical element alone is insufficient to achieve return to work. Most successful interventions also addressed beliefs in one way or another, and many of them included some kind of occupational intervention. Most of the programmes that did not explicitly address these latter two elements were unsuccessful in achieving return to work. The balance of the evidence does seem to support the hypothesis that a rehabilitation intervention is more likely to produce successful vocational outcomes if it addresses all three bio-psycho-social elements of disability and obstacles to recovery.
(Weir & Nielson 2001) Review of reviews	**Interventions for disability management** The objective of the review was to determine how effective modified work programs, work hardening, and work conditioning are in the management of chronic pain disability. The literature search identified two systematic literature reviews to provide the evidence about these interventions for disability management. Studies of work conditioning showed methodological variability, heterogeneous subjects, variable definitions of modified work, and limited outcome measures. Using return-to-work outcomes, 8 of the 11 studies of adequate methodological quality reported positive effects of modified work programs, mostly light duty. For work conditioning and work hardening, studies showed methodological variability combined with heterogeneous subjects, including varying times out of work and varying work ethics from different countries. Most study results were uncertain, though results of three of the four medium-quality studies were positive. Modified work programs may improve return-to-work rates of workers with work-related injuries for 6 months or longer. There is inadequate evidence to determine what particular aspects of modified work programs are helpful. Work conditioning and work hardening may or may not improve the return to work of more chronically disabled workers.

TABLE 3: MUSCULOSKELETAL DISORDERS

(Williams & Westmorland 2002) Narrative review	**Perspectives on workplace disability: a review of the literature** Many employers recognize the importance of workplace disability management approaches and are assuming greater responsibility for preventing and minimizing work-related disability. This review looks at the effectiveness of these interventions for the rehabilitation of injured workers with musculoskeletal work injuries. The literature suggests that employer participation, a supportive work climate and cooperation between labour, and management are crucial factors in facilitating return to work. Given the complexity of the disability management process and the numbers of individuals involved, it is essential that all workplace parties work together to achieve the goal of safe and early return to work.
(Williams et al. 2004) Systematic review	**Effectiveness of workplace rehabilitation interventions in the treatment of work-related upper extremity disorders: a systematic review** The reviewers started from the standpoint that workplace rehabilitation interventions should enable injured workers to carry out their employment duties (help with sustained, safe return to pre-injury work). Methodological considerations reduced 53 initially selected papers to 8 for analysis. The findings indicate there is insufficient evidence to identify effective workplace rehabilitation interventions for work-related upper extremity disorders. Although the evidence may be poor, it tends to favour a positive impact for several workplace interventions such as ergonomic modifications in keyboard designs, rest and exercise breaks, nurse case managers' training on accommodations, and exercise programmes. *(Only 2 of the positive studies actually reported absence-related outcomes).*
(Williams et al. 2007) Systematic review	**Effectiveness of workplace rehabilitation interventions in the treatment of work-related low back pain: a systematic review** Evaluation of the effectiveness of workplace rehabilitation interventions for injured workers with low back pain. 15 articles, consisting of 10 studies that were of sufficient quality to be included in the review. The best evidence was that clinical interventions with occupational interventions was effective in returning injured workers with low back pain to regular work faster and decreasing pain and disability. Early return to work/modified work was effective in decreasing the rates of back injuries as well as lost-time back injuries, and reducing pain and disability. It is interesting to note that these studies also included early contact with the worker by the workplace and a health care provider intervention at the workplace. Ergonomic interventions such as participatory ergonomics and workplace adaptation, adaptation of job tasks and adaptation of working hours were effective in returning injured workers to work.
(Zampolini et al. 2007) Quasi-systematic review	**RTW in back conditions** The purpose of this review is to analyse the components involved in return to work (RTW). The evidence is moderate and the meta-analysis failed to show strong indications of efficacy. The better interventions to facilitate RTW are multidisciplinary, not necessarily intensive but taking into account a biopsychosocial approach - direct intervention alone on the impairment is not the best program to facilitate RTW; a task specific and behavioural approach seem to be efficacious, which could explain the apparent paradox of the better results of low intensity exercises of 'back school' compared to high intensity ones; focusing the intervention on the person and the context is the modality to improve RTW. The predictor of RTW does not only concern impairment (pain, stiffness etc.); the self-estimation of ability is important to forecast RTW. Intervention seems to be cost-effective if we calculate the saving cost in terms of pensions. Comprehensive bio-psycho-social approaches seem to be the better modality of intervention to facilitate the RTW.

[LBP = low back pain; MSD = musculoskeletal disorder; RTW = return to work]

TABLE 4: REVIEWS AND REPORTS ON MENTAL HEALTH CONDITIONS

Table 4a: Anxiety and depression (common mental health problems)

TABLE 4a: ANXIETY AND DEPRESSION (COMMON MENTAL HEALTH PROBLEMS)

Authors	Key features *(Reviewers' comments in italic)*
(Abbass et al. 2006) Cochrane Review	**Short-term psychodynamic psychotherapies for common mental disorders** Included 23 studies (1431 patients) with common mental disorders - anxiety disorders, depression, stress-related physical conditions, certain behaviour disorders and interpersonal or personality problems mixed with symptom disorders. The main outcomes included general psychiatric symptoms, measures of depression, measures of anxiety, somatic symptom measures and 4 used measures of social adjustment. Outcomes for most categories of disorder suggested significantly greater improvement in the treatment versus the control groups, which were generally maintained in medium and long term follow-up. However, only a small number of studies contributed data for each category of disorder, there was significant heterogeneity between studies, and results were not always maintained in sensitivity analyses. 4 studies gave occupational outcomes and all showed improvements but these were too heterogeneous to draw any firm conclusions.
(Barbui & Tansella 2006) Narrative review	**Identification and management of depression in primary care settings: a meta-review of evidence** A 'review of reviews' summarising effectiveness evidence in three areas: (1) Screening for depression in primary care: Screening alone does not improve the recognition, management and outcome of depression in primary care settings. (2) Managing depression in primary care employing specific management strategies: Management strategies, including (a) training primary care staff, (b) consultation-liaison, (c) collaborative care, (d) replacement/referral are supported by insufficient evidence to provide a definite answer as to the clinical effectiveness of individual models. (3) Treating primary care depressive patients with antidepressants: Robust evidence exists to encourage doctors to prescribe effective doses of antidepressants in patients with moderate to severe depression who seek treatment in primary care settings. The authors concluded that population-level screening campaigns have a negative ratio of costs to benefits. However, at an individual-level of care increasing the ability of primary care physicians in recognising depression remains a relevant factor. Primary care physicians should consider whether depression is mild, moderate or severe. This patient categorisation should guide appropriate management and therapeutic strategies.
(Bilsker et al. 2006) Conceptual review	**Managing depression-related occupational disability: a pragmatic approach** Objective of this paper was to identify issues that arise for psychiatrists and other physicians when dealing with occupational disability in patients with depression and to suggest practical strategies for responding more effectively to the challenges of this aspect of patient functioning. The authors suggest that to successfully manage issues of occupational disability, psychiatrists and other physicians must understand the distinction between impairment and disability. They acknowledge that the research literature concerning optimal strategies for managing depression-related disability is sparse.

TABLE 4a: ANXIETY AND DEPRESSION (COMMON MENTAL HEALTH PROBLEMS)

(Binks et al. 2006) Cochrane review	**Psychological therapies for people with borderline personality disorder** Included 7 studies of 262 people. This review suggests that some of the problems frequently encountered by people with borderline personality disorder may be amenable to talking/behavioural treatments but all therapies remain experimental and the studies are too few and small to inspire full confidence in their results. *(No occupational outcomes).*
(Bisson & Andrew 2007) Cochrane review	**Psychological treatment of post-traumatic stress disorder (PTSD)** Included 33 studies of trauma-focused cognitive behavioural therapy/exposure therapy (TFCBT); stress management (SM); other therapies (supportive therapy, non-directive counselling, psychodynamic therapy and hypnotherapy); group cognitive behavioural therapy (group CBT); eye movement desensitization and reprocessing (EMDR). With regards to reduction of clinician assessed PTSD symptoms, there was evidence that individual TFCBT, EMDR, stress management and group TFCBT are effective in the treatment of PTSD, compared with waiting list or usual care. Other non-trauma focused psychological treatments did not reduce PTSD symptoms as signifcantly. There was some evidence that individual TFCBT and EMDR are superior to stress management in the treatment of PTSD at between 2 and 5 months following treatment, and also that TFCBT, EMDR and stress management were more effective than other therapies. *(No occupational outcomes).*
(Boardman et al. 2003) Editorial	**Work and employment for people with psychiatric disabilities** Work is something that many of us take for granted, but many people with mental illness are excluded from work and are unlikely to gain or sustain open employment. This is despite the fact that the majority of people with mental illness wish to be engaged in meaningful activity. Being 'in work' has important implications for the personal well-being, social status and civil rights of those with mental illness, as well as for their use of health and social services. Work offers considerable personal and economic benefits for users of mental health services. The authors discuss the problems faced by those with long-term mental illness, and barriers to employment such as disincentives in the benefit system, stigma, and employer reluctance. They suggest there is widespread ignorance of the existing evidence about services and approaches that are effective in helping people, and that there is a need to develop a range of effective vocational services that will cover the spectrum of disability. *(The extent to which these opinions and suggestions apply to common mental health problems is not clear, since the majority of the editorial addresses severe problems. The only evidence presented on work outcomes dealt exclusively with severe mental problems and is used to argue for supported employment schemes).*
(Bower & Rowland 2006) Cochrane review	**Effectiveness and cost-effectiveness of counselling in primary care** Eight trials were included (n = 772). Counselling is associated with modest improvement in short-term clinical outcomes (reduced psychological symptoms) compared to usual care, but provides no additional advantages in the long-term. Patients are satisfied with counselling. Although some types of health care utilisation may be reduced, counselling does not seem to reduce overall healthcare costs. There was no effect in social functioning. *(No data on vocational outcomes)*

TABLE 4a: ANXIETY AND DEPRESSION (COMMON MENTAL HEALTH PROBLEMS)

(Canadian Senate 2004) Narrative review and expert consensus	**Mental health, mental illness and addiction: issues and options for Canada**

[Standing Senate Committee On Social Affairs, Science And Technology, Canada]

Individuals with mental illness may have access to help in dealing with their problems at some workplaces. However, with or without these supports, they may still feel compelled to keep their personal struggle to themselves. This may be due to fear of losing one's job, or of being stigmatised. It may prevent that person seeking treatment. This can have negative consequences for their well-being, their productivity, and ability to remain at work.

The relationship between mental illness and work is bidirectional. On the one hand, mental illnesses are a major cause of absenteeism from work, under-performance, employee turnover and reduced productivity. On the other hand, the workplace can be a cause of stress affecting mental health and work performance. Possibly, some forms of workplace stress may even trigger the onset of mental illnesses. Whatever the direction of causality between mental illness and work, there is general consensus that the workplace is a critical environment for the promotion of mental health, the early detection of mental illness, and the accommodation/integration of employees suffering from mental disorders. The attributes of a healthy workplace may benefit the individual, the employer, and society as a whole by enhancing productivity and reducing the overall economic burden of mental illness.

For those affected by mental illness, employment is an important contributor to recovery. It may aid recovery and reduce the frequency and severity of episodes of acute illness by providing structure, the opportunity for social connections and a fuller life. Through regular remuneration, employment can end or reduce dependence on social assistance and reduce individual need for mental health services and supports.

In contrast, loss or lack of employment due to mental illness may jeopardize a person's recovery. Income and standard of living are reduced, resulting in economic dependence and low self-esteem. Inadequate employment also leads to the loss of personal relationships with fellow workers, social marginalization and changed relationships with family and friends.

Many individuals with mental illness succeed in their employment without any assistance being provided to them; recent advances in treatment and drug therapy have increased their capacity to join the mainstream and live independently. Those who participate in the labour force contribute to productivity and competitiveness. Others, however, need assistance to get and keep a job. In this context, the issue of mental illness, addiction and work can be explored from three different perspectives. The first addresses the issue of making employment accessible to individuals who never had a job. The second emphasizes mental illness and addiction that may affect currently employed individuals. The third focuses on individuals who have lost their job due to mental illness or addiction and wish to reintegrate the labour market.

For those who do find work, periods outside the labour force caused by their mental illness often impede re-entry into the labour force. Three key barriers apply. First, individuals may be subject to discrimination by their employer and/or work colleagues. Second, they may require flexible work arrangements that employers are unwilling, or do not know how to provide. And third, those who have been outside of the labour force for extended periods are unlikely to possess the type of credentials, skills and employment experiences that make them attractive to employers.

Two main factors make mental illness specifically a workplace issue. First, mental illness usually strikes younger workers. Second, many mental illnesses are both chronic and cyclical in nature, requiring treatment on and off for many years. There is a vital role for employers and government to play in addressing mental illness and addiction in the workplace, including through accommodation policies, return to work programs and disability management.

There is a compelling case for employers to address mental illness and addiction in the workplace. In the global economy, information and innovation have become the keys to competitive success. And using these keys requires skilled, motivated, reliable workers. Human capital – motivation, knowledge, perspective, judgement, the ability to communicate, share ideas and have relationships – drives the global economy. In short, it is mental performance that drives competitive success in the worldwide economy.

TABLE 4a: ANXIETY AND DEPRESSION (COMMON MENTAL HEALTH PROBLEMS)

	Given the burden of mental illness and addiction on society and on individual workers, and given the rising cost of occupational disabilities, employers must help to enhance the level of awareness about mental illness and addiction in their organizations; they also must devote more attention to improving access to treatment and rehabilitation services for workers through their EAPs. Employers must also place greater emphasis on work flexibility and accommodation for employees who suffer from mental illnesses. Accommodation refers to any modification of the workplace, or in the workplace procedures, that makes it possible for a person with special needs to do a job. Just as individuals with physical disabilities may require physical aids or structural changes to the workplace, individuals with mental disorders most often require social and organizational accommodations to be made. These generally involve changes to the way things have traditionally been done in a particular workplace. Permitting someone with a mental illness to work flexible hours, for example, provides him or her access to employment in the same way that a ramp does for an individual in a wheelchair. Such accommodation does not constitute preferential treatment. Accommodation means equitable treatment for individuals with disabilities. One study suggests that the cost of accommodating an employee with a mental illness is fairly low, usually well under $500. Roadmap to Mental Disability Management which unifies physical and mental health within a single environmental, health and safety system. The Roadmap also provides standards for governing return-to-work policy. More precisely: • Employers do not need to know the nature of the diagnosis of the disabling illness that is involved in any given case. This information is private and confidential. • Employers do need to understand, support and participate in return-to-work plans which will inevitably involve customized adjustments in the content of the employee's job or hours of work in order to make the transition go smoothly. • Employers need to know that while the employee is coming back, he/she is not 100 per cent and gradual return-to-work is necessary to help the individual catch up with things, get up to speed and build tolerance and endurance. *(This report make a strong moral and business case for helping people with mental illness (of any type) to engage in work. It emphasises early detection and access to relevant support (such as EAP), along with appropriate workplace accommodations).*
(Churchill et al. 2001) Systematic review	**A systematic review of controlled trials of the effectiveness and cost-effectiveness of brief psychological treatments for depression** [Health Technology Assessment] Patients receiving any variant of psychotherapy were significantly more likely to improve to a degree where they were no longer considered clinically depressed, exhibited fewer symptoms post-treatment and experienced greater symptom reduction from baseline than those receiving treatment as usual. Patients receiving CBT were significantly more likely than those receiving other forms of psychotherapy (interpersonal therapy, psychodynamic therapy or supportive therapy) to improve to a degree where they were no longer considered clinically depressed. It was not possible to draw any firm conclusions from the limited follow-up and economic data available, but there was tentative evidence that psychotherapy was more efficient than usual care and a modest cost-effective advantage in favour of CBT. *(No occupational outcomes).*
(Curran et al. 2007) Narrative review and survey	**Mental health and employment: an overview of patterns and policies across Western Europe** Conducted a questionnaire survey to collect data on employment of people with mental health problems and related economic issues in 17 countries participating in the Mental Health Economics European Network (MHEEN). Objective was to explore the relationship between mental health problems and employment across Europe due to the cost of lost productivity. Narrative data was collected that indicated the impact of mental health problems on lost productivity is substantial and growing. A range of policies have been developed to address this challenge, covering the spectrum of issues from workplace interventions promoting positive mental health to anti-discrimination laws to enable participation in the workforce. The authors concluded much more work needs doing. *(Evidence of the impact or effectiveness of policy changes is not provided).*

TABLE 4a: ANXIETY AND DEPRESSION (COMMON MENTAL HEALTH PROBLEMS)

(Davis & Rinaldi 2004) Narrative review	**Using an evidence-based approach to enable people with mental health problems to gain and retain employment, education and voluntary work** Employment provides an economic means, gives social status and promotes social inclusion. While people with mental health problems attach a high priority to gaining employment, they face many barriers that inhibit their ability to gain and retain employment. This paper describes how a mental health trust actively promoted vocational rehabilitation through implementing evidence-based principles within the clinical teams. It reports how the trust acknowledged the unique contribution of occupational therapy in partnership with vocational services to enable its clients to access competitive employment, mainstream education and voluntary work. Their conclusions from a narrative review are: (a) Approaches to work are more important in determining vocational success than the diagnostic and demographic characteristics of clients. Reviews have found that client characteristics have little impact on vocational outcomes. Employment history is a robust predictor of work outcomes, but motivation and self-efficacy appear to be more important (b) Research into models and approaches indicates that evidence-based supported employment has been demonstrated to be more effective in enabling people with mental health problems to gain and retain employment than prevocational training. The principles of evidence-based supported employment are: 1. Vocational rehabilitation as an integral component of the work of clinical teams 2. A primary goal of open employment in integrated settings 3. Rapid job-search and minimal prevocational training 4. Initial and continuing assessment and adjustment 5. Time-unlimited support and workplace interventions 6. Attention to client preferences and choice *(Approaches to work are more important than diagnosis and demographics).*
(den Boer et al. 2005) Cochrane review	**Paraprofessionals for anxiety and depressive disorders** Rationale for the review is that the established mental health care system does not have the resources to meet the extensive need for care of those with anxiety and depressive disorders. Paraprofessionals partially replacing professionals may be cost-effective. The objectives were to investigate the effectiveness of any kind of psychological treatment for anxiety and depressive disorders performed by paraprofessionals compared with professionals, waiting list or placebo condition; and, to examine whether the results apply to clinically significant anxiety and depressive disorders of referred patients with a psychiatric history and/or whose illness has lasted two years or more. Five RCTs were identified, all using self-report measures. These reported five comparisons of paraprofessionals versus professionals (N=106) and five comparisons of paraprofessionals versus control condition (N=220). No differences were found between paraprofessionals and professionals. Studies comparing paraprofessionals versus control indicated no significant difference in effect between paraprofessionals and professionals, and a strongly significant pooled effect for three studies (N=188; women only) favouring paraprofessionals over the control condition. The authors concluded that the small number of studies precludes definitive conclusions, but there are indications that treatment programmes for anxiety and depressive disorders could incorporate paraprofessionals for female patients.

TABLE 4a: ANXIETY AND DEPRESSION (COMMON MENTAL HEALTH PROBLEMS)

(Dewa et al. 2007) Narrative review	**An international perspective on worker mental health problems: who bears the burden and how are costs addressed?** This review discusses the burden of poor mental health in workers, who currently bears it, and how the associated rising costs are being addressed, from an international perspective. The authors identified stakeholder groups and the costs they incur as a result of problems related to mental health in 6 different domains: • Unemployment • Early retirement • Productivity - Absenteeism, Presenteeism, and Short-Term Disability • Spillover Effects on Coworkers and Supervisors • Spillover Effects on Families • Health Services Costs Results indicated that mental illness is associated with a wide range of costs distributed across multiple stakeholders including government, employers, workers and their families, and the health care system. The costs incurred by the groups are interrelated; an attempt to decrease the burden for one group of stakeholders will inevitably affect other stakeholders. Thus the answer to the question of who bears the costs of poor mental health is 'everyone'. The authors concluded that everyone can therefore benefit from investment in improved mental health in the workplace. However, because the benefits associated with improved worker mental health are often distributed among several stakeholders, the incentives for any single stakeholder to pay for additional services for workers may be diluted. As a consequence, no one invests. Nevertheless, there is a role for all stakeholders, just as there are potential benefits for all. Along with government, employers, employees, and the health care system must invest in promoting good workplace health. (*This article makes two important points: First, costs are borne by everyone. Second, benefits from improvements are spread across stakeholders and therefore diluted, meaning each stakeholder perceives less incentive to invest in mental health outcomes*).
(DH 2001) Evidence based clinical practice guideline	**Treatment choice in psychological therapies and counselling: evidence based clinical practice guideline** [UK Department of Health] Developed from evidence review and professional consultation with consensus approach. Addresses depression, including suicidal behaviour; anxiety, panic disorder, social anxiety & phobias; post traumatic disorders; eating disorders; obsessive compulsive disorders; personality disorders, including repetitive self harm; four physical conditions: chronic pain, chronic fatigue, gastrointestinal disorders (e.g. irritable bowel syndrome), and gynaecological presentations (e.g. pre-menstrual syndrome, pelvic pain, menopausal vasomotor symptoms). Excluded topics were: disorders in childhood and adolescence, psychoses including schizophrenia, mania and bipolar disorder, alcohol and other drug addictions, sexual dysfunction & paraphilias, organic brain syndromes and acquired brain injury, and, learning disability. • <u>Depressive disorders:</u> Psychological treatment is effective in general adult and older adult populations, including inpatient care (Ia). CBT and interpersonal therapy in particular have been found efficacious, with best evidence for cognitive behaviour therapy. (Ia). Behavioural therapy, problem-solving therapy, group therapy and marital and family interventions have all shown some evidence of efficacy (Ib). For brief psychotherapy, CBT variants were most efficacious compared with other therapies. Psychodynamic-interpersonal therapy has also shown evidence of effectiveness (Ib). Time-limited depression-targeted psychotherapies are efficacious when transferred from psychiatric to primary care settings (Ia).

TABLE 4a: ANXIETY AND DEPRESSION (COMMON MENTAL HEALTH PROBLEMS)

- Panic disorder with/without agoraphobia: Exposure-based treatment and CBT have shown efficacy in the treatment of agoraphobia, although exposure may be less effective on measures of panic (Ia). Applied relaxation may also be effective (Ia).

- Social phobia: Exposure and cognitive therapy are effective for the treatment of social phobia (Ia

- Generalised anxiety disorder (GAD): CBT is effective in treating GAD (Ia).

- Post traumatic stress disorder: Psychological treatment may have an impact on PTSD but this may be limited, and may reduce symptoms of depression and anxiety more than primary PTSD symptoms (Ia). Differential efficacy of particular treatments has not been established; relatively little research evidence is available. Best evidence of efficacy was reported for exposure and other CBT methods (stress inoculation and eye movement desensitisation and reprocessing - EMDR) (Ib), with some evidence for hypnotherapy and psychodynamic therapy (II). The efficacy of critical incident debriefing as a preventative intervention is not supported by current research evidence (Ia), but many of the published studies showing negative results for critical incident debriefing do not assure the quality of the intervention.

- Obsessive Compulsive Disorder (OCD): Behaviour therapy (or exposure with response prevention) and cognitive therapy appear to be efficacious in the treatment of OCD (Ia), although there is disagreement over which is more effective according to the available evidence. These psychological treatments appear to produce results similar to those achieved by drug treatments (Ia). Behavioural treatment may be less effective in treating depressive symptoms than anxiety symptoms in OCD (Ia).

- Eating disorders: For the treatment of bulimia, evidence suggests that psychological therapy is efficacious (Ia). The efficacy of cognitive therapy and CBT has been established (Ia); less research has been carried out on other forms of therapy, but there are indications that family therapy and interpersonal approaches may be effective (II). There was little evidence available from high-quality research reviews on the effectiveness of treatments for anorexia nervosa, but best evidence is for family therapy and broadly based individual therapy for patients with early onset and late onset of illness respectively (II).

- Somatic complaints – General: There is evidence for family and marital therapies in the treatment of psychosomatic disorders and physical illness (II). Patients with functional somatic symptoms, in the initial acute phase may respond to individual therapy if they are willing to participate (II).

  o Somatic complaints - Gastrointestinal. Evidence for IBS is not conclusive, but suggests psychological treatments may be useful (Ib). In treatment resistant GI disorders, psychodynamic-interpersonal therapy and hypnosis showed effectiveness (Ib).

  o Somatic complaints - Chronic fatigue. There is little high quality research on treatment of chronic fatigue syndrome. One Cochrane review indicates that CBT is more effective than controls in improving physical functioning and experience of fatigue (Ia). Other psychological treatments have not been reviewed. RCT evidence shows benefits of behaviour therapy (including graded exercise therapy) and some evidence for cognitive therapy (Ib).

  o Somatic complaints - Chronic pain. Cognitive and behavioural therapies, including biofeedback, show evidence of being effective in the treatment of chronic pain (Ib). There is little evidence of effectiveness on vocationally relevant outcomes.

  o Somatic complaints - Gynaecological. No high quality review evidence was identified, but there is growing evidence from recent RCTs that psychological approaches have utility. CBT and Rational Emotive Therapy (RET) are effective for pre-menstrual syndrome (Ib). Pelvic pain benefited from a cognitive behavioural approach. Vasomotor symptoms in menopause were reduced by applied relaxation therapy.

TABLE 4a: ANXIETY AND DEPRESSION (COMMON MENTAL HEALTH PROBLEMS)

	• Personality Disorders: There is little comparative outcome research on the treatment of personality disorders with psychotherapy, and no high quality reviews were identified. • Deliberate self-harm: Some evidence of efficacy in reducing self-harm using problem-solving therapy, the provision of an emergency card, and from behaviour therapy (Ib). However, the authors concluded that there were too few studies to make firm recommendations. *(This report is a little dated. A text search of the report revealed there is no information about work, productive activity, or vocational outcomes - other than the statement listed above about chronic pain).*
(DH 2007a) Practice guide	**Commissioning a brighter future: improving access to psychological therapies – positive practice guide** [UK Department of Health] Outlines the Improving Access to Psychological Therapies (IAPT) programme for the NHS. This is intended to raise standards of recognition of, and treatment for, the mass of people who suffer from depression and anxiety disorders. The programme is at the heart of the Government's drive to give greater access to, and choice of, talking therapies to those who would benefit from them. Talking therapies is a broad term covering a range of therapeutic approaches, which involve talking, questioning and listening to understand, manage and treat people's problems. The treatment includes counselling, cognitive behavioural therapy (CBT), psychoanalysis and psychodynamic therapies. Specific techniques included in this programme are: Bibliotherapy (the prescription of free, self-help books, from local libraries can help people 'narrow down' what reading materials may help them to manage their anxiety or depression. It also offers opportunities for community engagement. Offering telephone support with the recommended books will enhance the effectiveness of the outcomes); Psychological therapies (face-to-face therapy such as counselling, CBT, interpersonal psychotherapy, psychodynamic therapy, and other forms of psychotherapy; Guided self-help, or psycho-education (using booklets and information to help people); Computerised CBT (delivery of CBT via an interactive computer program such as Fear Fighter for treating people who have phobias or suffer from panic attacks, and Beating the Blues for treating people with mild to moderate depression); Information and support (information, assistance and guidance to help people find out about training, education and job opportunities and access to appropriate support); Telephone support (a brief intervention of cognitive behavioural therapy and other evidence-based approaches delivered by appropriately trained staff); Prescribed activity (e.g. exercise, social activity, participation in the arts or education). The key principles for psychological services are: 1. Right number of patients seen: understanding the level of need across your community and maximising services to meet those needs. 2. Right services: providing effective treatments and interventions within a stepped care framework delivered by an appropriate and competent workforce. 3. Right time: improved access to services for people with depression and anxiety disorders – both in terms of the numbers of people being treated and the waiting times they can expect from service providers. 4. Right results: collecting and delivering routine outcome data across the four domains of improved Health and well-being, social inclusion and employment, improved choice and improved patient experience. It is noted that while treatments vary according to the individual's condition, the stepped care approach advocates that a person should start with the least intensive treatment that offers a reasonable prospect of success, and, if necessary, should then 'step up' to a more intensive treatment. This is based on the Kaiser Permanente risk stratification model outlined in the following figure: The stepped care approach is advocated to enable local services to determine the correct therapeutic interventions for each step, the professional input required, as well as the ideal skills mix and it is believed this assists the efficient management of resources. *(There is no information on vocational rehabilitation or occupational outcomes).*

TABLE 4a: ANXIETY AND DEPRESSION (COMMON MENTAL HEALTH PROBLEMS)

(DH 2007b)	**Improving access to psychological therapies (IAPT) programme: computerised cognitive behavioural therapy (cCBT) implementation guidance**
Guidance	[UK Department of Health] Cognitive behavioural therapy is based on the premise that there is a close connection between cognition (how we think), our emotions (how we feel), and our behaviour (how we act). There is a strong scientific and research base to support the effectiveness of 'therapist delivered' cognitive behaviour therapy (CBT), in the management of people with depression, anxiety disorders, obsessive compulsive disorder, schizophrenia and bi-polar disorder. There is also a strong research base to support the use of 'therapist delivered' CBT in the management of a number of long-term conditions such as chronic obstructive pulmonary disease and diabetes. cCBT is a generic term that is used to refer to a number of methods of delivering CBT via an interactive computer interface. It can be delivered on a personal computer, over the Internet or via the telephone using interactive voice response (IVR) systems. As with CBT, pre-therapy assessment is recommended to ensure that people are suitable for therapy, and individuals require ongoing monitoring and support. It is suggested that a wide range of health or social care personnel could be used to facilitate the sessions. cCBT may be indicated for: 1) depression; 2) panic and anxiety disorders; 3) phobias; 4) obsessive compulsive disorder; 5) severe mental disorders (schizophrenia, bipolar disorder). *(Mentions that cCBT may be used in an occupational health setting, but there is nothing else on vocational rehabilitation or occupational outcomes).*
(DHC 2006)	**A vision for change: report of the expert group on mental health policy**
Government report	[Ireland Department of Health and Children] The DHC in Ireland appointed an Expert Group in August 2003 to prepare a comprehensive mental health policy framework for the next ten years, and to recommend how the services might best be organised and delivered. *A Vision for Change* proposes a holistic view of mental illness and recommends an integrated multidisciplinary approach to addressing the biological, psychological and social factors that contribute to mental health problems. It proposes a person-centred treatment approach which addresses each of these elements through an integrated care plan, reflecting best practice, and evolved and agreed with service users and their carers. Interventions should be aimed at maximising recovery from mental illness, and building on the resources within service users and within their immediate social networks to allow them to achieve meaningful integration and participation in community life. Specialist expertise should be provided by community mental health teams (CMHTs) – expanded multidisciplinary teams of clinicians who work together to serve the needs of service users across the lifespan. CMHTs should serve defined populations and age groups and operate from community-based mental health centres in specific sectors throughout re-configured mental health catchments areas (serving populations of 250-400,000). Some of these CMHTs should be established on a regional or national basis to address the complex mental health needs of specific categories of people who are few in number but who require particular expertise. *(The whole report emphasises the importance of social inclusion and especially employment. There is a whole chapter on rehabilitation and vocational rehabilitation, though this is focused on people with severe mental illness).* People with mental health problems are particularly vulnerable to social exclusion as the nature of these problems often means they are recurring, so that an individual may have repeated periods of illness and these may result in hospitalisation. Absence from work can lead to unemployment. The loss of a job is crucial, as it means both a loss of income and also loss of a social network and access to the wider social world. Loss of income can lead to debt and even homelessness.

TABLE 4a: ANXIETY AND DEPRESSION (COMMON MENTAL HEALTH PROBLEMS)

The benefit of work for individuals with mental health problems has long been recognised by mental health professionals. Mental health services in Ireland operate several models of supported employment, including sheltered workshops, 'train and place' models, social firms and peer-provided services, such as the Clubhouse model. Supported employment programmes are focused on immediate job search and help finding mainstream employment, with ongoing 'low-level' support (e.g. advice). IPS is also based on immediate job search and open employment, but has a very intensive support programme, e.g. ongoing time-unlimited support once in work, with workplace interventions provided when necessary to enable job retention.

There is evidence that supported employment models can greatly improve vocational and psychosocial outcomes for service users. These models put an emphasis on placing the service user in open employment, with high levels of support from members of the mental health team. Studies of the IPS model have shown increased rates of competitive employment. Given the evidence for supported open employment and individual placement and support, these approaches should be given preference.

Recommendations:

1. The flexible provision of educational programmes should be used to encourage young people to remain engaged with the education system and to address the educational needs of adults with mental health problems.

2. Measures to protect the income of individuals with mental health problems should be put in place. Health care access schemes should also be reviewed for this group.

3. Mental health services should take account of local deprivation patterns in planning and delivering mental health care.

4. Evidence-based approaches to training and employment for people with mental health problems should be adopted and such programmes should be put in place by the agencies with responsibility in this area.

(Dong et al. 2002) Conceptual review	**Mental illness and workplace absenteeism: exploring risk factors and effective return to work strategies** [Ontario Medical Association Committee on Work and Health] The importance of work: The relationship of work to personal identity, esteem and function is well understood through research on the impact of job loss and unemployment. The cumulative economic impact of mental illness is enormous. There is also increased demand for visits to the doctor, increased hospital stays, medical tests, prescription drugs, and other healthcare providers. Risk factors: Generally speaking, the longer a person is away from a job, the less likely it is that he or she will ever return to a productive working life. Statistics show that an individual has a 50 per cent probability of returning to work after six months on disability leave, 20 per cent after one year, and only 10 per cent after two years. Therefore, a return to work plan is essential to maintaining patient employability. Not doing so may have a negative impact on a person's physical health, as well as social and economic circumstances. RTW Process: Although the specific mechanics of RTW are variable, it is well known that early intervention is critical to improving the likelihood of a timely return to work. Further, a modified work strategy is one of the most important factors in improving RTW outcomes when a return to full duties is not possible. While there is a large volume of research on barriers to RTW, it is difficult to isolate one or two factors. In many cases, there is a complicated interaction between an array of factors that will influence how and when a person returns to the worksite. The contributing factors that may affect return to work can arise from a variety of sources: employee; employer; insurer, physician, societal.

TABLE 4a: ANXIETY AND DEPRESSION (COMMON MENTAL HEALTH PROBLEMS)

(Donohue & Pincus 2007) Systematic review	**Reducing the societal burden of depression: a review of economic costs, quality of care and effects of treatment** Included 113 studies in the review. It was noted that depression is a highly prevalent condition that results in substantial functional impairment, and that advocates have suggested there is a 'business case' for investing in quality improvement efforts in depression care, particularly in primary care settings. This business case suggests that the costs of depression treatment may be offset by gains in worker productivity and/or reductions in other healthcare spending. The objective of the review was to consider the evidence in support of this argument for improving the quality of depression treatment, and therefore the impact of depression on two of the primary drivers of the societal burden of depression was examined: healthcare utilisation and worker productivity. The results indicated the following: the economic burden of depression is substantial; depression leads to higher healthcare utilisation and spending, most of which is not the result of depression treatment costs; depression is also a leading cause of absenteeism and reduced productivity at work. It is clear that; however, critical gaps in the literature remain and need to be addressed; the economic burden of untreated and/or inappropriately treated depression is not known; there are considerable problems with access to and quality of depression treatment; progress has been made in terms of access to care, but quality of care is seldom consistent with national treatment guidelines; a wide range of effective treatments and care programmes for depression are available, but rigorously tested clinical models to improve depression care have not been widely adopted by healthcare systems. Barriers to improving depression care exist at the patient, healthcare provider, practice, plan and purchaser levels, and may be both economic and non-economic. Studies evaluating interventions to improve the quality of depression treatment have found that the cost per quality-adjusted life year (QALY) associated with improved depression care ranges from a low of $US 2519 to a high of $US 49,500. The authors concluded that effective treatment of depression is cost effective, but that evidence of a medical or productivity cost offset for depression treatment remains equivocal.
(Druss & von Esenwein 2006) Systematic review	**Improving general medical care for persons with mental and addictive disorders: systematic review** The objective was to review of studies of interventions designed to improve general medical care in persons with mental and addictive disorders. Six randomized trials were included. The interventions spanned a continuum of approaches for improving treatment, ranging from on-site medical consultation, through team-based approaches, to models involving facilitated referrals to primary care. Results indicated there was a substantial positive impact from these interventions on linkage to primary care (defined as one or more appointments with a GP), and on the quality of medical care provided. There was evidence of health improvement and improved abstinence rates in patients with worse health and/or greater medical comorbidity at baseline. The authors noted that although primary care is important for all populations, its effects are most visible in individuals with the greatest unmet health needs. Three studies assessed expenditures, and found the programmes to be cost-neutral from a health-plan perspective. It was concluded there is evidence that a range of models can improve these patients' health and healthcare, at a relatively modest cost. *(Work outcomes were not included in the review).*
(Egan et al. 2007) Systematic review	**The psychosocial and health effects of workplace reorganisation: 1. a systematic review of organisational-level interventions that aim to increase employee control** Identified 18 studies, no RCTs, 12 nonrandomised controlled studies that investigated the health and psychosocial effects of increasing employee participation and control through workplace reorganisation, with reference to the 'demand-control-support' model of workplace health. Eight controlled and three uncontrolled studies found some evidence of health benefits (especially beneficial effects on mental health, including reduction in anxiety and depression) when employee control improved or (less consistently) demands decreased or support increased. Two studies of participatory interventions occurring alongside redundancies reported worsening employee health. The authors concluded there is evidence suggesting that some organisational-level participation interventions may benefit employee health, as predicted by the demand-control-support model, but may not protect employees from generally poor working conditions. *(Absenteeism was not analysed by the authors, however they provided results in their tables: Absenteeism improved in 3 nonrandomised controlled studies, and 1 case series, and remained the same in 1 nonrandomised controlled study).*

TABLE 4a: ANXIETY AND DEPRESSION (COMMON MENTAL HEALTH PROBLEMS)

(Furukawa et al. 2007) Cochrane review	**Combined psychotherapy plus antidepressants for panic disorder with or without agoraphobia** Identified 23 randomised comparisons (representing 21 trials, 1709 patients), 21 of which involved behaviour or cognitive-behaviour therapies. In the acute phase treatment, the combined therapy was superior to antidepressant pharmacotherapy or psychotherapy. The combined therapy produced more dropouts due to side effects than psychotherapy. After the acute phase treatment, as long as the drug was continued, the superiority of the combination over either monotherapy appeared to persist. After termination of the acute phase and continuation treatment, the combined therapy was more effective than pharmacotherapy alone and was as effective as psychotherapy. The authors concluded that either combined therapy or psychotherapy alone may be chosen as first line treatment for panic disorder with or without agoraphobia, depending on patient preference. *(No data on occupational outcomes).*
(Gava et al. 2007) Cochrane review	**Psychological treatments versus treatment as usual for obsessive compulsive disorder (OCD)** Meta-analysis of seven RCTs (n = 241) showed that patients receiving any variant of cognitive behavioural treatment exhibited significantly fewer obsessive compulsive symptoms (SMD -1.24, 95% CI -1.61 to -0.87) and anxiety symptoms (SMD -0.52, 95% CI -0.92 to 0.11) and fewer depressive symptoms (SMD -0.30, 95% CI -0.58 to 0.03) post-treatment than those receiving treatment as usual. Different types of cognitive and/or behavioural treatments showed similar differences in effect when compared with treatment as usual. The overall treatment effect appeared to be influenced by differences in baseline severity. *(Only one study considered quality of life (borderline significance) and there was no data on occupational outcomes).*
(Gates 2000) Conceptual review	**Workplace accommodation as a social process** The main benefit of Employee Assistance Programmes, specifically in relation to job retention, is that they provide a source of early intervention for people with mental health problems while they are still working, that is, before they are lost in a downward spiral of time off work, decreasing mental health and potential job loss. Highlights the importance of social support and four roles for a job retention worker: 1) A source of *information* to the workplace about the nature of mental health problems, the functional effects of symptoms and medication, and (in)-capacity; 2) An *interpreter* of workplace policies and procedures to workers with mental health problems; 3) A *negotiator* helping to secure adjustments that meet the needs of both the worker with mental health problems and the demands of the employer; 4) A *trainer* to supervisors and relevant others in the organisation on how to accommodate people with mental health problems so that they have the skills to manage such issues.
(Goetzel et al. 2002) Conceptual review	**The business case for quality mental health services: why employers should care about the mental health and well-being of their employees** Argues that employers are appropriately concerned about rising mental healthcare costs, and that they want to know whether healthcare spending is improving the health of workers, and whether there is a productivity payback from providing good mental healthcare. Depressed individuals exert a significant cost burden for employers, and evidence is mounting that worker depression may have its greatest impact on productivity losses, including increased absenteeism and short-term disability, higher turnover, and suboptimal performance at work. There is no conclusive evidence that physical healthcare costs decrease when depression is effectively treated, there is growing evidence that productivity improvements occur as a consequence of effective treatment, and those improvements may offset the cost of the treatment. *(Evidence cited are case series, which are indicative only).*

TABLE 4a: ANXIETY AND DEPRESSION (COMMON MENTAL HEALTH PROBLEMS)

(Goetzel et al. 2005) Narrative review	**Return on investment in disease management** 8 depression RCTs were included, with average sample size of 289 intervention subjects, and average study duration of 1.1 years. Per-participant programme expenses averaged $1,479 and ranged from $51 to $5,549, indicating much variation in what was termed a depression management programme. None of the studies found a medical cost-offset for appropriate treatment of depression patients using pharmacological agents and/or psychotherapy. Quite uniformly across the various studies examined, good treatment of depression cost more money (about $500 more a year). The aggregate Return on Investment for depression management programmes was therefore negative, averaging a loss of $0.35 per dollar spent on the programme. The author suggested this may be different if productivity and functionality outcomes (e.g., absence, disability, on the-job-productivity, and performing activities of daily living) were also considered. *(The only evidence offered in support of this contention was the author's own article (Goetzel et al, 2002 – see above), which cited only case series).*
(Goldner et al. 2004) Narrative review	**Disability management, return to work and treatment** There are few research studies of disability management or return to work in people with less severe mental health problems. Evidence based treatment for major depression has been shown to yield corresponding improvement in occupational function, and employees with substantial improvement in symptoms after treatment rate themselves as much more able to function effectively in work. Furthermore, improvement in major depression appears to be associated with greater likelihood of remaining employed and with less sickness absence due to depression. Several studies suggest that CBT has a beneficial effect on work function over and above anti-depressant medication. Overall, as depression resolves, work function improves, and most of the improvement occurs within a few months of starting treatment. There is some emerging evidence that a disability management approach, similar to that used in musculoskeletal injuries, may yield significantly improved work function for depression-related work impairment. *(Most of the rest of the paper is about disability management approaches to musculoskeletal conditions and severe mental illness, and research methodology).*
(Grove 1999) Narrative review	**Mental health and employment: shaping a new agenda** Argues the case that employment should be given high priority as a realistic and legitimate aim of secondary mental health services for patients with severe mental illness. Summarises a consensus view on the principles underpinning service provision and suggests these should be viewed through the conceptual framework of the social model of disability. Services should be: • Needs-based – designed and operated around the clearly identified needs of individuals with mental health problems rather than programme-led or funding-led • Accessible – to all groups in the community, particularly those who are commonly under-represented (e.g. people from minority ethnic backgrounds or those with childcare responsibilities) • Orientated to the local 'market' reflecting the characteristics of the local economy and labour market • User-driven – meeting each user's unique requirements and giving them as much control as possible over the timing, pace and intensity of the services they receive • Offering choice – in terms of programmes, settings skill areas and levels • Providing support for individuals to find and keep jobs and/or to participate in education and training programmes • Offering security in a safe and supportive environment • Offering continuity and availability on a long-term basis and permitting re-access after a period of illness

TABLE 4a: ANXIETY AND DEPRESSION (COMMON MENTAL HEALTH PROBLEMS)

	• Allowing progression to employment or education if users so wish • Flexibility in moving towards a wide range of possible outcomes • Empowering users, building upon the strengths and abilities of users and involving them directly in service planning, operation and evaluation • Promoting integration in ordinary community settings which are socially valued and supporting the usage of community facilities and the development of wider relationships • Directed towards an ordinary working life – ordinary jobs and mainstream training opportunities • Quality driven and producing outcomes that are valued by consumers • Cost-effective – meeting needs effectively and efficiently Also pointed out that it is important for employment support services to think about employers in a more constructive way, not as part of the problem to be 'educated' or coerced into non-discriminatory attitudes. Rather as part of the solution – as potential partners in a reciprocal, negotiated arrangement that will help prevent wastage of lives (and resources) through mental ill-health.
(Harnois & Gabriel 2000) Report	**Mental health and work: impact, issues and good practices** [World Health Organization/International Labour Organization report] The central themes of this monograph are: to address the importance of work for people with mental health problems; to discuss the different vocational strategies and programmes for people with a mental health disorder; and to consider the role of the workplace in promoting good mental health practices for employees. The authors start with the premise: All of us have the right to decent and productive work in conditions of freedom, equity, security and human dignity. For persons with mental health problems, achieving this right is particularly challenging. There is growing evidence of the global impact of mental illness, and there is growing awareness of the role of work in promoting or hindering mental well-being and its corollary – mental illness. Most mental health professionals agree that the workplace environment can have a significant impact on an individual's mental well-being (both positively and negatively). Mental health problems are the most common cause of illness, sickness, disability and loss of productivity. 15-30% of people will experience some form of mental health problem at some time in their lives. Even if work is not the primary cause of mental illness, mental illness impacts on work and is therefore an occupational health issue. Considers major myths about mental illness in the workplace and the evidence that they are untrue: • Myth 1: Mental illness is the same as mental retardation. • Myth 2: Recovery from mental illness is not possible. • Myth 3: Mentally ill employees tend to be second-rate workers (even after effective treatment). • Myth 4: People with psychiatric disabilities cannot tolerate stress on the job. • Myth 5: Mentally ill individuals are unpredictable, violent and dangerous (even after effective treatment).

TABLE 4a: ANXIETY AND DEPRESSION (COMMON MENTAL HEALTH PROBLEMS)

	Argues that the workplace is an appropriate environment in which to educate individuals about, and raise their awareness of, mental health problems *(but does not address the key issue of who might perform this task, with what resources)*; to promote good mental health practices; for the recognition and early identification of mental health problems; and to establish links with local mental health services for referral, treatment and rehabilitation. Provides examples of good practice in mental health promotion in the workplace; management of workers who develop mental health problems; and vocational rehabilitation models/programmes for workers with long-term mental health problems. Mental health at work should encompass individual and organizational dimensions. *(This report appears to be aimed at policy makers, but maybe more particularly at employers. There is a strong assumption throughout that employers have both the responsibility and the ability to implement the recommendations. However, the business case for this is not advanced.)*
(Henderson et al. 2005) Editorial	**Long term sickness absence: Is caused by common conditions and needs managing** Noted the large rise in sickness absence and incapacity benefit claims due to psychological disorder that has occurred in the U.K. since the mid-1990's (when back pain was the predominant problem); and, that common mental health problems such as depression and anxiety, rather than complex psychoses, that contribute most to this rising sickness absence. These are managed almost entirely in primary care. However, not uncommonly, a position develops where an individual has recovered sufficiently to consider returning to work but perceives that exposure to one's employers, colleagues, or other aspects of work will lead to a relapse. General practitioners can have difficulty linking with employers to effect vocational rehabilitation and, as the patient's advocate, may feel uncomfortable recommending returning to work in this situation. The authors suggest that occupational physicians may be the best equipped to manage these cases, but are in short supply within the U.K. They also noted that patients often prefer psychological therapies to medications, but that psychological services in primary care are also in short supply.
(Huibers et al. 2007) Cochrane review	**Psychosocial interventions by general practitioners** Ten studies were included in the review, which addressed different psychosocial interventions for five distinct disorders or health complaints. There is good evidence that problem-solving treatment by general practitioners is effective for major depression. The evidence concerning the remaining interventions for other health complaints (reattribution or cognitive behavioural group therapy for somatisation, cognitive behavioural therapy for unexplained fatigue, counselling for smoking cessation, behavioural interventions to reduce alcohol reduction) is either limited or conflicting. *(Clinical outcomes only; no occupational outcomes).*
(Hunot et al. 2007) Cochrane review	**Psychological therapies for generalised anxiety disorder** Generalised anxiety disorder (GAD) is a highly prevalent condition, characterised by excessive worry or anxiety about everyday events and problems. Objective: To examine the efficacy and acceptability of psychological therapies, categorised as cognitive behavioural therapy (CBT), psychodynamic therapy and supportive therapy, compared with treatment as usual/waiting list (TAU/WL) and compared with one another, for patients with GAD. 25 studies (1305 patients) were included. Based on thirteen studies, psychological therapies, all using a CBT approach, were more effective than TAU/WL in achieving clinical response at post-treatment (RR 0.64, 95%CI 0.55 to 0.74), and also in reducing anxiety, worry and depression symptoms. No studies conducted longer-term assessments of CBT against TAU/WL. Six studies compared CBT against supportive therapy (nondirective therapy and attention-placebo conditions). No significant difference in clinical response was indicated between CBT and supportive therapy at post-treatment. Authors' conclusions: psychological therapy based on CBT principles is effective in reducing anxiety symptoms for short-term treatment of GAD. The body of evidence comparing CBT with other psychological therapies is too small and heterogeneous to draw any conclusions about which form of psychological therapy is more effective. *(Primary outcome was reduced anxiety symptoms, measured by clinical improvement or an anxiety scale. There was limited data on social functioning and quality of life. The authors of the review looked for occupational outcomes or cost-effectiveness but no studies provided any data).*

TABLE 4a: ANXIETY AND DEPRESSION (COMMON MENTAL HEALTH PROBLEMS)

(Kaltenthaler et al. 2004) Systematic review	**Computerized cognitive behaviour therapy: A systematic review** Identified 16 studies comparing computerized cognitive behavioural therapy (CCBT) with therapist led CBT (TCBT) or with treatment as usual. 11 were RCTs and the other 5 were cohort studies. Results indicated that cCBT is potentially useful in the treatment of anxiety disorders, depression and phobias. One RCT was identified with absenteeism as the primary outcome, and several used the Work and Social Adjustment (WSA) scale. *(The reviewers only provide data and analysis of symptoms as outcomes, and occupational outcomes were not included).*
(Kates & Mach 2007) Narrative review	**Chronic disease management for depression in primary care: a summary of the current literature and implications for practice** The objective of this review was to evaluate RCTs of chronic disease management models for depression in primary care in Canada. The results indicated most studies have demonstrated improved outcomes in terms of symptom reduction, relapse prevention, functioning in the community, adherence to treatment, community and workplace involvement, and satisfaction with care received. The authors concluded there is conclusive evidence for the benefits of changing systems of care delivery to support the more effective management of depression in primary care. A single RCT used work outcomes, and found significantly increased work productivity and reduced absenteeism *(this study compared usual care with an intervention that included training primary care providers in the model, guideline-based pharmacotherapy, guideline-based psychotherapy, and case managers who provided assessments, feedback, patient education, telephone follow-up. Cost data not available).* Their main recommendations for clinical practice were: primary care practices need to be able to regularly monitor individuals both during and after treatment of an episode of depression; and, psychiatrists can play important and effective roles by visiting primary care settings to discuss and assess individuals who suffer from depression. *(A description of method is not provided, even the number of included trials is not available).*
(Keane et al. 2006) Narrative review	**Posttraumatic stress disorder: etiology, epidemiology, and treatment outcome** Posttraumatic stress disorder (PTSD) results from exposure to a traumatic event that poses actual or threatened death or injury and produces intense fear, helplessness, or horror. Exposure to potentially traumatic events is quite common, but development of PTSD is rare in comparison. U.S. population surveys reveal lifetime PTSD prevalence rates of 7% to 8%. Potential reasons for varying prevalence rates across gender, cultures, and samples exposed to different traumas are discussed. Risk factors for PTSD are characteristics of the trauma, particularly peri-traumatic response and related cognitions, and post-trauma social support. Outcome studies indicate the most effective treatments are exposure therapies and anxiety management training as first-line treatment for PTSD. Among psychopharmacological treatments, selective serotonin reuptake inhibitors evidence the strongest treatment effects, yet these effects are modest compared with psychological treatments.
(Krupa 2007) Narrative review	**Interventions to improve employment outcomes for workers who experience mental illness** The objective was to review employment interventions for individuals who experience mental illness. The reviewer noted 7 distinct individual-level employment interventions (early identification, diagnosis, and treatment; assessment and planning; self-awareness counselling; coping skills training; work hardening; reasonable job accommodations; and, social network development) as well as interventions directed at the employer and at workplace organization. The reviewer noted there is a lack of high-level evidence for these employment interventions when used for mental illness. *(A description of method is not given. The number of included trials is not available).*

TABLE 4a: ANXIETY AND DEPRESSION (COMMON MENTAL HEALTH PROBLEMS)

(Layard 2006)	**The depression report: a new deal for depression and anxiety disorders**
Report	[London School of Economics]
	A report from the Centre for Economic Performance at the London School of Economics and Political Science. The report describes the problem that crippling depression and chronic anxiety are the biggest causes of misery in Britain today, and offers a solution. The argument advanced can be summarised as follows: One in six of the population can be diagnosed as having depression or a chronic anxiety disorder *(no evidence of severity is offered, beyond the statement that "we are not talking about the 'worried well'. We are talking about people whose lives are crippled by their distress". However, this view appears incongruous with the point-prevalence estimate that one-sixth of the population is affected, and therefore 'crippled').* This means that one in three families are affected. GPs offer medication, and some offer counselling, but only a quarter of people with depression or anxiety receives any kind of treatment *(this conclusion rests on the assumption that all individuals assessed by lay-interviewers should attract a medical diagnosis, and require treatment by a healthcare provider. Evidence to support this assumption was not provided. The alternative hypothesis that common mental health problems have become progressively 'medicalised' and destigmatised does not appear to have been considered). This is* partly due to people being unwilling to take medication due to disliking side effects, or because they want to control their own mood *(no evidence to support these statements is proffered. There is no exploration of potential interventions that might enhance willingness to take medications). The* situation is described as a tragedy and an expensive waste of people's lives. This is because depression and anxiety make it difficult or impossible to work *(given that 1 in 6 of the adult population is not off work due to these disorders, it seems clear that the majority do in fact continue to work, therefore the term 'impossible' seems overly strong).* There are now a million people on Incapacity Benefits (IB) because of mental illness, which is more than unemployment *(it is assumed that these cases will meet diagnostic criteria for depression or anxiety, yet no data is provided. The alternative explanation that many have entered under a general rubric such as 'stress' was not considered).* The solution offered is as follows: CBT is as effective as medication, and should be available to all people with depression or anxiety disorders according to NICE guidance, unless the problem is very mild *(the statement of equivalence between CBT and medication may not hold true if it were applied to one-sixth of the adult population each year. Again, evidence is not offered and this issue appears not to have been considered).* These could be cured at a cost of about £750, which is less than paying someone to be on IB for a month when extra benefits and lost taxes are taken into account *(the concept of a 'cure' alludes to abolition of symptoms, without their return. Major depression is considered to be self-limiting but often recurrent. The idea that 100% of cases might experience an outright cure appears naïve).* Therefore if the person works just a month more as a result of the treatment, the treatment pays for itself *(no information on work outcomes following treatment of depression and anxiety is provided; there is no discussion of cost-benefit for scenarios where less than 100% success rate is achieved).* A major expansion of NHS psychotherapy services is suggested, estimated as an additional 10,000 therapists, with the emphasis on cognitive-behavioural therapists *(no consideration is given to potential problems such as medicalising one-sixth of the adult population, and any problems such as dependency that might ensue).* Half would be 'clinical psychologists', and half would be trained from among the 60,000 nurses, social workers, occupational therapists and counsellors already working on mental health in the NHS. The report ends with a request for each reader to write to his or her MP to demand implementation of the solution outlined *(this emphasises the political nature of the report).*
(Leff 2001)	**The state of the evidence: mental health services and barriers to implementation**
Narrative review	Report completed from the Ministerial Round Tables meeting of 2001 at the 54th World Health Assembly, held under the title Mental Health: A Call For Action by World Health Ministers. Contains summaries of the 'state of the evidence' on four topics, including one about implementation barriers by Julian Leff (pages 23-37). This contains a section on the therapeutic value of work: Work is a crucial factor in the social reintegration of psychiatric patients. However, in developed countries it is very difficult to find a job if you have a history of mental illness... In order to improve the quality of life of people with mental illness living in the community, it is essential to forge strong links between mental health services and departments of employment, welfare and housing.

TABLE 4a: ANXIETY AND DEPRESSION (COMMON MENTAL HEALTH PROBLEMS)

(Lelliott et al. 2008) Report	**Mental health and work** [Report by the Royal College of Psychiatrists for the UK National Director for Work and Health]. Wide ranging report on the prevalence of mental health problems, impact and cost, stigma and discrimination, mental health and employment, mental health problems and worklessness, systems services and policy, and the research evidence about what works. Concluded that, despite their high prevalence in the workplace, there has been relatively little research about the effectiveness of interventions that assist people with common mental disorders to remain in work or return to work after a sickness absence. Summarised broadly similar conclusions from two recent reviews (Seymour & Grove 2005, Hill et al 2007) • For people who have common mental disorders that are affecting their work, brief individual therapy, mainly cognitive behavioural therapies, in short courses of up to eight weeks may be beneficial *(for clinical outcomes)*. Interventions should be comprehensive and address both individual and organisation-level factors. There is little evidence on organisation-level interventions alone and what there is shows mixed results. • When people are off work due to mental disorders an early return to work is aided by line managers keeping in touch at least once every two weeks. • Stress management techniques may improve people's ability to cope with stress and to avoid stressful situations at work. However, there is no firm evidence that stress management techniques reduce the prevalence of common mental illness or of sickness absence. Also, no studies have been conducted of the use of stress management in people who have already developed a common mental disorder. • Few of the many studies that demonstrate the effectiveness of a range of pharmacological and psychological treatments in treating common mental disorders have measured their impact on employment status, work performance or absenteeism. The few exceptions, which were mostly conducted in the United States, suggest that the overall gain in labour output is much less marked than the reduction in symptoms. • The conclusion of a systematic review, that counselling is effective in alleviating the symptoms of anxiety, stress and depression, and reduces sickness absence rates by 25–50% (McLeod 2001), has been challenged (Henderson et al. 2003; McLeod & Henderson 2003). Its critics contend that most of the studies reviewed have major methodological limitations and that the only true randomised controlled trial showed no benefit of counselling. There is at best an absence of evidence that workplace counselling improves occupational outcomes.
(Löthgren 2004a) Systematic review	**Economic evidence in affective disorders: a review** Six studies for depression were included in the review, three for bipolar disorder, and none for dysthymia. The reviewer noted one obvious conclusion is there is a paucity of literature regarding the costs of mood (affective) disorders in Europe. Of the six studies found for depression, four were from the UK, one from Spain and one from Sweden. Extrapolation of results is inadvisable. Estimates of direct costs are reasonably consistent between the few available studies, but are not consistent for the two studies that estimated indirect costs from short-term absence (neither included early retirement or mortality). *(The lack of research makes it difficult to draw conclusions).*
(Löthgren 2004b) Systematic review	**Economic evidence in anxiety disorders: a review** Only two studies were found for GAD, one from France and one from Hungary. One Spanish study was found for panic disorder. No studies were found for the other anxiety disorders. *(The lack of research makes it difficult to draw conclusions).*

TABLE 4a: ANXIETY AND DEPRESSION (COMMON MENTAL HEALTH PROBLEMS)

(McDaid et al. 2005) Narrative review	**Promoting mental well-being in the workplace: a European policy perspective** Across the European Union there is a trend of increasing absenteeism and early retirement due to mental health problems, particularly stress and depression. The social and economic costs of lost productivity in Europe are substantial. Moreover, the sustainability of social protection systems may be challenged further by increases in the levels of disability benefits paid to people who have left work on grounds of poor mental health. Yet despite these significant consequences, at both national and pan-European levels, decision-makers have been slow to recognise the importance of promoting mental health within the workplace, although recently there have been some positive developments. This paper outlines some of the socio-economic arguments for the promotion of good mental well-being in the labour force and identifies how they link with different national and European policy agendas around four key issues: economic growth and development, the promotion of a high level of public health, sustainability of social welfare systems and social inclusion. The role and activities to promote mental well-being in the workplace undertaken by both national and international organizations in Europe are outlined along with important gaps and challenges that need to be addressed. *(No evidence of the effect or impact of policy change is provided).*

(Mancuso 1990)
 	
Narrative review
	Reasonable accommodation for workers with psychiatric disabilities
	
	This article was originally written in response to the requirement contained in the Americans with Disabilities Act of 1990 for employers to make 'reasonable accommodations' for workers with disabilities. Beyond the legal and definitional discussion, the author attempts to outline practical guidance for workplace accommodations *(that may facilitate SAW/RTW)*. These cover four key areas of worker function:
	
	1. Changes in communication
	  • Arrange for work requests to be put in writing for a worker who becomes anxious and confused when given verbal instructions
	  • Train a supervisor to provide positive feedback along with criticisms of performance, for an employee re-entering the work force who needs to be reassured of their abilities after a long psychiatric hospitalization
	  • Allow a worker who personalizes negative comments about their work performance to provide a self-appraisal before receiving feedback from a supervisor
	  • Schedule daily planning sessions with a co-worker at the start of each day to develop hourly goals for someone who functions best with a clear time structure
	2. Modifications to the physical environment
	  • Provide room dividers for a worker who has difficulty maintaining concentration (and thus accuracy) in an open work area
	3. Job modifications
	  • Arrange for someone who cannot drive or use public transport to work at home
	  • Restructure a receptionist job by eliminating lunchtime switchboard duty
	  • Exchange problematic secondary tasks for part of another employee's job description
	4. Schedule modification
	  • Allow a worker with poor physical stamina to extend their schedule to allow for additional breaks or rest periods during the day
	  • Allow a worker to shift their schedule to attend psychotherapy appointments
	(This is a pre-2000 publication but has been retained because it contains highly practical recommendations, and these have not been superseded to date).

TABLE 4a: ANXIETY AND DEPRESSION (COMMON MENTAL HEALTH PROBLEMS)

(McIntosh et al. 2004)	**Clinical guidelines and evidence review for panic disorder and generalised anxiety disorder**
	[UK National Institute for Clinical Excellence]
Clinical guideline	Stepped care:

Step 1: Recognition and diagnosis of panic disorder and generalised anxiety disorder

- The diagnostic process should elicit necessary relevant information such as personal history, any self-medication, and cultural or other individual characteristics that may be important considerations in subsequent care. (See also 'Which NICE guideline', page 12).

Step 2: Offer treatment in primary care

- There are positive advantages of services based in primary care practice (for example, lower drop-out rates) and these services are often preferred by patients.
- The treatment of choice should be available promptly.

Panic disorder

- Benzodiazepines are associated with a less good outcome in the long term and should not be prescribed for the treatment of individuals with panic disorder.
- Any of the following types of intervention should be offered and the preference of the person should be taken into account. The interventions that have evidence for the longest duration of effect, in descending order, are:

  1. psychological therapy (cognitive behavioural therapy [CBT])
  2. pharmacological therapy (a selective serotonin reuptake inhibitor [SSRI] licensed for panic disorder; or if an SSRI is unsuitable or there is no improvement, imipramine or clomipramine may be considered)
  3. self-help (bibliotherapy – the use of written material to help people understand their psychological problems and learn ways to overcome them by changing their behaviour – based on CBT principles).

Generalised anxiety disorder

- Benzodiazepines should not usually be used beyond 2–4 weeks.
- In the longer-term care of individuals with generalised anxiety disorder, any of the following types of intervention should be offered and the preference of the person with generalised anxiety disorder should be taken into account. The interventions that have evidence for the longest duration of effect, in descending order, are:

  1. psychological therapy (CBT)
  2. pharmacological therapy (an SSRI)
  3. self-help (bibliotherapy based on CBT principles).

Step 3: Review and offer alternative treatment

- If one type of intervention does not work, the patient should be reassessed and consideration given to trying one of the other types of intervention.

Step 4: Review and offer referral from primary care

- In most instances, if there have been two interventions provided (any combination of psychological intervention, medication, or bibliotherapy) and the person still has significant symptoms, then referral to specialist mental health services should be offered.

Step 5: Care in specialist mental health services

(Nothing on vocational rehabilitation or occupational outcomes).

TABLE 4a: ANXIETY AND DEPRESSION (COMMON MENTAL HEALTH PROBLEMS)

(McLeod 2001; McLeod & McLeod 2001) Report	**Counselling in the workplace: the facts** **How effective is workplace counselling? A review of the research literature** [British Association for Counselling and Psychotherapy Report] *(Although described as a systematic review, it does not meet the generally accepted definition).* Workplace counselling was defined as brief psychological therapy for employees who feel under stress at work, provided by the employer. An 'external' service, such as an Employee Assistance Programme (EAP), typically comprises face-to-face counselling, a telephone help-line, legal advice and critical-incident debriefing. In an 'in-house' service, counsellors may be directly employed by the organisation. The review included more than 80 pieces of work covering the experiences of over 10,000 clients over more than 45 years: controlled studies, naturalistic studies in which reliable pre- and post-counselling data were collected, and case studies. Employees who received counselling were highly satisfied, and believed it had helped them resolve their problem. Work-related symptoms returned to normal in more than half of all clients. Clinically significant improvement in levels of anxiety and depression was reported in 60-75% of clients. Counselling was associated with more than 25% reduction in sickness absence and improvement in other organisational outcomes such as more positive work attitudes, fewer accidents and enhanced work performance. The results were presented as clear and unequivocal: that counselling is an effective treatment for anxiety, depression and substance misuse, as well as 'stress'. *(This review has been subject to severe scientific criticism: (Henderson et al. 2003; Lelliott et al. 2008; McLeod & Henderson 2003)* Most of the studies had major methodological weaknesses. The studies were limited by small sample sizes, short follow-up periods and wide variation in the form and content of the therapy given. Even in the 'best evidence' section only 5 out of 19 studies had a form of non-treatment control group: of these, two used controls who were not seeking any form of help at all and one used those who dropped out at the first session as controls. There was only one randomised controlled trial and that showed no benefit of counselling. Workplace counselling does appear to give employee satisfaction, but there was insufficient data to conclude that it produced meaningful clinical improvement or consistent employment objectives such as reduced absenteeism. The Royal College of Psychiatrists (2008) concluded that 'There is at best an absence of evidence that workplace counselling improves occupational outcomes'.
(Michie & Williams 2003) Systematic review	**Reducing work related psychological ill health and sickness absence: a systematic literature review** The primary focus of this review was the association between work factors and psychological ill health among health care staff. However, because of the paucity of evidence in health care, evidence was reviewed across all work settings, although presented separately for health care workers. 40 studies were included in the review, including some prospective and longitudinal. Results indicated that key work factors associated with psychological ill health and sickness absence in staff are long hours worked, work overload and pressure, and the effects of these on personal lives; lack of control over work; lack of participation in decision making; poor social support; and unclear management and work role. There was some evidence that sickness absence is associated with poor management style. Six of the included studies were intervention studies (using 2519 subjects), three of which were RCTs. Successful interventions that improved psychological health and levels of sickness absence used training and organisational approaches to increase participation in decision making and problem solving, to increase support and feedback, and to improve communication. The authors concluded that many of the work related variables associated with high levels of psychological ill health are potentially amenable to change, as shown in intervention studies that have successfully improved psychological health and reduced sickness absence. However, only 2 of these six intervention studies had work outcomes: one *(quasi-experimental)* an individual-level intervention where communication skills development was found to have a positive influence on the absence rates of direct care psychiatric staff; the other *(a case series)* an organisational-level intervention to reduce referral time to occupational health from 6 to 2-3 months for local authority staff, which reduced sickness absence 40 weeks in the control period to 25 weeks in the intervention period. *(This review indicates the potential for uncomplicated interventions to reduce sickness absence, but the level of evidence is low from a single quasi-experimental study (n=65) and a case series (n=604)).*

TABLE 4a: ANXIETY AND DEPRESSION (COMMON MENTAL HEALTH PROBLEMS)

(Neumeyer-Gromen et al. 2004) Systematic review	**Disease management programs for depression: a systematic review and meta-analysis of randomized controlled trials** Identified 10 randomised controlled trials on disease management programmes (DMP) for depression in adults. They defined DMP by use of evidence-based practice guidelines, patient self-management education and provider education, population-screening process. DMP is a population-based care strategy for highly prevalent chronic diseases with major care deficits of economic relevance. Depression meets these relevance criteria. The included studies were graded with all but one awarded high quality rating. Meta-analysis results indicated: Depression severity: RR=.75 (95% CI .70-.81) for DMP compared to usual care, assessed dichotomously by at least 50% improvement, n=3928 Patient satisfaction: RR=.57 (95% CI .37-.87) for DMP compared to usual care, n=1077 Adherence to treatment regimen: RR=.59 (95% CI .46-.75) for DMP, n=3618 Health-related quality of life (HRQOL): 4 studies corroborated significantly better intervention effect of DMP, n=2544 Employment status: significantly more likely to be still employed at 12 months, n=1356 Provider satisfaction: all primary care providers preferred DMP, one study only, n=370 Economic evaluations: In all studies DMP increased costs compared to usual care, n=2784. Authors noted that costs for DMP are well within range of accepted medical/public health interventions. Authors concluded use of DMP for depression significantly enhanced the quality of care for depression.
(NHS 1999) UK National Service Framework	**National Service Framework for mental health** [UK National Health Service] The introduction states that mental illnesses are common, affecting one in six adults at any point in time, and that the UK government is determined to give mental health a much higher priority. The National Service Framework for Mental Health spells out national standards for mental health, what they aim to achieve, how they should be developed and delivered and how to measure performance in every part of the country. This National Service Framework sets out standards in five areas; each standard is supported by the evidence and knowledge base, by service models, and by examples of good practice. Local milestones are proposed; time-scales need to be agreed with NHS Executive regional offices and social care regions, and progress will be monitored. • Standard one addresses mental health promotion and combats the discrimination and social exclusion associated with mental health problems. • Standards two and three cover primary care and access to services for any one who may have a mental health problem. • Standards four and five encompass the care of people with severe mental illness. • Standard six relates to individuals who care for people with mental health problems. • Standard seven draws together the action necessary to achieve the target to reduce suicides as set out in Saving lives: Our Healthier Nation Advice is provided on local implementation, ensuring progress, and national support for local action. *(Mentions work as a cause of stress and mental ill-health, but nothing significant on vocational rehabilitation or occupational outcomes).*

TABLE 4a: ANXIETY AND DEPRESSION (COMMON MENTAL HEALTH PROBLEMS)

(NICE 2004a; NICE 2007) Clinical guideline & amendments	**Management of depression in primary and secondary care** [UK National Institute for Clinical Excellence] 'People who have had severe or chronic depression may require special help in returning to work. Work provides a number of protective factors for depression including structure to a day, social contacts and self-esteem.' 'Where a Patient's depression has resulted in loss of work or social disengagement from other social activities over a longer term, a rehabilitation programme addressing these difficulties should be considered. (Recommendation grading C / evidence level IV – Expert committee reports or opinions and/or clinical experience of respected authorities).' *(No further detail on vocational rehabilitation interventions or evidence on effectiveness).*
(NICE 2006) Technology appraisal	**Computerised cognitive behavioural therapy for anxiety and depression** [UK National Institute for Clinical Excellence] Fourteen studies (six RCTs, two non-RCTs and six non-comparative studies) were identified for the five packages included in the review. Some of trials had considerably more female than male participants, particularly in the case of depression. In most studies, the mean age of patients was in the range 30–45 years. In the majority of trials, patients were included who were also taking medications for their particular disorder. Multiple outcomes using multiple measures were collected. In summary, the technology appraisal recommended the following packages for the management of people with common mental health conditions for whom this type of intervention is appropriate: • *Beating the Blues* ® as an option for delivering computer-based cognitive behavioural therapy (cCBT) in the management of mild and moderate depression (Statistically significant improvement in Beck Depressive Inventory score (effect size 0.65) compared with treatment as usual). • *FearFighter*™ as an option for delivering computer-based cognitive behavioural therapy (cCBT) in the management of panic and phobia (Statistically significant improvement, comparable to Therapist CBT). The cost benefit analysis assumed that 64% of CBT would be provided using a computer. This would translate into significant cost savings of between £116 million and £136 million per annum in England compared to therapist face to face provision. *(Nothing on vocational rehabilitation or occupational outcomes).*
(NICE 2008) Evidence review	**Workplace interventions that are effective for promoting mental wellbeing: synopsis of the evidence of effectiveness and cost-effectiveness** [UK National Institute for Clinical Excellence] This evidence review was conducted for the public health intervention advisory committee because NICE was asked by the Department of Health (DH) to develop guidance for employers on promoting mental wellbeing through productive and healthy working conditions. The review considered studies that assessed the effectiveness of workplace interventions aimed at either promoting or improving mental wellbeing. <u>Organisational Level Interventions</u> (a) Changing working/organisational practices: insufficient…*[about]*…organisational participatory interventions in the workplace to improve mental wellbeing (b) Training Supervisors and Managers: insufficient evidence…*[about]*…the impact of different types of supervisory training on the mental wellbeing in subordinate workers

TABLE 4a: ANXIETY AND DEPRESSION (COMMON MENTAL HEALTH PROBLEMS)

(c) Altering Shift or Work Practices: there is evidence that taking a vacation or changing the shift system has an impact on mental wellbeing and burnout, but this may be short-term and last only 3 weeks

(d) Support or training to improve skills or job role: Psychosocial Intervention courses can have a positive impact on burnout in the short term. The longer term impact is unknown

Stress Management Interventions (individual-level)

(a) Training to cope with stress: a number of approaches do have a positive impact on mental wellbeing including Affect School, Cognitive Training, group sessions, face-to-face feedback, and paper-based approaches, rather than web-based training or mail-shots followed up by telephone calls

(b) Counselling and therapy: Acceptance and Commitment Therapy, an Innovation Promotion Programme about changing sources of stress and a computerised Cognitive Behavioural Therapy programme had an effect on anxiety and depressive symptoms in the short term

(c) Exercise and relaxation interventions: results in two [of three] studies indicate that aerobic exercise has a positive effect on mental wellbeing; but, there is insufficient research available at the moment to state whether relaxation training has a positive or negative impact on mental wellbeing.

(d) Health promotion interventions: using health promotion methods which included aspects of improving mental wellbeing, can improve mental wellbeing in the individuals being assessed. However, one of the difficulties with the use of broader health promotion approaches is singling out which part of a multiple intervention is having the impact

Economic analyses

With respect to costs, the reviewers reported: There appears to be no research published since 1990 reporting the cost-effectiveness, cost-utility or cost-benefit of worksite interventions that directly promote mental wellbeing in the workplace. NICE generated a hypothetical economic model to generate cost estimates, based on results from three stress-management studies. This model suggested work-site interventions to promote the mental wellbeing of employees can reduce absence costs…[and]…save employers between £495 and £5,160 per affected employee per year; and, the net-benefit to employers of implementing interventions to promote the mental wellbeing of employees ranges from negative £220 to positive £1,155 per affected employee participating in the programme, incorporating solely the intervention-induced reductions in absence costs. Including the intervention-induced reductions in presenteeism as well, the net-benefit to employers ranges from positive £130 to positive £5,020 per affected employee participating in the programme.

(This review focused on the effect of interventions to promote mental health in the workplace, and did not consider vocational rehabilitation. However, the findings have relevance for the latter in as much that SAW/RTW approaches may be facilitated by the presence of a 'healthy' workplace or undermined by a 'toxic' one).

TABLE 4a: ANXIETY AND DEPRESSION (COMMON MENTAL HEALTH PROBLEMS)

(Nieuwenhuijsen et al. 2008) Cochrane review	**Interventions to improve occupational health in depressed people** Depressive disorders have a negative effect on work functioning. The objective of this review was to evaluate the effectiveness of interventions aimed at improving occupational health in employees with depressive disorders. 9 RCTs and 2 cluster-randomised trials were included. However no studies directed at the workplace were identified, all interventions were aimed at the individual level. Interventions included antidepressant medication, psychological interventions, a combination of these, and enhanced primary care. Only one study specifically addressed work issues during treatment (by occupational therapy), the others just presented occupational health outcome measures. One study (n=57) found that psychodynamic therapy in combination with Tricyclic Antidepressant medication was more effective in reducing the number of days of sickness absence than medication alone. Four studies found no difference between various different medications for sickness absence. Two single studies found no difference between cCBT or problem-solving therapy compared to usual primary care for sickness absence. Two studies found no significant effect of enhanced primary care for sickness absence. The reviewers concluded that: Limited evidence is available for the lack of effect of most interventions that aim to improve occupational health in depressed workers. We can cautiously conclude that those interventions alone do not enhance the occupational health of depressed workers. Evidence from one trial showed that the combination of psychodynamic therapy and antidepressant medication has a positive effect compared to medication alone. A combination of interventions seems to yield the best chance of increasing occupational health of depressed workers. *(Given that no studies directed at the workplace were identified, this review is in fact a review of vocational outcomes for interventions aimed at the individual. Therefore, the findings demonstrate that symptomatic treatment of depression by either medication, psychotherapy, or a combination of both, do not by themselves enhance vocational outcomes).*
(Ofman et al. 2004) Systematic review	**Does disease management improve clinical and economic outcomes in patients with chronic diseases?** Stated that 20 studies on depression were included in the review, but no summary of results was provided. In the discussion it was reported: Disease management programmes for patients with depression had the highest percentage of comparisons (48% [41/86]) showing substantial improvements in patient care. *(This referred to a simple count of the number of comparisons that were statistically significant, without any information about design of the studies, effect sizes, type of subjects, outcomes measured, etc. No information about work, or costs).*
(Olsheski et al. 2002) Conceptual review	**Disability management and psychosocial rehabilitation: considerations for integration** The authors argue that while disability management has been successful in accommodating physical disabilities in the workplace, this is not true for psychological/mental health related disabilities. Suggests that integration of the principles and strategies of psychosocial rehabilitation into disability management programmes should help to protect these individuals' employability and control sickness absence costs. Suggested principles include: • Joint employee-management steering committee for programme development, implementation and operation. • Job analysis: functional limitations due to mental health problems are different from physical disabilities. Adjustments are less tangible and harder to plan and implement. Individual mental functional capacities need to be linked to work performance, e.g. understanding and memory, concentration, social interaction and adaptation. • Supervisors need to be educated about the individual's strengths, limitations and the nature of adjustments required. • Transitional return to work programmes: but the goal of such transitional programmes is to return to the original job. • Supported employment: however, due to the stigma attached to mental illness, job coaching functions may have to be more discrete and subtle to protect confidentiality.

TABLE 4a: ANXIETY AND DEPRESSION (COMMON MENTAL HEALTH PROBLEMS)

	• Suitable mental health professionals could evaluate the worker's functional limitations from their mental health problem, analyse the mental and psychological requirements of the job, recommend specific job adjustments, and monitor the worker's progress. • Staff development and training: developing understanding of their role in supporting a 'return to work / stay at work' philosophy. • Case management, to provide essential communication and coordination. • Employers can create an organisational climate that allows for the integration of psychosocial rehabilitation into the return to work process. • In conclusion, although psychosocial rehabilitation interventions have been used primarily for severe mental health conditions, many of the principles and services could be integrated into disability management programmes to assist workers with common mental health problems.
(Pirraglia et al. 2004) Systematic review	**Cost-utility analysis studies of depression management: a systematic review** Identified 9 cost-utility analyses of depression management from a registry of 539 studies published between 1976 and 2001, reflecting a relative paucity of literature on the topic. Objective was to identify cost-utility of depression screening, pharmacologic treatment, nonpharmacologic therapy, and case management. Results indicated that pharmacologic interventions generally had lower costs per quality-adjusted life year than nonpharmacologic interventions. Nearly all studies reported less than $50,000 per quality-adjusted life year *(authors pointed out that the often-used cutoff is $50,000)*. Psychotherapy alone ($34,000), case management alone ($24,000 to $76,000), and psychotherapy plus case management ($24,000) all had lower costs per quality-adjusted life year than usual care. Depression screening and treatment appeared to fall within the cost-utility ranges accepted for common nonpsychiatric medical conditions. One-time screening in primary care had a favourable cost-utility ratio, but screening every 5 years was a marginally high cost per quality-adjusted life year ($55,000), and annual screening cam at a high cost ($210,000). *(These results suggest that regular depression screening is expensive, but may have a acceptable cost for one-time applications. Both psychotherapy and case management can add utility to the management of depression at reasonable expense)*
(Rinaldi & Perkins 2007) Narrative review	**Vocational rehabilitation for people with mental health problems** The majority of people with mental health problems want to work, yet they have the lowest employment rate for any disabled group of people in the UK. Research shows that unemployment is linked to worsening physical and mental health, whilst having a job is good for a person's physical and mental health and can lead to a reduction in symptoms, fewer hospital admissions and reduced service use. Mental health professionals have an important role in promoting employment opportunities for people with mental health problems, in terms of helping them to both gain and retain employment. However, evidence suggests that all too often the advice and guidance given by mental health professionals is not in line with the research evidence available for helping people with mental health problems gain and retain employment. There is currently a range of vocational rehabilitation services for people with mental health problems provided or commissioned by mental health services, though few are evidence-based in their approach. Over the last decade there have been significant developments in an evidence-based approach within vocational rehabilitation for people with severe mental health problems which have demonstrated that people can gain and retain employment. The Department of Health has published guidance on vocational services for people with severe mental health problems. In addition, there is an emerging evidence base identifying factors and interventions that promote job retention. The extent to which mental health services promote confidence in work is critical if success is to be achieved. *(The main focus is on severe mental illness).*

TABLE 4a: ANXIETY AND DEPRESSION (COMMON MENTAL HEALTH PROBLEMS)

(Royal College of Psychiatrists 2002) Narrative review	**Employment opportunities and psychiatric disability** Key findings: • Work plays a central role in people's lives and is a key factor in social inclusion. • Work is important in maintaining and promoting mental and physical health and social functioning. Being in work creates a virtuous circle; being out of work creates a vicious circle. • Work is important in promoting the recovery of those who have experienced mental health problems. • Barriers to work for people with severe mental illness include structural factors, stigma and prejudice, attitudes and approaches of the mental health services and the lack of well-run employment schemes. • Partnerships and interagency working are crucial to developing employment services for people with psychiatric disabilities. • Key factors for putting partnerships into practice include: developing a user focus, finding partners, communication, oiling the wheels, commitment from the top, addressing boundary problems, achieving a professional approach, being tuned in, understanding the local business scene, and evaluation of schemes. • General practitioners (GP), through their clinical management and provision of advice on fitness to work, are in a key position to influence and sometimes determine a patient's trajectory through the employment system. • The longer that a person is off work for illness reasons, the less chance he or she has of returning to work. • It is likely that a rapid response and assistance into rehabilitation can help the return to work. • Attitudes of mental health services and lack of effective schemes act as barriers to getting people with psychiatric disabilities into work. • Community mental health teams (CMHTs) and specialist rehabilitation services are the main components of the mental health services that have a role to play in assisting users into work and supporting them there. • Mental health services currently place insufficient emphasis on returning people to work and there is no specific provision for work schemes or work liaison schemes in CMHTs. • CMHTs are ideally placed to take the lead in coordinating the vocational rehabilitation of those with psychiatric disabilities, but they presently lack sufficient expertise in welfare advice and vocational work. Specialist vocational workers are required in CMHTs. Since March 2002 the Care Programme Approach has had to include plans to 'secure suitable employment or other occupational activity'. • Vocational services must be supported by other suitable, quality mental health services to improve the functioning of those with mental illnesses and to offer a spectrum of in-patient, day patient and other community services. • Maintaining people in work is important, and close liaison between employers and CMHTs plays a key role in achieving good employment outcomes. • Communication and liaison between GPs, mental health professionals and occupational health staff is an essential part of keeping people with psychiatric disabilities in work or getting them back to work. General practitioners should: • always consider how clinical management would support a patient back into work; • review the patient before the first 6 weeks of certified incapacity, to reduce the chances of long-term sickness; • try to keep positive expectations about patients' return to work; • emphasise progress and offer appropriate therapy where possible; • differentiate between the risk of losing an existing job and the problems of getting back into work after a long absence; • communicate as clearly as possible with the employer within the constraints of ethics and confidentiality.

TABLE 4a: ANXIETY AND DEPRESSION (COMMON MENTAL HEALTH PROBLEMS)

| (Rose 2006)

Conceptual review | **A model of care for managing traumatic psychological injury in a workers' compensation context**

Conceptual discussion and pragmatic model of care that attempts to describe a best practice approach with the 'right service at the right time' suitable for psychological sequelae to workplace traumas (including robberies, assaults, motor vehicle accidents, severe physical injuries, and witnessing fatalities). Delivery based in Alberta workers compensation environment, includes integrated case management. The authors provide discussion about important debates such as provision of critical incident debriefing, use of medications for acute stress disorder and post-traumatic stress disorder. Their model suggests:

- Pre-trauma preparation interventions such as training for high risk workers
- Acute stress management, from the day of trauma for up to 2 weeks, with aim to prevent chronic problems. Suggest techniques should (1) normalise reactions through providing information, (2) encourage uptake of suitable interventions, and accessing normal social supports, (3) stress management techniques, (4) identify high levels of distress for selected referrals, (5) provide debriefing opportunity, and (6) relief of irrational guilt by counselling.
- Work site reintegration to commence within 8 weeks.
- Medical management from day of trauma lasting up to 26 weeks including treatment of physical injuries, initial pharmacological treatment for acute stress, pharmacological treatment of post traumatic stress disorder and any comorbid conditions, ongoing medical management of comorbid physical injuries.
- Psychological screening provided at about 2 to 4 weeks post injury. Goal is to identify acute stress disorder with aim of preventing progression, or ameliorating severity of post traumatic stress disorder.
- Psychotherapy from 2 weeks following injury. Suggest cognitive-behavioural therapy (CBT) for 8 to 12 weeks, or eye movement desensitisation and reprocessing (EMDR) for up to 12 sessions.
- Comprehensive psychological assessment 12 to 16 weeks after injury, but suggest earlier if mild traumatic brain injury also involved. Determine effectiveness of psychotherapy and medications to date, psychiatric referral if necessary.
- Case manager, plays key role in transition points between different phases of care.

Noted there is little data on long-term follow-up for psychotherapies or medications, but suggest there may be a role for some 'booster session' over the next 1 or 2 years. Pilot implementation noted this model is feasible and effective in obtaining better outcomes *(assumed to be return to work)*, with challenges such unwillingness to participate due to mental health stigma, and fear of escalating claim costs. |
| (Roth & Fonagy 2005)

Book | **What works for whom? a critical review of psychotherapy research**

Depression. 1-year prevalence in age 18-54 for Major Depressive Disorder (MDD) is 4.5%, and Dysthymia is 1.6%. Prevalence among women is bout double that among men. Relapse occurs in 75% within 10 years, and 85% within 15 years. 80% of those with Dysthymia will develop MDD. The effectiveness of treatment needs to be judged by capacity to manage the index episode and ability to maintain remission. Depression treatment effectiveness: The best quality studies demonstrate effectiveness of both Interpersonal Psychotherapy (IPT) and CBT, and these have equivalent effectiveness. It is reasonable to conclude they are both as effective as medication. For the less severely depressed 8 sessions are needed, but 16 are needed for the more severely depressed. There is some suggestion of benefit from combining therapies, but this is hard to demonstrate. Predicting relapse in individual patients is difficult, but 'booster' sessions for those considered vulnerable are effective, but it is costly. In primary care, CBT, IPT and nondirective counselling all seem reasonably effective but in the short-term. Treatment for Dysthymia: There is much less research. Available evidence suggests that adding psychotherapy to medication confers little advantage. |

TABLE 4a: ANXIETY AND DEPRESSION (COMMON MENTAL HEALTH PROBLEMS)

Bipolar Disorder. 1-year prevalence rate of 1%, with men and women equally affected. It is usually a recurrent disorder, with more than 80% of those having one manic episode going on to have further episodes. Both the manic and depressive episodes are more frequent than depressive episodes in MDD. In 5-15% there are four or more episodes within one year. Rapid cycling is associated with poorer prognosis. The majority return to functioning between episodes, but 20-30% continues to have difficulties. Psychological interventions will almost certainly be adjunctive to medication. Lithium provides a prophylactic response in about two-thirds.

Anxiety Disorders

Specific Phobia. Lifetime prevalence is 11.3%, 1-year prevalence is 8.8%. 70-85% respond well to exposure treatments.

Social Phobia. 6-month prevalence is between 1% and 2.6%. CBT and variants of CBT, including exposure.

Generalised Anxiety Disorder (GAD). 1-year prevalence is between 2.3% and 6.4%. Relaxation therapy, and CBT are the most effective. Applied relaxation, exposure and variants of CBT are treatments of choice. Relatively brief treatments of 12-15 sessions appear to be effective. Effect sizes for cognitive and behavioural interventions tend to be larger than for medication.

Panic Disorder with and without Agoraphobia. 6-month prevalence is 6% for agoraphobia, and 3% for panic disorder.

The prevalence for all these disorders is considerably higher in women than in men: 60% higher for panic, 30% higher for agoraphobia, and 50% higher for social phobia. In community surveys it is usual to find that >50% of identified cases are untreated. Between 30 and 80% with a principal diagnosis of anxiety have at least one other anxiety disorder. The highest rates of comorbidity with a current mood disorder are with GAD (26%). Anxiety disorders are usually chronic and persistent. Applied relaxation, exposure, and variants of CBT are effective, using about 12 to 15 sessions.

Obsessive-Compulsive Disorder (OCD). Lifetime prevalence is 2.2% to 3.0%, 6-month prevalence is 1.5%. The disorder appears to be chronic. Nearly 50% of OCD patients have a phobic disorder, 31% a major depressive disorder, and 24% substance abuse. Exposure and response prevention (ERP), and other cognitive and behavioural approaches are treatments of choice. Patients with comorbid depression present a therapeutic challenge.

Post-traumatic Stress Disorder (PTSD). Lifetime prevalence is between 1% and 2.6%. Often associated with significant comorbidity. Many individuals exposed to trauma do not develop PTSD. Once present, it can be a disabling and persistent condition. Some form of 'psychological debriefing' is often provided, but this appears to be ineffective. Psychological treatments are effective for PTSD, and this includes CBT and eye movement desensitisation and reprocessing (EMDR).

Eating Disorders:

Anorexia Nervosa. Prevalence is between 0.5% and 1% in women in late adolescence and young adulthood.

Bulimia Nervosa. Prevalence is between 15 and 3%.

Prevalence for eating disorder is lower in men than in women., and this is more pronounced for anorexia. CBT has large effect sizes, but a combination with medication appears to of benefit.

Schizophrenia. Annual incidence is 0.01%, and lifetime prevalence is 0.34%. The course is chronic usually. Neuroleptic medication is the treatment of choice, a substantial proportion of patients will remain troubled by symptoms. Psychosocial interventions, of a wide variety may be helpful. *(Substance abuse and dependence, sexual dysfunction have been omitted from this summary since they are not the focus of this report).*

TABLE 4a: ANXIETY AND DEPRESSION (COMMON MENTAL HEALTH PROBLEMS)

(Sanderson & Andrews 2006)) Systematic review	**Common mental disorders in the workforce: recent findings from descriptive and social epidemiology**
	The objective was to review the recent descriptive and social epidemiology of common mental disorders in the workplace, including prevalence, participation, work disability, and impact of quality of work, as well as to discuss the implications for identifying targets for clinical and preventive interventions. The reviewers identified epidemiologic studies in community settings (that is, in the general population or in workplaces). Findings were as follows:
	Descriptive Epidemiology - Prevalence and Participation
	Depression and simple phobia were found to be the most prevalent disorders in the working population.
	The limited data on rates of participation suggested higher participation among people with depression, simple phobia, social phobia, and generalized anxiety disorder.
	Descriptive Epidemiology - Work Disability
	Depression and anxiety were more consistently associated with 'presenteeism' (that is, lost productivity while at work) than with absenteeism, whether this was measured by cutback days or by direct questionnaires.
	Social Epidemiology
	3 workplace cohort studies involving a total of more than 30 000 participants, jobs with low autonomy (skill discretion) and those with high demands increased the psychiatric risk by 24% to 63%. Two of these studies used middle-aged respondents from specific industries (the civil service and the gas and electricity sector)
	Seven longitudinal studies, with an average sample size of 6264, showed a strong association between aspects of low job quality and incident depression and anxiety. There was some evidence that atypical work was associated with poorer mental health, although the findings for fixed-term work were mixed.
	The authors concluded there is strong evidence that an unfavourable psychosocial work environment is an independent risk factor for depressive and anxiety symptoms, and therefore mental health risk reduction in the workplace is an important complement to clinical interventions for reducing the current and future burden of depression and anxiety in the workplace.

(SCMH 2007) Policy Paper	**Mental health at work: developing the business case** [Sainsbury Centre for Mental Health]
	Outlines the business costs of mental ill health in UK:
	• £8.4 billion per year in sickness absence. Average employee takes 7 days off sick each year, of which 40% are for mental health problems
	• £15.1 billion a year in reduced productivity
	• £2.4 billion a year in replacing staff who leave jobs due to mental health problems
	Simple steps to improve management of mental health in the workplace include prevention and early identification should enable employers to save at least 30% or more of these costs – at least £8 billion per year. These are:
	• Take action to promote mental wellbeing among staff – e.g. awareness training for line managers
	• Give better help to those experiencing distress – especially access to evidence-based psychological treatments
	• Support those who need time off to come back to work – e.g. maintain regular contact.

TABLE 4a: ANXIETY AND DEPRESSION (COMMON MENTAL HEALTH PROBLEMS)

(Schneider 2003) Briefing document	**Employment for people with mental health problems** [UK Department of Health] The aim of this study was to add to the knowledge yielded by the Cochrane review on vocational rehabilitation for people with severe mental illness. It included a review of 225 additional studies published since 1991. The reviewers found strong evidence that service users are more likely to get jobs and keep them if they are not impeded by poor social skills and 'negative' symptoms (e.g. withdrawal, lethargy), but also if they: have worked before; have positive attitudes towards work; are placed as soon as possible in a job of their choice; receive preparation targeted at work rather than general training; receive ongoing support in their job; actively participate in an occupational intervention; and, are not worse off financially as a result of working. They also concluded that vocational services seem to be more effective at getting people into work when integrated with mental health teams. The Individual Placement and Support (IPS) model of supported employment has strong evidence in its favour, but it was noted that it may not suit everyone at all times. IPS can be delivered through job brokers, Workstep or existing voluntary and statutory employment schemes. Integration with the community mental health team is a critical requirement in doing so. *(Based mainly on evidence from severe mental illness, though some of the argument appears generally applicable to common mental health problems).*
(Seymour & Grove 2005) Report	**Workplace interventions for people with common mental health problems: evidence review and recommendations** [British Occupational Health Research Foundation report] This report defined common mental health problems as those that: occur most frequently and are more prevalent; are mostly successfully treated in primary rather than secondary care settings; and, are least disabling in terms of stigmatising attitudes and discriminatory behaviour. Concluded that for the: 1. Job retention of employees at risk: *** individual approaches to stress reduction, management and prevention for a range of health care professionals are effective and are preferable to multi-modal approaches. 2. Rehabilitation of employees with sickness absence associated with mental health problems: *** cognitive behavioural (CBT) interventions are effective and they are more effective than other intervention types. CBT is most effective for workers in high-control jobs. ** brief (up to 8 weeks) therapeutic interventions such as individual counselling are effective for employees with job-related or psychological distress *(This review did not distinguish clinical and occupational outcomes. Checking their original sources for the effectiveness of CBT, suggests that most of their conclusions are primarily about clinical outcomes and are not accurate for work outcomes).* Round Table Discussions at the launch of the Report supported these conclusions and expanded upon several points: 1. Common health problems (CMP) at work are generally labelled 'stress' but the same problems outwith work tend to be given different diagnoses. 2. Health professionals need to take a more balanced approach to CMPs. E.g. GPs need to be informed that work can have positive therapeutic effects (evidence shows that work is more often good for mental health than bad for it). 3. Practical tools need to be developed to implement evidence-based individual level interventions.

TABLE 4a: ANXIETY AND DEPRESSION (COMMON MENTAL HEALTH PROBLEMS)

4. Good quality research is needed into organisational level interventions.

5. Good cost-benefit studies are required to establish the business case and persuade employers and others to invest in better management of CMPs.

6. The question was raised whether the findings in this Report were compatible with the HSE Stress Management Standards. The response was that these were really looking at two different things. The stress management standards focus specifically on workplace issues and interventions, and acknowledge that there is currently a lack of evidence on some of these issues. Even if workplace issues were resolved, there would still be a lot of CMPs and these would impact on work. This Report focuses on the management of these CMPs.

(Simon et al. 2001) Narrative review	**Depression and work productivity** The authors conducted a literature search *(they did not provide any information on the method, or the number of studies they identified)*. They found that cross-sectional naturalistic studies indicated major depression is one of the health conditions associated with the greatest work loss and work cutback. The longitudinal naturalistic studies, conducted mostly in primary care, provided consistent evidence that work performance is responsive to change in depression symptoms *(lack of control group means causal relationship remains uncertain)*. Uncontrolled treatment studies (case series) indicated that work impairment reduces following successful treatment, although the remission of serious work impairment tended to lag behind symptom improvement. Randomised controlled trials have demonstrated significant reductions in self-reported work impairment with active treatment. Other randomised studies have noted similar benefits to social functioning. A limited amount of data is available on cost savings due to reduced work impairment. *(This review provides evidence that work impairment due to depression can be reduced through successful treatment of the disorder, but it did not address the issue of work causing symptoms).*
(Simon 2003) Narrative review	**Social and economic burden of mood disorders** Social and economic effects of mood disorders include functional impairment, disability or lost work productivity, and increased use of health services. Evidence for these impacts includes cross-sectional studies, longitudinal studies, and randomized trials of specific treatments or treatment programs. With respect to unipolar depression, strong evidence demonstrates that depression is associated with significant functional impairment and that effective treatment helps to restore function. Studies of the effect of depression on work disability and health care costs show strong cross-sectional associations (i.e., greater disability and higher costs among those with depression) and longitudinal associations (i.e., improvement in depression is associated with reduced disability and lower costs). All of these findings regarding unipolar depression seem as consistent in the subgroup of patients with comorbid chronic medical illness as in the total population with depressive disorders. Fewer data are available regarding social and economic burden of bipolar disorder, but available data show cross-sectional associations between mood symptoms and functional impairment, disability, and health care costs. *(The social and economic effects of depression, including work loss and productivity, that is comorbid with chronic medical conditions appears similar to those due to depression in the general community, but evidence is currently limited to cross-sectional studies. Note, this review differs from Simon (2001), it focuses on unipolar depression in people with comorbid chronic medical conditions, not just the general population of depressed).*

TABLE 4a: ANXIETY AND DEPRESSION (COMMON MENTAL HEALTH PROBLEMS)

(Steffick et al. 2006) Narrative review	**Worksite disease management programmes for depression: potential employer benefits** Reviewed the academic and business literature, identifying 205 articles *(it is not clear how many of these were included, since the bibliography contains only 84 citations in total)*. Disease management defined as utilisation of strategies to control healthcare costs while simultaneously improving outcomes and quality of care. The authors concluded there is substantial evidence that depressive disorders have significant impact on work performance and days lost, and that there is wide variation in quality of treatment making it a natural candidate for disease management. They discuss evidence from RCTs indicating that successful or improved treatment leads to significant reductions in work loss, some of which is equivocal, but conclude that most academic evidence shows treatment leads to symptom improvement that can restore workers productivity and attendance. They provide case studies from businesses that have evaluated depression management approaches, and found benefit. Overall, the authors conclude that while there is evidence supporting the components of depression disease management programmes, there is a lack of evidence and few worksite programmes have been developed to date.
(Social Exclusion Unit 2004) UK Government Report	**Mental health and social exclusion** Reviewed the reasons why employment is important for people with mental health problems and for social inclusion. Primary care: GPs can have a crucial role in facilitating job retention, through suggesting work adjustments or referring to a vocational adviser. Vocational advisers based in primary care can be an accessible source of information on managing the return to work or finding a new job. They can give advice on benefits, liaise with the employee and employer to manage their return, or help with other issues that might impact on work such as housing or financial concerns. Cognitive behavioural therapy and specific work counselling can be useful in the first months of sickness absence. Occupational Health: Occupational health (OH) services should support job retention and remove unnecessary barriers to work for people with disabilities or health problems. It is important that there is an effective dialogue, with the individual's consent, between GPs and the workplace (including OH services) to ensure that all available support is mobilised to improve job retention and access to employment. Secondary care: Broadly speaking, it is only in recent years that mental health trusts have started to consider employment as a realistic option for people with mental health problems. There is still great variation in available support. 35 per cent of respondents to the Social Exclusion Unit consultation felt that health and social care services placed a low priority on employment, and only 6 per cent felt it was a high priority. Even now, 'vocational services' can too often include a succession of training courses that are designed to fill people's time but do not provide a platform for moving into open employment. However, the best projects bring together key partners to meet clients' health, employment and other needs. They can have a critical role in persuading clients to interact with Jobcentre Plus and overcome fears about benefit loss, both of which can be barriers to work. A cost-effectiveness study commissioned for the Social Exclusion Unit concluded that Supported Employment and Individual Placement and Support projects were significantly more effective than other approaches in enabling people with *(severe)* mental health problems to find and keep open employment. *(The report also summarised various government services and initiatives, including JobCentre Plus, NHS Plus, Pathways, JRRPs, Safe and Healthy Working Scotland and various local and private initiatives).*

TABLE 4a: ANXIETY AND DEPRESSION (COMMON MENTAL HEALTH PROBLEMS)

(Sullivan 2005) Conceptual review	**Promoting health and productivity for depressed patients in the workplace** Conceptual argument for enhanced disease management in the workplace for depressed employees. Observes that the majority of costs associated with depressive illness are due to lost productivity and therefore the employer bears most of the burden. Suggest that efforts to improve employee health are hampered by compartmentalisation of medical costs, pharmacy costs, behavioural health costs, and productivity measures. A reintegration is required, and believes this can be achieved through employers conducting health risk assessments, proactively minimising risk factors, and ensuring depressed workers get access to good healthcare including suitable medication. (*Conceptual arguments, but supporting evidence not provided*).
Teasdale & Deahl 2007) Book chapter	**Mental health and psychiatric disorders** There should be a focus in the workplace on health and well-being, with a well thought through, proactive approach to mental health and an organised way of dealing with mental ill health. In practice, the more common mental health problems encompass stress, anxiety, depression and their manifestation in the workplace; stigma and discrimination are major issues. A successful return to work is perhaps one of the most meaningful yet least used measures of health outcome in addition to being an important positive prognostic indicator, irrespective of psychiatric diagnosis. Assessment of capacity for work should focus on abilities, disability and functional capacity, not diagnosis. Disability depends on the interaction between the individual's mental health problems and impairments and the workplace obstacles including attitudes, working practices, policies, and the working environment that might exclude the individual with a mental health problem from working. Health care and the workplace should take steps to facilitate return to work rather than passively waiting for the patient to 'get better'. Close liaison is required between GPs, psychologists &/or psychiatrists, and occupational physicians. Line managers can be very useful in identifying where (poor) working arrangements or relationships may have been contributory, and in facilitating successful return to work and arranging appropriate adjustments or modifications. However, 'there is little evidence to demonstrate whether particular types of services or interventions are effective in getting the mentally ill back to work'. GPs, employers and even mental health professionals have typically poor expectations of the capabilities of the mental well as well as over-estimating the risk to employers of employing individuals with mental health problems. Moreover, mental health professionals often have a very poor understanding of the workplace, and poor communication with the workplace.
Thomas et al. 2002) Narrative review	**Job retention and mental health: a review of the literature** The external obstacles to (return to) work for unemployed people with mental health problems include: • Stigmatisation of mental illness within society, including in particular employers. There is a perception that people with (a history of) mental health problems may be less productive, have more sickness absence, and be less likely to remain is sustained employment. • Disclosure and fear of discrimination • The Disability Discrimination Act (1995) requires the employer to make *reasonable adjustments* (termed *accommodations* in the US) but these may be less obvious and less readily available for people with mental health problems (e.g. additional support, modified psychosocial aspects of work, or some kind of flexible scheduling) than for those with physical disabilities (e.g. modified physical demands and work environment) • Lack of support services in the workplace • Negative attitudes and low expectations of mental health providers. Attitudes and practices in UK mental health services that do not consider or support (return to) work as a realistic option for people with mental health problems or the concern of health care.

TABLE 4a: ANXIETY AND DEPRESSION (COMMON MENTAL HEALTH PROBLEMS)

Job retention models and services for people with mental health problems (*which may be equally applicable to rehabilitation and return to work*) include: employee assistance programmes; the social process model; and a case management approach. (Return to) work and job sustainability for people with mental health problems may be promoted by comprehensive mental health services, organisational factors and a better person-environment fit. The main principles include:

* Promoting positive and realistic perspectives on mental illness and employment among people with mental health problems.
* Considering the individual's job preferences and job satisfaction.
* Promoting healthy workplaces for all employees.
* Facilitating natural supports in the workplace.
* Providing supportive and well-trained management/supervision.
* Promoting modified work programmes and facilitating workplace adjustments.
* Facilitating early intervention and minimal time off work programmes.

Work has the potential to be part of the recovery process. Mental health providers and the health system more widely, need training to become more aware of the impact that employment, loss of employment and unemployment have on people with mental health problems, In addition,. Specialist services are urgently required to ensure that employment issues are on the agenda and correctly managed for people with mental health problems.

(No evidence on effectiveness or occupational outcomes).

Timbie et al. 2006) Meta-analysis	**A meta-analysis of labor supply effects of interventions for major depressive disorder** The authors noted that depressive disorders can be very disruptive to labour market activities. They identified 4 randomised controlled trials published between 1980 and 2004, that included work outcome measures in depressed patients undergoing treatments, with the goal of estimating effects of interventions on 'labor supply' *(ie time missed from work, or employment status)* and comparing this with clinical outcomes. One study was an efficacy trial comparing an antidepressant with placebo, while the other three were primary-care quality improvement studies aimed at improving quality of care. These included mixed treatment modalities including medication and psychotherapy. Results were pooled. An improvement of 0.34 standard deviations was found in the clinical effect of interventions compared to placebo or usual care, and 0.12 standard deviations for the effect on labour supply. The authors concluded that treatment for depression resulted in significant reductions in symptom severity, and hence clinical benefit was obtained. However, the overall gain in labour output was only a third as large as the reductions in symptom severity. It was noted that a possible reason for this finding is extrinsic factors that affect labour supply. *(This review supports the conclusion that while symptomatic improvement can be achieved for mental health problems such as depression, the clinical interventions themselves are unlikely to influence return-to-work rates without the addition of a work-focused approach).*
(Tse & Walsh 2001) Narrative review	**How does work work for people with bipolar affective disorder?** Bipolar disorder is a chronic, relapsing disorder that leads to long-term psychosocial disability. These reviewers identified 10 studies (6 longitudinal, 4 cross-sectional) that used employment rates as outcome variables. They concluded that while employment rates amongst individuals with bipolar disorder may improve over time, and is relatively better compared to some other chronic mental disorders, employment prospects do not match pre-onset levels of achievement. For those with bipolar disorder, clinical recovery does not necessarily mean functional recovery, and the usual early age of onset may further reduce an individual's preparedness for employment.

TABLE 4a: ANXIETY AND DEPRESSION (COMMON MENTAL HEALTH PROBLEMS)

(Wewiorski & Fabian)
 	
Review and meta-analysis
	Association between demographic and diagnostic factors and employment outcomes for people with psychiatric disabilities: a synthesis of recent research
	
	A literature review was conducted, followed by a meta-analysis of 17 studies. The objective was to identify relationships between employment outcomes and sociodemographic and illness variables. Literature review indicated that: younger age is associated with better employment outcomes; gender does not have an association; race may not be important; history of prior employment is a strong predictor of outcome, and the pattern of that employment may be more important; influence of educational background is uncertain; symptoms of the illness are important predictors of vocational outcomes rather than the diagnostic label, and negative symptoms and skills deficits appear to be the most important.
	
	Meta-analysis results were consistent with findings from the literature review
	
	• Sociodemographic Variables
	  o Being employed is associated with being younger
	  o Attaining employment is not associated with age
	  o Gender is not related to employment status
	  o Race does not influence employment status, but does influence employment attainment (Caucasians more likely to attain)
	• Illness Variables
	  o Diagnosis of affective disorder significantly more likely than schizophrenia to be employed, and remain employed
	  o Attaining competitive employment less likely with schizophrenia than all other disorders
	  o Attaining competitive employment more likely with affective disorder than all other disorders
	
	Authors concluded the process of obtaining and sustaining employment is complex and this may not be uniform across demographic and diagnostic subgroups within the population of individuals with psychiatric disabilities.
	
	(Indicates that the most important predictors of outcome are history/pattern of prior employment and the symptoms of the illness are rather than the diagnostic label, with negative symptoms and skills deficits key).

(WHO 2005) Guidance	**Mental health policies and programmes in the workplace: mental health policy and service guidance package** [World Health Organisation] This document provides guidance for policy-makers and planners on: developing policies and comprehensive strategies for improving the mental health of populations; using existing resources to achieve the greatest possible benefits; providing effective services to persons in need; and, helping people with mental disorders to reintegrate into all aspects of community life, thus improving their overall quality of life. Obstacles to the introduction of a mental health policy in the workplace re outlines, with possible solutions: Concern that mental health policy will reduce profits • Provide information to employers on mental health and productivity • Encourage employer organizations to become involved in mental health activities • Explore opportunities for external funding

TABLE 4a: ANXIETY AND DEPRESSION (COMMON MENTAL HEALTH PROBLEMS)

Belief that the workplace is too small for a mental health policy

- Encourage employer organizations to provide assistance to small workplaces
- Encourage links between small workplaces and primary health care services

Resistance from stakeholders

- Provide information to stakeholders
- Use influential people in the workplace to champion mental health
- Arrange demonstration project

Insufficient resources

- Develop low-resource strategies
- Explore opportunities for redirecting resources from other activities

Employers are afraid that focusing on mental health problems will have unforeseeable consequences

- Provide relevant information on the impact of mental health issues in the workplace.
- Provide evidence of effective mental health interventions
- Show how other businesses have successfully implemented mental health programmes
- Introduce activities slowly

Stigma: some employers and employees may feel that employees with mental health problems are weak, unreliable, potentially dangerous and less productive than other employees.

- Show evidence that challenges the myths of mental illness.
- Invite a speaker who has had experience of a mental illness to speak with staff to educate the workforce

Employers do not want to employ people with mental health problem

- Provide information to employers on mental health problems
- Make sure that employers know about their legal responsibilities
- Use experiences from other businesses to illustrate positive impact of employing people with mental health problems

Employees do not attend activities

- Make sure that the activities reflect employees concerns
- Involve employees in the planning of activities
- Ensure that information about the programmes is distributed to employees
- Ensure that employees are given the time to attend the programme

TABLE 4a: ANXIETY AND DEPRESSION (COMMON MENTAL HEALTH PROBLEMS)

(Wittchen & Jacobi 2005) Systematic review and meta-analysis	**Size and burden of mental disorders in Europe – a critical review and appraisal of 27 studies**
	Identified 27 studies of epidemiological data (over 150,000 subjects from 16 European countries) on a wide range of mental disorders from community studies conducted in European countries to determine the availability and consistency of prevalence, disability and treatment findings for the EU.
	Prevalence: On the basis of meta-analytic techniques as well as on reanalyses of selected data sets, it is estimated that about 27% (82.7 million) of the adult EU population, 18-65 of age, is or has been affected by at least one mental disorder in the past 12 months. Taking into account the considerable degree of comorbidity (about one third had more than one disorder), the most frequent disorders are anxiety disorders, depressive, somatoform and substance dependence disorders. When taking into account design, sampling and other methodological differences between studies, little evidence seems to exist for considerable cultural or country variation.
	Disability and treatment: despite very divergent and fairly crude assessment strategies, the available data consistently demonstrate (a) an association of all mental disorders with a considerable disability burden in terms of number of work days lost, and (b) generally low utilization and treatment rates. Only 26% of all cases had any consultation with professional health care services, a finding suggesting a considerable degree of unmet need. However, the reviewers noted that since prevalence estimates could not simply be equated with defined treatment needs, studies are needed to determine the degree of met and unmet needs for services by taking into account severity, disability and comorbidity.
	Most disorders were associated with a loss of three times more work days compared to having no 12-month disorder. Neurological disorders (22% workdays lost during past 30 days) were found to have the strongest work days lost impact, followed by panic disorder, specific phobias, and post-traumatic stress disorder (all 11%), depressive disorder (9%) and social phobia (8%). Alcohol abuse/dependence, in contrast, revealed lower values (3%). Using identical measures in an aggregate six-country-comparison, we found mental disorders usually to reveal a stronger work days lost association than many somatic disorders (e.g. diabetes: 2% WLD loss, lung disease: 4%, heart disease: 7%).

[CBT = cognitive behavioural therapy; DMP = disease management program; RCT = randomised controlled trial; RTW = return to work]

Table 4b: 'Stress'

TABLE 4b: 'STRESS'	
Authors	**Key features** (Reviewers' comments in italic)
(Arthur 2000) Descriptive review	**Employee assistance programmes: the emperor's new clothes of stress management?** Employee assistance programmes (EAPs) have a long history in the US, but are a relatively recent service in the UK. They usually involve counselling provided by employers, both private and public, that allow psychologically distressed employees, and sometimes their dependants, free and confidential access to qualified mental health professionals. The common group of core components includes free, confidential access to a contracted, affiliate network of mental health practitioners who provide assessment, counselling and therapeutic services for employees experiencing a wide range of personal, emotional and psychological problems, with a telephone help-line for information and advice on domestic, legal, medical and financial matters. The reviewer noted that while evidence of effectiveness is thin, with methodological weaknesses, overall it suggests that employees who use broadly based EAPs have significant mental health problems, experience symptom reduction, are satisfied with the counselling-type interventions they receive, appreciate the provision of the service by their employer, and may (but not necessarily) have fewer absences as a result. It is concluded: EAPs, and to a lesser extent stress management techniques, have a role to play in supporting employees who experience or may experience symptoms of psychological distress; they are not in themselves effective enough to counter the effects of stressful work environments; providing them for cost saving and improved productivity reasons alone may result in disappointment. *(This article is not a comprehensive review. It mixes a discussion of stress management with EAPs. Stress management is an intervention, whereas EAPs are not strictly an intervention but a system for delivering intervention(s), usually counselling. This means, questions about effectiveness of stress management can be answered by clinical trials. However, questions about 'effectiveness of EAPs' are significantly more complex. With respect to effectiveness of the intervention, the question should really be whether counselling works. Questions about the process of delivering through EAPs are more appropriately focused on questions such as whether they facilitate access for workers who may otherwise never have sought help, whether they facilitate earlier access than other systems, and whether significant mental health disorders are detected by EAP providers and appropriate referrals made. It should also be noted the privacy policy of EAPs means conducting RCTs is virtually impossible.)*
(Caulfield et al. 2004) Systematic review	**A review of occupational stress interventions in Australia** 6 studies were included, all from the public sector, though only one was an randomised controlled trial and one other had a control group. Most interventions were at the individual level, despite the preponderance of research identifying the importance of work environment stressors. None of the studies had any occupational outcomes. The authors concluded that there is a paucity of published evidence on effective occupational stress interventions in Australia.

TABLE 4b: 'STRESS'

(Cox et al. 2000b) Report	**Research on work-related stress** [European Agency for Safety and Health at Work] Most 'stress management' interventions target the individual rather than the organisation (the former is usually seen as cheaper and less cumbersome), are often off-the-shelf designs, and are entirely divorced from the process of diagnosis of the problems - if diagnosis takes place at all. Three common types of intervention on stress management are found in the literature: Primary (some form of organisational or work development to reduce stressors, including work design and ergonomics); Secondary (worker training, either in form of health promotion or psychological skills); Tertiary (employee assistance, focused on provision of counselling). The relative effectiveness of such programmes has been difficult to determine (largely for methodological reasons). The scientific literature suggests that organisational-level interventions (or at least, intervention programmes that target the organisation as well as the individual employees) may be the most beneficial for both individuals and organisations. The available evidence suggests that, although few in number, organisational-level interventions that aim to eliminate or control the hazards within the work environment have significant advantages and represent the best way forward. *(These reviewers have emphasised the significant limits to the common assumption that ill health invariably follows the experience of stress. They also highlight the lack of evidence for management of work-related stress. Despite this they advocate organisation-level intervention rather than individual-level. However, this recommendation states only that it 'could' be useful).*
(Cox et al. 2000a) Research report	**Organisational interventions for work stress: a risk management approach** [UK Health & Safety Executive Research Report] This report presents a risk management approach to the reduction of work stress. Describes the origins and logical basis of a risk management approach to the reduction of work stress, and the strategy that frames its processes and procedures. The basic health and safety equation of Hazard–Risk–Harm is proposed as the conceptual framework for understanding the nature and management of work stress. The experience of stress is then the link between employees' exposure to the hazards of work and any subsequent and related harm to their health, in a direct causal chain. Defines psychosocial and organisational hazards as 'those aspects of work design and the organisation and management of work, and their social and environmental context that have the potential for causing psychological, social or physical harm'. Defines stress as 'an emotional experience that is complex, distressing and disruptive'; stress can arise from two different sources at work: a) anxiety about exposure, or the threat of exposure, to the more tangible and physical hazards of work, or b) exposure to problems in the psychosocial environment and with their social and organisational settings i.e. psychosocial and organisational hazards. Stress can be dealt with primarily at source, by reducing exposure to hazards that are regarded as stressful, or at the individual level by treating the experience of stress itself or its health effects. This report is primarily concerned with the former strategy, though the case examples used demonstrate that most interventions involve both organisational and individually-focused elements. Argues that the priority is prevention but in practice control strategies tend necessarily to be a mixture of approaches. States that existing research into the nature and effects of work stress is neither appropriate nor adequate as an assessment of the associated risks. Lays out the logic of a risk assessment strategy framed by current thinking in health and safety management: <u>Hazard identification:</u> reliable identification of stressors and degree of exposure for specific groups of employees. Argues that 'since many of the exposures that give rise to the experience of stress at work are chronic in nature, the proportion of employees that reporting a particular aspect of work as stressful may be a 'good enough' exposure statistic'.

TABLE 4b: 'STRESS'

	Assessment of harm: Evidence that exposure to these hazards is associated with impaired (sic) health, in a wide range of health-related outcomes. Identification of likely risks: explore the association between exposure to hazards and likely risks, to make some estimate of the size and/or significance of the likely risks. (Acknowledges later that this is based on associations between stressors and health outcomes but argues that is 'good enough evidence' for the overall risk management process). Description of the underlying mechanisms: understand and describe the possible mechanisms by which hazards are associated with (sic) health related harms.'. Admits that all of these steps are 'challenging' and largely based on employees' subjective perceptions but argues this constitutes 'employees' expert knowledge of work', their experience of work and of stressors, and can be cross-checked by psychometric properties, face, conceptual and concurrent validity, and consensus. Concedes that 'the scientific literature on risk reduction in relation to work stress is sparse'. (This report travels the well-trodden hazard-risk-harm approach. However, evidence for its effectiveness in the work stress area is not provided).
(Damiani et al. 2004) Systematic review	**Do occupational stress management programmes affect absenteeism rates?** Of 53 experimental and quasi-experimental studies targeting a working population and using individual and /or organisational interventions, 5 used absenteeism as an outcome measure. In the short-term, three out of five studies reported a larger (absolute) reduction in the frequency of sickness leave in the intervention compared with the control group. The reduction was only in workers with >6 days sick leave per year. One year after the intervention, three out of four studies showed no evidence of absenteeism reduction. (That is, the evidence suggests absenteeism rates are not influenced by occupational stress management programmes).
(Edwards & Burnard 2003a) Systematic review	**A systematic review of stress and stress management interventions for mental health nurses** The reviewers' aim was to identify stressors, moderators and stress outcomes for mental health nurses, and also to determine the effectiveness of stress management interventions for the same group. 77 articles were included in the review, 58 from the U.K. 69 studies focused on stressors, moderators and stress outcomes (study type and methodology was not reported, but these appear to be cross-sectional surveys). Eight papers were identified that evaluated stress management techniques (study type and methodology was not reported, but these appear to be case series). The interventions considered as successful for mental health nurses by the reviewers included: relaxation techniques, training in behavioural techniques, stress management workshops and training in therapeutic skills. The reviewers noted methodological flaws. One study (appears to be a case series) included a work-related outcome measure (Milne et al., 1986), and found that training in behavioural techniques improved work satisfaction and levels of sickness and reduced strain. (This review is highly limited by the methodological weakness of the studies included).
(Edwards & Burnard 2003b) Systematic review	**A systematic review of the effects of stress and coping strategies used by occupational therapists working in mental health settings** Focus of this systematic review was the effectiveness of stress management interventions provided for occupational therapists working in mental health settings, but the authors reported a lack of any such literature. However, they found 14 studies that identified sources of stress at work, how to measure stress, and the impact of stress. Most of these studies appear to have been cross-sectional surveys. The authors concluded there is a lack of evidence about effectiveness of stress management interventions for this population of mental health workers. (A major weakness of this review was that the authors did not classify the methodology used for each study they included. Hence it is not possible to gauge the strength of evidence).

TABLE 4b: 'STRESS'	
(Giga et al. 2003) Systematic review	**The UK perspective: a review of research on organisational stress management interventions** 16 studies conducted in the UK were included: 6 RCTs, 5 non-randomised control group, 4 case series, and 1 cross-sectional survey. Most interventions were at the individual level and some mixed, but only 3 were purely organisational. The authors identified 14 different types of interventions used, the most common were relaxation, CBT and employee assistance programmes (EAPs). Most studies had short follow up of 6 months or less, with only 5 reporting 1-year data and 2 of these giving 2-year data. Only 5 of the reviewed studies included work outcome measures: 1 RCT reported beneficial effects on absenteeism, and 1 RCT reported no effect; 1 non-randomised controlled study reported significant improvements in absenteeism rates; and, 2 case series reported improvements in self-reported work functioning. The reviewers concluded that interventions at both the individual and organisational level can yield human and/or organisational benefits, but suggested those at the individual level are less sustained. The authors noted serious methodological shortcomings in much of the research, including the following conclusions: all interventions were found to contribute to, or be associated with some positive outcomes, including those at the individual level (e.g. reductions in anxiety and depression) and organisational level (e.g. improved productivity and reduced absenteeism). *(These conclusions appear to be an optimistic interpretation of available results. For absenteeism the evidence is equivocal from RCTs, but supported by 1 non-randomised controlled study. For productivity or work functioning, evidence is limited to 2 case series using subjective measures).*
(Hannigan et al. 2004) Systematic review	**Stress and stress management in clinical psychology: findings from a systematic review** 7 studies included in the review. Objective was to identify factors that contribute to stress, burnout and job satisfaction for qualified UK clinical psychologists; to identify the various coping strategies that are employed; to identify stress management interventions that have been used by members of the clinical psychology profession in the UK *(the authors began from the premise that occupational stress is a major problem for individuals and organizations, and that stress can cause burnout, ill-health, high workforce turnover, absenteeism, lowered morale and reduced efficiency and performance).* Reported sources of stress for clinical psychologists included client characteristics, excessive workloads, professional self-doubt and poor management. Coping strategies included talking with colleagues, and other 'active' approaches to personal stress management. Up to 40% of UK clinical psychologists participating in studies were found to be experiencing 'caseness' levels of distress. Conclusions: Mental health work is stress-provoking. However, organizational and professional factors may militate against psychologists seeking and receiving support at work. (*No review of study method/quality was used. This was in fact a review of seven surveys, using self-report questionnaires completed by clinical psychologists. The results therefore represent an overview of the perceptions held by this group of healthcare professionals. They do not provide information about the relationship between work and development of stress problems, or about the effectiveness of interventions).*

(HSE 2004a) Systematic review	**Management standards for tackling work-related stress**
	[UK Health & Safety Executive]
	
	The HSE approach is developed from the concept that 'good management is the key to managing the causes of work-related 'stress'.
	An analysis tool covers six standard areas:
	Demands- includes issues like workload, work patterns, and the work environment.
	    Standard: employees indicate that they are able to cope with the demands of their jobs.
	Control – How much say the person has in the way they do their work
	    Standard: employees indicate that they are able to have a say about the way they do their work.
	Support – Includes the encouragement, sponsorship and resources provided by the organisation, line management and colleagues.
	    Standard: employees indicate that they receive adequate information and support from their colleagues and superiors.

TABLE 4b: 'STRESS'	
	Relationship – includes promoting positive working practices to avoid conflict and dealing with unacceptable behaviour.
	Standard: employees indicate that they are nor subjected to unacceptable behaviours, e.g. bullying at work.
	Role – Whether people understand their role within the organisation and whether the organisation ensures that the person does not have conflicting roles.
	Standard: employees indicate that they understand their role and responsibilities.
	Change – How organisational change (large or small) is managed and communicated in the organisation,
	Standard: employees indicate that the organisation engages them frequently when undergoing an organisational change.
	And, in each area, – Systems are in place locally to respond to any individual concerns.
	(Based on the hazard-risk-harm approach. However, evidence for its effectiveness in the work stress area is not provided).
(IIAC 2004)	**Stress at work as a prescribed disease and post-traumatic stress disorder**
	[Industrial Injuries Advisory Council]
Position paper	The Industrial Injuries Advisory Council advises the Secretary of State for Social Security on the scientific evidence for the Industrial Injuries Disablement Benefit (IIDB) scheme. This paper considered whether work-related stress met the legal requirements of a prescribed occupational disease: i.e. that it is a recognised risk of particular work, and its link with occupational exposure can be established or reasonably presumed in individual cases. IIAC highlighted a number of problems:
	• The term 'stress' is used in different senses by different people to include stressful exposures or circumstances (stressors) and stress-related outcomes and illnesses.
	• Diagnosis is usually based on symptoms, which are common in the general population, and reporting is heavily influenced by personal, societal and cultural factors. There is no clear medical consensus on specific diagnosis, how to assess the severity or impact on functioning, or on management of stress-related mental illness (though some specific mental illnesses can be defined).
	• Risk factors are subjectively reported and influenced by individual personal perceptions. There is no agreement at present on how to confirm that important stressors have been present, or to define their time course and the extent of exposure.
	• There is no robust body of epidemiological evidence that makes it possible to say on the balance of probabilities that an individual case of a particular illness in a given occupation was due to work.
	In view of these difficulties, IIAC concluded that stress does not meet the legal requirements, and recommended that it should not be accepted as a prescribed occupational disease. *(IIAC considered PTSD separately, concluded it was a recognized psychiatric disorder, and recommended that under specific conditions it should be accepted as a prescribed occupational disease).*
(Lunt et al. 2005)	**HSE review of the risk prevention approach to occupational health: applying health models to 21st century occupational health needs – health models information pack**
	[UK Health & Safety Executive and Health & Safety Laboratory: Workshop, 20 September 2005]
Workshop materials	Occupational health is defined as: 'a state of physical, mental, and social well-being at work, and not merely the absence of disease and disability, that is influenced by factors within and outside the work place'. The traditional risk assessment approach to health and safety is based on a biomedical model, regards work as a hazard, and aims at the primary prevention of work injury and industrial disease. This approach was developed for and remains appropriate for accidents (e.g. on building sites or with machinery), exposure to hazardous material (e.g. asbestos) or the prevention of occupational diseases (e.g. deafness or asthma).

TABLE 4b: 'STRESS'

However, that approach is not appropriate and may even be counter-productive for some common health problems (e.g. 'stress', mild/moderate mental health problems, or musculoskeletal conditions) which have a high prevalence in normal people whether they are working or not, where risk factors are complex, where there is often no 'injury' or 'disease', where causation is multifactorial and ambiguous, and where primary prevention may be unrealistic. In these conditions, there is an argument that the focus should be more balanced and include improving management (both clinical and occupational) and the secondary prevention of (long-term) disability and sickness. These conditions can only be understood and managed, both clinically and at work, by addressing *all* of the personal/psychological, health-related and social/occupational factors that influence illness, disability and incapacity for work (the 'biopsychosocial model'). It is important to consider an organisational as well as an individual perspective on health at work.

Traditional risk assessment underpins occupational safety and is widely understood and accepted. It is essential to work within the current legislation and regulatory framework and not to undermine the risk assessment process. The occupational health framework must address emerging issues around health, work and well-being, but the way forward should be by evolution, enhancement and consistency. Thus, the Health and Safety strategy for the 21st century should incorporate both risk assessment and prevention *and* the broader health at work agenda. That will require a multi-disciplinary approach, which includes organisational interventions and does not only emphasise the individual. There needs to be broader collaboration between the Dept of Health, the Department for Work and Pensions, and the Health & Safety Executive/Health & Safety Commission.

Key messages are that health problems are part of everyday life and occupational health should be viewed in the wider context of health, work and well-being. It is important to emphasise the benefits and not just the hazards of work for (physical and mental) health: work may be part of the solution rather than the problem. The suitability of the person for the job ('person-job fit') is important. People of working age need to be encouraged and helped to deal with common health problems both in the occupational and non-occupational context. Messages about health and work should be framed carefully, and take a balanced approach to the relative risks and benefits.

(Murta et al. 2007)

Systematic review

Process evaluation in occupational stress management programs: a systematic review

The reviewers identified 84 studies that included either individual- or organisational-level stress management interventions at the workplace, with an outcome evaluation. This was restricted to 52 studies that presented data on at least one component of process evaluation, which involves systematic measurement to determine the extent to which a particular programme is implemented. There were 32 experimental studies, 16 quasi-experimental, and 4 case series. The most commonly reported process evaluation components were recruitment, dose received, participants attitudes toward interventions, and reach. The authors concluded the incomplete reporting of information relevant to process evaluation makes it difficult to identify reliable determinants of effective intervention implementation or outcomes; and the implementation of more rigorous and broader process evaluation should be a priority for future research. They also note a number of trends: the greater the involvement and support from supervisors and managers, the better the intervention implementation and likely outcomes achieved; the smaller the intervention dose delivered, the smaller the chances of altering organisational climate; the more positively participants perceived the sessions to be and the context in terms of 'warmth' and 'safe climate', the greater the likelihood of altering job-related stress; the more frequent the monitoring of participants' attitudes toward intervention and its effects, the more awareness is raised about personal stress. *(This study highlights the current evidence base on workplace stress management interventions is undermined by the lack of information about the extent to which each intervention studied was delivered as planned. This is analogous to a study of exercise as an intervention for musculoskeletal disorder where no attempt was made to determine if the patient actually did the exercises).*

TABLE 4b: 'STRESS'	
(Mimura & Griffiths 2003) Systematic review	**The effectiveness of current approaches to workplace stress management in the nursing profession** 7 RCTs and 3 prospective cohort studies were included, though the quality was poor. There is more evidence for the effectiveness of programmes based on providing personal support than environmental management to reduce stressors. However, given the small number and poor quality of the studies, it was not possible to draw any conclusions about the most effective interventions. *(Work outcomes were not included).*
(Semmer 2006) Narrative review	**Job stress interventions and the organisation of work** Author proposes that organization-level interventions should be more effective than those at individual-level, based on theory. The review is not intended to be comprehensive, but to focus on issues from this perspective. There is need for methodological improvement in studies. It is concluded that a combination of person-focused and organization-focused approaches is the most promising. *(The issue of case definition for stress is not considered. Most of the studies reviewed are case series. A very wide range of outcome variables was reported, mostly self-report. Some studies included work-related outcome variables, such as perception of workload, but none used vocational outcomes such as sickness absence or RTW).*
(Spurgeon 2007) Proceedings	**Stress as an occupational disease** [Industrial Injuries Advisory Council] The Health & Safety Executive defines stress as 'the adverse reaction people have to excessive pressure or other types of demand placed upon them'. This definition was developed in the context of management guidance for prevention and control and represents a consensus expert view. Within this definition several categories of work 'pressure' (demands, control, support, relationships, role, change) have been identified. Individuals may respond to these pressures with adverse physiological, psychological and behavioural reactions. An example of physiological responses would be an increased heart rate and elevated blood pressure. Psychological responses would include the development of conditions such as anxiety and depression, while changes in behaviour might include altered patterns of eating and sleeping or abuse of substances such as drugs and alcohol. Possible outcomes of these responses together or alone might be demonstrable effects on physical or mental health, on social behaviour or on performance at work. Defining a health outcome in relation to stress-related conditions poses a number of challenges for IIAC. There is poor consensus on case definition and on the assessment of severity of stress-related disorders. The nature of the conditions makes quantitative or objective testing of the disablement difficult. There is a general reliance on symptoms which makes independent verification of the conditions difficult. There are differing opinions on whether stress can be labelled as a disease. Mental health problems such as anxiety or depression may be more readily identifiable but even there, there is frequently disagreement between experts on diagnosis. Stress may occur at work or at home and these may interact. While a number of triggers have been identified, there is no agreement on a reliable method by which to confirm with consistency, the presence or absence of particular stressors, or the degree of exposure to these. The attribution of a stress-related condition to occupation is difficult, not least because these conditions are very common in the general population and are not unique to any particular occupation. In addition these conditions do not have distinctive clinical features when related to occupation; the causes are often multi-factorial; risk factors may be influenced by personal perceptions and most importantly from the Industrial Injuries Advisory Council's point of view, there is no strong evidence to identify a doubling of risk for the condition in specific occupations. For these reasons, the Industrial Injuries Advisory Council have been unable to recommend that any adverse health outcomes ascribed to stress at work be included on the schedule of prescribed diseases. *(Also briefly summarises PTSD and why it has been accepted as a Prescribed Disease).*

TABLE 4b: 'STRESS'

(Thomson et al. 2003) Narrative review + case studies	**Best practice in rehabilitating employees following absence due to work-related stress** [Used case studies from 14 organisations to identify current practices of job retention and vocational rehabilitation after a period of ill health stemming from work-related stress, and to review the evidence of their effectiveness. This was used to describe the elements of best current practice. These were: • Early contact with the employee • Early health assessment • Quality of the health assessment, emphasising accurate assessment and diagnosis • Developing an agreed rehabilitation plan, agreed by all stakeholders • Therapeutic interventions: Current evidence suggests that approaches based on cognitive behavioural therapy are most effective in relation to work-related stress. However, the evidence also shows that other forms of therapy, such as counselling and psychotherapy, are more effective than no intervention. • Flexible return to work interventions, with typical graded returns lasting 4 to 6 weeks • Work adaptations and adjustments Elements of best practice in company policy include: written policy or guidelines; monitoring sickness absence; case management; stress and rehabilitation awareness in line managers.
(van der Klink et al. 2001) Meta-analysis	**The benefits of interventions for work-related stress** The authors conducted a review and meta-analysis of 48 studies, using 3736 subjects, to investigate the effectiveness of occupational stress-reducing interventions and the populations for which such interventions are most beneficial. Four types of interventions were distinguished: cognitive-behavioural interventions (18 studies), relaxation techniques (17 studies), multimodal programmes (8 studies), and organization-level interventions (5 studies). A small but significant overall effect was found. A moderate effect was found for cognitive-behavioural and multimodal interventions, and a small effect for relaxation techniques. The effect size for organization-level interventions was non-significant. Effects were most pronounced for complaints, psychological resources and responses, and perceived quality of work life. Overall, cognitive-behavioural interventions were more effective than other types of intervention. None of the interventions had any significant effect on absenteeism. The reviewers concluded that stress management interventions are effective, and that cognitive-behavioural interventions are more effective than the other intervention types. *(There are some major limitations in the quality of this evidence. All included studies had control groups, but most were quasi-experimental rather than RCTs. The better quality studies compared two types of treatment, and did not have no-treatment control groups. Most studies were conducted with volunteer samples rather than clinically referred samples. The only work-related outcome variable was the subjective 'perceived quality of work'.)*
(van der Klink & van Dijk 2003) Narrative review	**Dutch practice guidelines for managing stress-related disorders in occupational and primary health care** The author noted that stress-related disorders, and especially adjustment disorders, are considered to be widespread among working populations and are responsible for high costs in terms of suffering, sick leave, disability, and economic losses. Yet, despite their high prevalence, there appears to have been relatively little research on the effectiveness of treatments, especially in occupational health settings. Clinical guidelines about mental health problems have been developed for Dutch occupational physicians and general practitioners, and these include a classification based on the diagnosis of adjustment disorder (*Guideline for Mental Health Problems, 2000, published by the Dutch Association of Occupational Physicians - NVAB. Dutch only*). Recommendations for treatment are based on cognitive-behavioural principles, using stress inoculation training and graded activity, and aim to enhance the problem-solving capacity of patients in relation to the work environment. *(The principal evidence base used appears to have been 'experience in adjacent fields', and expert consensus. A study by Rebergen et al (2006) found that 1 year after publication of these national guidelines Dutch occupational physicians held a positive attitude towards them and held a general intention to apply them in practice, but actual compliance with the guideline was minimal).*

TABLE 4b: 'STRESS'

(WCRCWA 2001)	**Stress, Compensation and the General Practitioner**
	[Workers' Compensation & Rehabilitation Commission of Western Australia]
Report	This report was prepared for WorkCover WA by the Royal Australian College of General Practitioners, and gives a summary of the role of the general practitioner in managing work-related stress. A narrative literature was conducted, and a qualitative study using interviews, both aimed at identifying barriers in general practice to the optimal management of work-related stress and to develop key recommendations for the effective and efficient management of work-related stress in general practice. The key recommendations were that:
	• Protocols for the diagnosis of stress claims need to be developed
	• Work-related stress claims should be administratively reviewed if the claimant has not returned at least partly to work within 14 days
	• WorkCover WA should develop clinical guidelines
	(It appears since publication of this report that neither protocols for diagnosis, nor clinical guidance has been forthcoming).

[CBT = cognitive behavioural therapy; PTSD = post-traumatic stress disorder; RCT = randomised controlled trial; RTW = return to work]

TABLE 5: REVIEWS AND REPORTS ON CARDIO-RESPIRATORY CONDITIONS

Table 5a: Cardiac/cardiovascular conditions

TABLE 5a: CARDIAC/CARDIOVASCULAR CONDITIONS	
Authors	**Key features** (Reviewers' comments in italic)
(Ades et al. 1997) Meta-analysis	**Cost-effectiveness of cardiac rehabilitation after myocardial infarction** Favourable outcomes of cardiac rehabilitation, measured by controlled clinical trials, include reduction in the frequency and duration of subsequent re-hospitalisations for cardiac diagnoses, reduction in total and cardiac-related mortality, reduction in the incidence of symptomatic coronary ischemia, improvement in physical work capacity and endurance, improvement in secondary risk factor profile, and improvement in perceived quality of life. The known economic benefits of cardiac rehabilitation are derived primarily from reduced secondary utilization of inpatient medical resources. This meta-analysis included 10 controlled clinical trials, mainly from the late 1980s, and updated costs to 1995. It concluded that cardiac rehabilitation participants had an incremental life expectancy of 0.202 years during a 15-year period. In 1988, the average cost of the programme was $1,485, partially offset by averted cardiac re-hospitalizations of $850 per patient. A cost-effectiveness value of 2,130 $/YLS was determined for the late 1980s, projected to a value of 4,950 $/YLS for 1995. A sensitivity analysis supported the results. *(No indirect costs or benefits included in the analysis). (Pre-2000 but retained since it is some of the best available economic evidence).*
(Ara 2004) Systematic review	**A literature review of cardiovascular disease management programs in managed care populations** Included 20 studies in managed care populations: 5 in patients with congestive heart failure (CHF), 9 in hypertensive patients, and 6 in hyper-lipidemia and/or coronary artery disease (hyperlipidemia-CAD) patients. The most common management strategies for congestive heart failure were case management and physician education, with an emphasis on close patient monitoring; however, these were all before and after studies and there were no randomised controlled trials (RCT). 9 studies of disease management in hypertension demonstrated significantly lower health care costs and significantly fewer hospitalizations. A number of cardiovascular disease management strategies reported promising results. Overall, however, there was a lack of rigorous study design. There was lack of agreement on appropriate economic and clinical outcomes: most outcomes were a combination of impact on health care resource utilization (i.e., hospitalizations, office visits, Emergency Room visits, drug utilization patterns, etc. [12 studies]), clinical markers (9 studies), cost or cost-effectiveness (4 studies), and functional status or Quality of Life (3 studies). *(No occupational outcomes).*
(Balady et al. 2007; Thomas et al. 2007) Scientific Statements	**Cardiac rehabilitation/secondary prevention programmes: core components (2007 Update) and performance measures** [American Heart Association] Definition: 'Cardiac rehabilitation services are comprehensive, long-term programs involving medical evaluation, prescribed exercise, cardiac risk factor modification, education, and counselling. These programs are designed to limit the physiologic and psychological effects of cardiac illness, reduce the risk for sudden death or re-infarction, control cardiac symptoms, stabilize or reverse the atherosclerotic process, and enhance the psychosocial and vocational status of selected patients.' Cardiac rehabilitation/secondary prevention programs are generally divided into 3 main phases: 1. In-patient cardiac rehabilitation (also known as Phase 1 cardiac rehabilitation): a program that delivers preventive and rehabilitative services to hospitalized patients following an index cardiovascular event, such as an MI/acute coronary syndrome;

TABLE 5a: CARDIAC/CARDIOVASCULAR CONDITIONS

2. Early outpatient cardiac rehabilitation (also known as Phase 2 cardiac rehabilitation): a program that delivers preventive and rehabilitative services to patients in the outpatient setting early after a cardiovascular event, generally within the first 3 to 6 months after the event but continuing for as much as 1 year after the event;

3. Long-term outpatient cardiac rehabilitation (also known as Phase 3 or Phase 4 cardiac rehabilitation): a program that provides longer term delivery of preventive and rehabilitative services for patients in the outpatient setting.

Currently, a minority of patients (in US) receive cardiac rehabilitation services and secondary prevention services due, in general, to a number of patient-, provider-, and health care system-related barriers. core components for cardiac rehabilitation/secondary prevention programmes were developed jointly by the American Heart Association and various interested American professional associations. Performance measures focus on 1) referral of eligible patients to a cardiac rehabilitation program and 2) delivery of cardiac rehabilitation services through multidisciplinary cardiac rehabilitation programs, using structure-based and process-based measures. The ultimate purpose of these programmes and performance measures is to help improve the delivery of cardiac rehabilitation in order to reduce cardiovascular mortality and morbidity and optimize health in persons with cardiovascular disease, including acute myocardial infarction. (The core components and performance measures relate entirely to clinical management and outcomes, with no mention of vocational rehabilitation and no occupational outcomes).

(Benz Scott et al. 2002) Systematic review	**Why are women missing from outpatient cardiac rehabilitation programs?** Included 23 studies. Nearly 40% of myocardial infarctions occur in women, who are more likely than men to face greater mortality and morbidity within the first year of recovery. There is evidence that participation in a cardiac rehabilitation program can improve these outcomes. Nevertheless, participation rates in cardiac rehabilitation are only 15-20% in women, compared with 25-30% in men. This review found (despite the limitations of the evidence) that age, personal resources, low rates of physician referral and weak recommendations to participate in rehabilitation may explain the low numbers of women participating in cardiac rehabilitation. Makes recommendations that practitioners caring for women with cardiac disease should be aware of the evidence on the effectiveness of cardiac rehabilitation and should improve advice and referrals.
(Beswick et al. 2005) Systematic review	**Improving uptake and adherence in cardiac rehabilitation** Outpatient cardiac rehabilitation is recommended for patients following acute myocardial infarction and revascularization. Uptake and adherence are low, particularly in women, older people, socially deprived and ethnic minority patients. Patient, service and professional barriers to rehabilitation uptake have been described. Six, 12 and five studies, respectively, provided adequate information on methods to improve uptake, adherence and professional compliance. A minority of studies were randomized controlled trials. Motivational and self-management strategies and use of lay volunteers showed some promise in improving rehabilitation uptake or lifestyle change. Nurse-led coordination of care after hospital discharge may have a role in improving rehabilitation uptake. Overall, however, there have been few studies of sufficient quality to make specific recommendations on methods to improve participation in cardiac rehabilitation. (No direct link to occupational outcomes, but attendance is fundamental to any benefit).
(Bjarnason-Wehrens et al. 2007) Narrative review	**Gender-specific issues in cardiac rehabilitation: do women with ischemic heart disease need specially tailored programmes?** Most studies of cardiac rehabilitation in the past included mainly men and only 1/3 analysed results separately by gender. Traditionally, cardiac rehabilitation was used mainly for patients aged <65-70 years, and women are on average 10 years older than men when they have a myocardial infarction. After a first cardiac event, women report greater distress and lower self-efficacy and self-esteem. In addition, older age, lower exercise levels and reduced functional capacity and co-morbidities are barriers to physical activity and participation in cardiac rehabilitation. However, studies of exercise-based cardiac rehabilitation show no major differences between men and women in terms of changes in medical risk factors, functional capacity and quality of life. The same is true for older vs. younger patients. (No discussion of vocational rehabilitation or occupational outcomes, perhaps because of the focus on older women).

TABLE 5a: CARDIAC/CARDIOVASCULAR CONDITIONS

British Heart Foundation

Coronary heart disease statistics website

Prevalence (%) of those who have or have had:

Male, age	**45-54**	**55-64**	**65-74**
Angina	2.4	7.5	17.4
Myocardial infarction	2.2	6.7	12.1
Abnormal heart rhythm (e.g. atrial fibrillation)	4.9	7.3	11.8

Female, age	**45-54**	**55-64**	**65-74**
Angina	1.5	5.0	7.9
Myocardial infarction	0.8	2.1	4.2
Abnormal heart rhythm (e.g. atrial fibrillation)	6.1	6.9	7.3

www.heartstats.org/uploads/documents%5C48160_text_05_06_07.pdf (accessed 10 January 2008)

(Cannon et al. 2002)

Systematic review

Critical pathways for management of patients with acute coronary syndromes

[US National Heart Attack Alert Program]

Critical pathways might improve quality of care and outcomes for patients with acute coronary syndrome by: increasing the use of guideline-recommended medications, targeting use of cardiac procedures and other cardiac testing, and reducing the length of stay in hospitals and intensive care units. Initial studies have shown promising results in improving quality of care and reducing medical costs. However, further research is needed to determine whether these changes in the process of care will translate into improved clinical outcomes. *(No occupational outcomes).*

(Clark et al. 2005a; Clark et al. 2005b)

Meta-analysis

Randomized trials of secondary prevention in coronary artery disease

[Agency for Healthcare Research and Quality Technology Report (US)]

Included 63 RCTs: to investigate the effectiveness of secondary prevention programmes with or without an exercise component.

46 RCTs on education/counselling: a) group education/counselling about risk factor management plus supervised exercise programme; b) group education/counselling about risk factor management without exercise; c) individual counselling and follow-up. Borderline significant reduction in recurrent MI, hospitalisation and mortality, with no significant difference between the three interventions. Eighteen of 30 trials evaluating health-related quality of life or functional status reported statistically significantly better outcomes in patients receiving interventions, although the effect sizes were generally small. Limited and inconclusive evidence on cost-effectiveness. *(HRQoL was based on subjective measures, related to symptoms. No evidence on occupational outcomes).*

(Cooper et al. 2002)

Systematic review

Factors associated with cardiac rehabilitation attendance

Not all eligible patients are referred for cardiac rehabilitation: elderly and female patients may be subject to referral bias. Of those who are referred, attendance rates at cardiac rehabilitation generally vary from 25-60%. Non-attenders are likely to be older, have lower income/greater deprivation, to deny the severity of their illness, less likely to believe they could influence outcome, or perceive that their physician recommends cardiac rehab. Job status, gender and health concerns play an indirect role in attendance behaviour.

A number of factors influence attendance, some of which are modifiable. Although further research is needed to establish the most effective mechanism and delivery for full psychological and physical cardiac rehabilitation, optimising attendance and adherence of future rehabilitation is important. *(No direct link to occupational outcomes, but attendance is fundamental to any benefit).*

TABLE 5a: CARDIAC/CARDIOVASCULAR CONDITIONS

(Cooper et al. 2007) Clinical guideline	**Clinical guidelines and evidence review for post myocardial infarction: secondary prevention in primary and secondary care for patients following a myocardial infarction** *(Produced by UK National Collaborating Centre for Primary Care and the Royal College of General Practitioners. Updates previous NICE 2001 Guideline on 'Prophylaxis for patients who have experienced a myocardial infarction')* Patients should be advised to undertake regular physical activity sufficient to increase exercise capacity (Moderate scientific evidence). Patients should be advised to be physically active for 20-30 minutes a day to the point of slight breathlessness. Those who are not achieving this should be advised to increase their activity in a gradual step by step fashion, aiming to increase exercise capacity. They should start at a level that is comfortable and increase the duration and intensity of activity as they gain fitness (Consensus). Cardiac rehabilitation should be equally accessible and relevant to all patients after an MI; particularly people from groups that are less likely to access this service (Consensus). *(Focuses entirely on clinical management and cardiac outcomes, with no mention of vocational rehabilitation or occupational outcomes).*
(Cortés & Arthur 2006) Systematic review	**Determinants of referral to cardiac rehabilitation programs in patients with coronary artery disease** 10 observational studies (5 US, 3 Canadian and 2 Australian) published between 1999-2004 included 30333 patients. The mean referral rate was 34% with a range from 10-60%. Major predictors of referral were English speaking, age <75years, male, prior myocardial infarction, being admitted to hospitals providing cardiac rehabilitation and having insurance coverage. This review highlights disparities in referral to CR and reveals a treatment gap in the secondary prevention of cardiovascular disease. *(No data on vocational rehabilitation or occupational outcomes).*
(Daly et al. 2002) Narrative review	**Barriers to participation in and adherence to cardiac rehabilitation programs** Despite the documented evidence of the benefits of cardiac rehabilitation in enhancing recovery and reducing mortality following a myocardial infarction, only about one third of patients participates in such programs. Adherence to these programs is an even bigger problem, with only about one third maintaining attendance in an exercise program after 6 months. Factors associated with non-participation include lack of referral by physicians, associated illness, specific cardiac diagnoses, various personal psychological factors, lack of perceived benefit of cardiac rehabilitation, distance and transport, reimbursement, family and social support, and occupation. Factors associated with non-adherence include being older, female, lower education, lack of perceived benefit from the program, persistent angina, and less physically active. *(No direct link to occupational outcomes, but attendance is fundamental to any benefit).*
(Day 2003) Narrative review	**Women and cardiac rehabilitation** Over the past 15 years, an increasing number of studies have looked at gender differences in cardiac rehabilitation participation and benefits. Women consistently have lower referral and participation rates, but those who do participate get equal benefits. Both men and women are most strongly influenced by physician recommendations, while men are influenced more by their spouse and women more by their adult children. Women are perceived as being less motivated to participate and quote multiple 'practical' reasons such as life and caring roles, transport and physical problems. Women are less tolerant of physical activity, have lower adherence to exercise regimes and higher dropout rates. Recommends that nurses should be aware of gender issues and women's needs when advising about cardiac rehabilitation. *(No vocational rehabilitation or occupational outcomes).*

TABLE 5a: CARDIAC/CARDIOVASCULAR CONDITIONS

(de Gaudemaris 2000) Narrative review	**Clinical issues: return to work and public safety** Advances in cardiovascular therapy mean that the cardiovascular function of many patients is restored to such an extent that returning to work is physically possible. However, psychological and social factors are more important than medical considerations when it comes to deciding whether or not to go back to work. These authors considered that, even with ideal medical treatment, many patients should not go back to work for a variety of medical, psychological and social reasons (e.g. risks of further MI or diminished ability to do the job). Therefore, the decision whether or not to go back to work with cardiovascular disease involves not only weighing medical considerations but also the patient's psychosocial profile and factors associated with his or her job. Work can only be resumed with the cooperation of several parties, i.e. the patient's personal physician, cardiologist, and employer. Physicians are often reluctant to send their patients back to work based on their concern about prognosis and risks. *(This paper takes a very traditional 'risk assessment' approach, based on theoretical possibilities rather than scientific evidence. Compare with Talmage & Melhorn 2005 (Table 5a). A large part of the paper considers issues of public safety. From the individual's perspective, the authors fail to take account of the physical, psychological and social benefits of return to work (RTW). This paper illustrates the potential, professionally-created barriers created by this approach).*
(ExTraMATCH Collaborative 2004) Meta-analysis	**Exercise training in patients with chronic heart failure** Exercise training for at least 8 weeks significantly reduced mortality in patients with cardiac failure (hazard ratio 0.65, 95% CI 0.46 – 0.92). There is no evidence that properly supervised medical training programmes for patients with heart failure might be dangerous. *(No occupational outcomes).*
(Falcone et al. 2003) Narrative review	**Peripheral arterial disease rehabilitation** Patients with intermittent claudication (IC) typically can walk less than a few blocks before needing to rest to alleviate symptoms. Daily physical activity is reduced up to 45% in patients with IC, as compared with healthy subjects of similar age. Assessment should include treadmill exercise testing or bicycle ergometry, and evaluation of functional status using validated community-based questionnaires. A supervised exercise rehabilitation program is an efficacious method for alleviating IC symptoms, and can increase the speed, distance, and duration walked in patients with intermittent claudication. There is limited evidence on resistance, strength training. Exercise rehabilitation has long been recommended as an effective first-line therapy to reduce symptoms and improve quality of life for patients with IC. However, despite its proven efficacy, exercise rehabilitation is not widely used as a primary therapeutic choice. *(No evidence on vocational rehabilitation or occupational outcomes).*
(Goetzel et al. 2005) Narrative review	**Return on investment in disease management** Included 12 studies of congestive heart failure, 7 of which were RCTs. Per-patient costs averaged $1,399 and savings averaged $3,884. The average return on investment (ROI) across studies was $2.78. Of the five RCTs examined, all but one produced a positive ROI. *(This review only covered direct medical costs and there were no data on indirect costs such as sickness absence). (See also Table 6c).*
(Holland et al. 2005) Systematic review	**Systematic review of multidisciplinary interventions in heart failure** Included 30 trials. Multidisciplinary interventions were defined as those in which management was the responsibility of a multi-disciplinary team including medical input plus one or more of: specialist nurse, pharmacist, dietician or social worker. Interventions included home visits, home physiological monitoring or televideo link, telephone follow-up link, and hospital or clinic interventions alone. Multi-disciplinary interventions reduced heart failure and all-cause hospital admissions and all cause mortality. The most effective interventions were delivered at least partly in the home. *(No occupational outcomes).*

TABLE 5a: CARDIAC/CARDIOVASCULAR CONDITIONS

(Jolliffe et al. 2001) Cochrane review	**Exercise-based rehabilitation for coronary heart disease** Exercise programmes alone reduced cardiac mortality by 31% and all cause mortality by 27%; the corresponding figures for comprehensive cardiac rehabilitation programmes including exercise were 26% and 13%. There was no effect on the recurrence rate for non-fatal MI. 11 trials showed small and variable effects on health-related quality of life, using a variety of subjective and psychological questionnaires. *(No evidence on occupational outcomes. Not updated since 2000).*
(Jolly et al. 2006) Meta-analysis	**Home- vs. centre-based cardiac rehabilitation** 18 trials of home-based vs. 'usual care' and 6 trials of home-based vs. supervised centre-based rehabilitation programmes. In post-MI patients, exercise capacity was significantly reduced in patients receiving home-based rehabilitation compared with usual care. There was no significant difference in cardiac related outcomes between home-based and centre-based rehabilitation programmes, though this was based on <750 patients total. *(No evidence on occupational outcomes).*
(Lee et al. 2007) Systematic review	**The economics of cardiac rehabilitation and lifestyle modification** Included 9 studies and two previous reviews *(including Ades 1997 – see Table 5a)*, but emphasised the variable quality of the evidence. Concluded cautiously that traditional, exercise-based cardiac rehabilitation programmes are economically advantageous: saving on re-hospitalisation costs and total medical costs, and that the net cost per quality-adjusted life year (QALY) was quite moderate. A single controlled but non-randomised trial from Sweden in 1977-80, showed that after 5 years, 52% of the treatment group were actively employed compared to 27% of the control group (based on intention to treat analysis, not just those participating). Including sick leave costs, the authors calculated a total benefit-cost ratio of 51:1
(Leng et al. 2000) Cochrane review	**Exercise for Intermittent claudication** Included 10 trials. Exercise therapy produced significantly improved maximal walking time (minutes) by approximately 150% (range 74% to 230%). *(No evidence on occupational outcomes. Not updated since 2000).*
(Lewin 1999) Editorial	**Return to work after MI, the roles of depression, health beliefs and rehabilitation** Following MI, 67-92% of patients return to work but 30% believe that their MI has damaged their capacity for work and 20% may take early retirement within 1 year. However, it has been estimated that 40-50% of failures to RTW cannot be explained by physical illness alone. The goal of exercise programmes is to improve this by: a) physiological –improve myocardial function to compensate for the infarct, and b) psychological - that patients' confidence and readiness to return to work would be enhanced if they were shown that it was safe to exercise and that they could become fitter and stronger. Results show that most patients do improve their strength and stamina but only two out of 11 RCTs *(up to 1995)* that measured work outcomes showed any improvement in RTW. Suggests that harmful beliefs play a major role in failure to return to work: 80% believe the main cause of their MI was 'stress' 'worry' or over-work'; beliefs about damage to their heart and risk of recurrent MI (often reinforced by thoughtless remarks by doctors); negative beliefs about illness; anxiety and depression. The problems for rehabilitation may be that: a) many patients do not regard (improved) physical fitness as a good measure of risk of premature death; b) patients' faulty understanding of the causal mechanisms of cardiac disease persist after MI; and c) unrecognized and untreated depression. Many rehabilitation programmes *(in 1999)* do not address these issues. It is important that rehabilitation programmes do address these issues. Asking patients *if* and then *why* they think their work might be to blame for their heart attack, how quickly *they* think they should go back to work, if they think they should reduce their effort and *why* need only take a few minutes. That is likely, in some patients, to reveal unnecessary fears or misconceptions about their illness that, if only for the sake of improved communication, should be laid to rest. However, it must also be recognized that some of the determinants of RTW are beyond the control of a rehabilitation programme. *(Pre-2000 but retained as key UK reference).*

TABLE 5a: CARDIAC/CARDIOVASCULAR CONDITIONS

(McAlister et al. 2004) Systematic review	**Multidisciplinary strategies for the management of heart failure patients at high risk for admission** Included 29 RCTs (5039 patients). Strategies that incorporated follow-up by a specialized multidisciplinary team (either in a clinic or a non-clinic setting) reduced mortality (risk ratio [RR] 0.75, 95% confidence interval [CI] 0.59 to 0.96), Heart failure (HF) hospitalizations (RR 0.74, 95% CI 0.63 to 0.87), and all-cause hospitalizations (RR 0.81, 95% CI 0.71 to 0.92). Programs that focused on enhancing patient self-care activities reduced HF hospitalizations (RR 0.66, 95% CI 0.52 to 0.83) and all-cause hospitalizations (RR 0.73, 95% CI 0.57 to 0.93) but had no effect on mortality (RR 1.14, 95% CI 0.67 to 1.94). Strategies that employed telephone contact and advised patients to attend their primary care physician in the event of deterioration reduced HF hospitalizations (RR 0.75, 95% CI 0.57 to 0.99) but not mortality (RR 0.91, 95% CI 0.67 to 1.29) or all-cause hospitalizations (RR 0.98, 95% CI 0.80 to 1.20). In 15 of 18 trials that evaluated cost, multidisciplinary strategies were cost-saving. Authors' conclusion: Multidisciplinary strategies for the management of patients with HF reduce HF hospitalizations. Those programs that involve specialized follow-up by a multidisciplinary team also reduce mortality and all-cause hospitalizations. (*No occupational outcomes*).
(Mital & Mital 2002) Narrative review	**Returning coronary heart disease patients to work: a modified perspective** Cardiac rehabilitation is the process by which CHD patients are restored to their optimal physical, mental, medical, psychological, social, emotional, vocational and economic status. This definition implies multidisciplinary rehabilitation involving medicine, physiology, psychology, vocational and ergonomics. Potential candidates for (*vocational*) rehabilitation generally have: i) assessment of physical demands for expected occupational and recreational activities after recovery from MI, and ii) an exercise test to determine current physical work capacity. Rehabilitating CHD patients to work is highly desirable from an economic and humanitarian standpoint. Thus, RTW or reemployment at the earliest possible time should be the ultimate goal of any cardiac rehab program. However, existing cardiac rehabilitation programs do not reduce lost time from work, and there has been no improvement in duration of sickness absence since 1970. The majority of cardiac patients, on the average, take 6 months to return to work. Psychosocial factors are also more closely related to RTW outcomes than medical ones. It is proposed that cardiac rehabilitation programmes should focus on simulating actual work activities to enhance the cardiac patient's physical, cognitive and occupational capacity. (*This review was combined with an individual study in which a job simulation program was devised and tested. Only conclusions from the review were extracted*).
(Mital et al. 2004) Narrative review	**Return to work after a coronary event** Coronary heart disease is the leading cause of premature, permanent disability in the US labour force, accounting for 19% of social security disability allowances. The cost is estimated to be $130 billion, including insurance, wage replacement and health care. Rehabilitating CHD patients to work is therefore highly desirable form both an economic and humanitarian perspective. Age, gender, physical work capacity, education level, type of occupation and societal factors, in addition to psychosocial factors, play a crucial role on determining successful return to work. Whether a patient will return to work after a major cardiac event is a complex question and not resuming work is not based solely on cardiac findings. Women, older workers (particularly those >60 years), blue collar workers with strenuous physical jobs and patients with psychological problems are less likely to return to work. However, the most important and decisive factors are psychosocial: depressed mood, motivation to work, lowered perceptions of workability, socioeconomic and availability of alternative financial security. Current cardiac rehabilitation programmes generally have inadequate clinical assessment of capacity for work and lack focus on vocational rehabilitation. Despite restoring many patients to their premorbid functional status, they have generally not reduced time off work nor improved occupational outcomes. The authors recommend that cardiac rehabilitation programmes should nor only use aerobic exercise to restore functional capacity, but should also incorporate a specific focus on return to work, actual job-related activities and assessment of physical strength, flexibility and dexterity. This approach needs to be replicated in other settings, including the workplace. Such programmes are expensive, and cost-effectiveness also needs to be demonstrated. Providing this is done, the job-simulation approach to cardiac rehabilitation would be worth pursuing. However, given the high costs of cardiac disease and the limited success of current cardiac rehabilitation programmes, provides strong motivation for trying other options.

TABLE 5a: CARDIAC/CARDIOVASCULAR CONDITIONS

(NACR 2007) Statistical Report	**National Audit of Cardiac Rehabilitation: annual statistical report 2007** [National Audit of Cardiac Rehabilitation] 39% of patients hospitalised for MI in UK in 2005-06 received cardiac rehabilitation: England 42%, Wales 34%, Scotland 26%, N Ireland 25%. Only a tiny fraction of the 66,000 people newly diagnosed with heart failure each year receive rehabilitation. There are around 345,000 new cases of angina each year and practically none attend rehabilitation. The average age of those attending cardiac rehabilitation was 65 years for men and 71 years for women. 22% were employed full-time and 4% part-time; 5% were self-employed. All patients took part in some kind of exercise or activity programme: Nearly 80% took part in group exercises, 27% had some form of individualized exercise and 32% had a home exercise programme. Around 60% took part in group talks, including discussions about diet. Less than 1% had a vocational assessment). *(NACR 2007 National Audit of Cardiac Rehabilitation Annual Statistical Report 2007 www.cardiacrehabilitation.org.uk/docs/NACR_2007.pdf)*
(NHS Centre for Reviews 1998) Healthcare bulletin	**Effective Health Care: cardiac rehabilitation** [UK National Health Service Centre for Reviews] RTW rates are fairly high following an acute cardiac event, but a substantial number subsequently stop work or retire early. Current provision *(in 1998)* of cardiac rehabilitation in UK is growing rapidly but there is a wide variation in practice, management, and organisation of services. Many patients who might benefit do not receive cardiac rehabilitation. Uptake is only 15-60%, with ~50% drop-out by 6-12 months – helps if doctor strongly recommends, when access is convenient, and when partner/spouse involved. Many of the problems experienced by people with heart disease are not due to physical illness but to anxiety and misconceptions about their health. The majority of programmes are exercise-based: exercise does not carry any increased risk, and has a positive impact on physical ability to exercise and physiological measures of cardiac function, but there is insufficient evidence to assess impact on RTW. Many programmes combine exercise with various forms of education and counselling, with improvement in cardiac mortality of 20-25% (at least for those with mild MI), inconclusive evidence of impact on exercise levels (at least in the short-term) and psychological well-being, but no proven impact on RTW. Limited evidence supports cost-effectiveness. *(UK Effective Health Care Bulletins are based on systematic review and synthesis of research; produced by methodologists with expert input. Limited information on RTW). (Pre-2000 but retained as key UK reference).*
(NHS 2000) UK National Service Framework	**National Service Framework for coronary heart disease** [National Health Service] This UK government (Dept of Health) initiative concerns how the NHS and others can best help people who have had a cardiac event maximise their chances of leading a full life and resuming their place in the community. It spells out national standards for coronary heart disease in 7 areas: 1) reducing heart disease in the population; 2) preventing coronary heart disease in high risk patients; 3) heart attack and other acute coronary syndromes; 4) stable angina; 5) revascularisation; 6) heart failure; 7) cardiac rehabilitation. Emphasises that it is important that cardiac rehabilitation is seen as an integral component of both the acute stages of care and of secondary prevention). Chapter 7: Cardiac rehabilitation: Standard twelve: NHS Trusts should put in place agreed protocols/systems of care so that, prior to leaving hospital, people admitted to hospital suffering from coronary heart disease have been invited to participate in a multidisciplinary programme of secondary prevention and cardiac rehabilitation. The aim of the programme will be to reduce their risk of subsequent cardiac problems and to promote their return to a full and normal life.

TABLE 5a: CARDIAC/CARDIOVASCULAR CONDITIONS

	(Focused mainly on clinical management, modification of cardiac risk factors and lifestyle modification and on cardiac outcomes). Exercise sessions: It is not clear which model of care is most effective and different models of service delivery seem to suit different patients. There is evidence, however, that structured, taught exercise sessions are most cost-effective in groups and that cost-effectiveness increases with group size. *(No guidance on vocational rehabilitation and no evidence on occupational outcomes, except that the audit tool includes the following three questions:)* • Do the notes indicate whether the patient has concerns about return to work? • If yes, has the patient been referred for vocational guidance? • Number of patients who express return to work problems who have been referred for vocational guidance? *(The chapter on cardiac rehabilitation does not include any hard evidence on vocational rehabilitation or outcomes. This NSF has not been updated since 2000. The suggested audit questions do not appear to have been implemented in NACR 2007).*
(NCCC 2006) Clinical guideline	**Hypertension** [UK National Collaborating Centre for Chronic Conditions] *(Focuses entirely on clinical management and does not provide any evidence on vocational rehabilitation or occupational outcomes).*
(NICE 2003) Clinical guideline	**Chronic heart failure** [UK National Institute for Clinical Excellence] *(Focuses entirely on clinical management and does not provide any evidence on vocational rehabilitation or occupational outcomes for chronic heart failure, but refers back to earlier review of cardiac rehabilitation in general - NHS Centre for Reviews 1998).*
(NZGG 2002) Guideline	**Cardiac rehabilitation: summary and resource kit** [New Zealand Guidelines Group] Cardiac rehabilitation is the coordinated sum of interventions required to ensure the best physical, psychological and social conditions so that patients with chronic or post-acute cardiovascular disease may, by their own efforts, preserve or resume optimal functioning in society and, through improved health behaviours, slow or reverse progression of disease. The main goals of cardiac rehabilitation are: 1. To prevent further cardiovascular events by empowering patients to initiate and maintain lifestyle changes 2. To improve quality of life through the identification and treatment of psychological distress 3. To facilitate the patient's return to a full and active life by enabling the development of their own resources. Comprehensive cardiac rehabilitation programmes have been shown to reduce mortality from coronary heart disease, re-infarction rates and hospital admissions and improve quality of life for the patient and their family. Meta-analysis of randomized controlled trials of cardiac rehabilitation have shown a 25% reduction in total mortality in those patients who combined multi-factorial risk factor counselling with exercise compared with exercise alone. Phases of cardiac rehabilitation *Phase I: Inpatient rehabilitation* Phase I rehabilitation in hospital includes early mobilisation and education helping the patient, spouse, partner, whānau and family begin to develop an understanding of heart disease. The patient should be given a discharge plan (with a copy sent to his/her general practitioner) usually offering medical follow-up, information and referral to Phase II programmes.

TABLE 5a: CARDIAC/CARDIOVASCULAR CONDITIONS

Phase II: Outpatient rehabilitation

Phase II rehabilitation is traditionally a supervised ambulatory programme beginning as soon as possible after discharge and referral. It usually involves:

- An exercise component (home activity and/or supervised exercise sessions)
- Education sessions aimed at increasing understanding of the disease process, risk factors, treatment, and nutrition advice
- Guidance for the resumption of physical, sexual and daily living activities, including work
- Psychosocial support.

On completion of the programme a summary letter should be written to the patients GP and specialist.

Phase III: Long term maintenance

Phase III promotes long term maintenance of the skills and behaviour changes learned within Phase I and II. In New Zealand, this phase is primarily the domain of independent community 'cardiac clubs' which act as support groups.

Work and vocational adjustment

Recommendations include: Comprehensive cardiac rehabilitation programmes should include vocational guidance to facilitate an appropriate and realistic return to work.

In addition to providing income, work is an important source of self-esteem. Most patients will return to work or productive activity following myocardial infarction. Return to work is associated with an improvement in emotional well-being. Vocational guidance as part of a comprehensive cardiac rehabilitation programme will enable a patient to consider when to return to work, or whether a modification of their work is desirable. Almost half of people that do not make it back to work do so because of psychological reasons, not physical factors. Efforts to facilitate a return to work should begin as early as possible, since patients who delay are less likely to resume work.

For those who see work as a potential barrier to participation in an outpatient based programme, options such as home based cardiac rehabilitation should be considered.

Cardiac rehabilitation staff should facilitate a discussion between employer and patients that allow a phased return to work, or time off to attend cardiac rehabilitation programmes.

Outcomes include return to work and quality of life. ***Audit*** includes % resumed previous work.

(Ofman et al. 2004) Systematic review	**Does Disease Management Improve Clinical and Economic Outcomes in Patients with Chronic Diseases?** Disease Management was compared with standard and usual care in 6 studies of patients with coronary artery disease. The most frequently used interventions were patient education, multidisciplinary team care, and patient reminders. Two studies showed no change in provider adherence to drug guidelines. Only one study reported a significant reduction in the number of patients having a non-fatal re-infarction during 10 year follow-up. There were 9 studies on patients with heart failure, with no significant effects on provider adherence to management guidelines. There were 9 studies on patients with hypertension, providing strong evidence of significantly greater improvements in blood pressure.

TABLE 5a: CARDIAC/CARDIOVASCULAR CONDITIONS

(Perk & Alexanderson 2004) Systematic review	**Sick leave due to coronary artery disease** At least 50% of patients *(who were previously employed)* can return to work following myocardial infarction. Several studies showed that duration of sick leave is influenced mainly by psychological and social factors such as depression, self-confidence, low educational level, physically demanding work, or low work satisfaction. There is limited and conflicting evidence that cardiac rehabilitation has any signifcant impact on RTW. *(Findings reported for myocardial infarction only. Much of this review is about patterns of sickness absence after strokes or major cardiac interventions, and only a small part is on vocational rehabilitation interventions).*
(Phillips et al. 2005) Narrative review	**Return to work and the person with heart failure** An extensive, systematic literature search *(in 2004)* revealed a paucity of literature on work-related issues for persons with heart failure. There was no evidence on their vocational rehabilitation, and no RCTs that measured RTW outcomes. *(The authors then attempted to develop guidance for nurses based on the general literature on cardiac rehabilitation).*
(Rees et al. 2004) Cochrane review	**Exercise-based rehabilitation for heart failure** 29 trials of patients with primary or secondary heart failure. Exercise training significantly increased VO2 max by 2.16 ml/kg/min (95% CI 2.82 to 1.49), exercise duration increased by 2.38 minutes (95% CI 2.85 to 1.9), exercise capacity by 15.1 Watts (95% CI 17.7 to 12.6) and distance on the six minute walk by 40.9 metres (95% CI 64.7 to 17.1). Improvements in VO2 max were greater for training programmes of greater intensity and duration. Health-related quality of life improved in seven of the nine trials that measured this outcome. Authors' conclusions: Exercise training improves exercise capacity and quality of life in patients mild to moderate heart failure in the short term. However, a) follow-up was generally < 12 months, and b) the findings of the review are mainly based on small-scale trials in predominantly male patients with relatively stable cardiac failure who are unrepresentative of the total population of patients with heart failure. *(No evidence on vocational rehabilitation or occupational outcomes).*
(SIGN 2002) Clinical guideline	**Cardiac rehabilitation** [Scottish Intercollegiate Guidelines Network] Describes 4 phases of cardiac rehabilitation: Phase 1 is the in-patient phase. The key elements are medical evaluation, reassurance and education, correction of cardiac misconceptions, risk factor assessment, mobilisation and discharge planning. A nurse counsellor can help to improve patient and partner knowledge and reduce anxiety and depression. Phase 2 is the early post-discharge period, when many patients feel isolated and insecure. A self-help programme has been shown to reduce anxiety, depression and hospital re-admission rates. Phase 3 has historically taken the form of a structured exercise programme in a hospital setting with educational and psychological support and advice on risk factors. Increasingly it is recognized this can be provided safely and effectively in the community. A 'menu-based approach' includes 'vocational rehabilitation to assist return to work or retirement'. Phase 4 involves the long-term maintenance of physical activity and lifestyle change. *(Focuses mainly on clinical management, exercise programmes, psychological lifestyle and behavioural issues, information and advice. No detail or evidence on vocational rehabilitation or occupational outcomes).*

TABLE 5a: CARDIAC/CARDIOVASCULAR CONDITIONS

(SIGN 2007b) Clinical guideline	**Risk estimation and the prevention of cardiovascular disease** [Scottish Intercollegiate Guidelines Network] *(Very medical, focused on primary prevention and no occupational outcomes).*
(SIGN 2007a) Clinical guideline	**Management of stable angina** [Scottish Intercollegiate Guidelines Network] *(Very clinical and surgical, nothing on rehabilitation (cross-refers to SIGN 2002) and no occupational outcomes).*
(Simpson & Pilote 2003) Systematic review	**Quality of life after acute myocardial infarction** Health related quality of life (HRQoL) is an important measure of a patient's recovery after an illness. Systematic review of 11 studies showed that the impact of an acute myocardial infarction on HRQoL appeared to be modest (among those who survived the MI and who did not drop-out of the studies – which may introduce a 'healthy survivor' effect). Severity of cardiac symptoms, need for invasive procedures, age (particularly those <65 years) and time since infarction had greatest impact on HRQoL. Physical capacity, work status, symptoms, functional status and general health perceptions declined most soon after MI, but the majority of those domains improved to normal levels within a year. The major exception was work status. Many patients were unable to perform the same level of tasks they could do pre-MI and many experienced significant reductions in the number of hours they were able to work. There was little improvement on long-term follow-up. Patients who returned to work tended to have higher overall HRQoL than those who did not return to work *(though the reviewers were unable to say if this was case selection or cause and effect).* However, the reviewers pointed out although MI had a significant impact on work status, many of these patients were near retirement age anyway at the time of their MI.
(Smidt et al. 2005) Systematic review	**Effectiveness of exercise therapy: a best-evidence summary of systematic reviews** <u>Intermittent claudication:</u> 7 systematic reviews (4 of reasonable quality, including Leng 2002) showed that exercise therapy is effective compared to no treatment. Exercise therapy consisted of (treadmill) training in walking, and lower limb strengthening exercises (e.g. stair climbing). Patients were encouraged to continue with daily walking exercises at home until they felt moderate pain. There were also indications that exercise therapy is more effective in improving maximal walking time than angioplasty and equally as effective as surgery. No conclusions could be drawn with regard to the effectiveness of a specific type of exercise therapy. <u>Cerebrovascular Accident (CVA):</u> 11 systematic reviews (3 of reasonable quality) provided insufficient evidence to support or refute the effectiveness of exercise therapy for patients who had suffered a stroke or for patients with hemiplegic shoulder pain, compared to no treatment or other conservative treatments. *(No occupational outcomes). (Other extracts in Tables 3 and 5b).*
(Talmage & Melhorn 2005) (Hyman 2005) Physician guidance	**A physician's guide to return to work: working with common cardiopulmonary problems** [American Medical Association] *(Guide book for primary care physicians and care providers to assist navigation of return to work issues, supported by science and consensus: the authors admit a firm belief that work is good for man).* Most myocardial infarctions or acute coronary syndromes occur unrelated to work: stress or vigorous physical exercise are only identifiable in 10-15%. In patients who are post MI and/or who have stable angina, sustained work demands of < 40% and infrequent work demands of <80% maximal exercise capacity (on treadmill measurement) are generally safe. Exercise at work may be more likely to protect rather than cause recurrent cardiac events. Reduced work tolerance when work capacity appears adequate appears to be mainly related to psychosocial factors.

TABLE 5a: CARDIAC/CARDIOVASCULAR CONDITIONS

	Cardiopulmonary conditions are common, and the physician should think through the issues of risk, capacity and tolerance. As a general principle, any known risk factors that may have contributed to the disease formation should be assessed and modified (in addition to rehabilitation and return-to-work support). As with other body system problems, patients with cardiopulmonary disease are rarely harmed by return-to-work recommendation. The considerable benefits of returning to work usually outweigh the risk. *(Provides a reasoned case for promoting and assessing capacity for return to work with cardiac conditions. No further information on vocational rehabilitation interventions, effectiveness or occupational outcomes). (Entries in respect of working with musculoskeletal conditions are in Table 3).*
(Taylor et al. 2004) Meta-analysis	**Exercise-based rehabilitation for patients with coronary heart disease** Included 48 trials with a total of 8940 patients. With a few exceptions, the trials examined exercise therapy delivered in a supervised manner, often in a formal health care setting, such as a hospital. Compared with usual care, cardiac rehabilitation was associated with reduced all-cause mortality (odds ratio [OR] = 0.80; 95% CI: 0.68 to 0.93) and cardiac mortality (OR = 0.74; 95% CI: 0.61 to 0.96). There were no significant differences in the rates of nonfatal myocardial infarction and revascularization, and changes in high- and low-density lipoprotein cholesterol levels and diastolic pressure. Health-related quality of life improved to similar levels with cardiac rehabilitation and usual care. *(No vocational rehabilitation interventions or occupational outcomes. This paper appears to be from the same group and the same review as the Cochrane review (Joliffe 2001) and the Canadian HTA (Brown et al 2003) on the same subject).*
(van Dixhoorn & White 2005) Meta-analysis	**Relaxation therapy for rehabilitation and prevention of ischaemic heart disease** 27 studies were included: 6 studies of 'abbreviated' therapy (3 hours or less), 13 studies of 'full' relaxation therapy (9 hours or more), and 8 studies of full relaxation therapy expanded with cognitive therapy. Intensive supervised relaxation practice enhances recovery from an ischaemic cardiac event and contributes to secondary prevention. It is an important ingredient of cardiac rehabilitation, in addition to exercise and psycho-education. Relaxation therapy can improve exercise tolerance, even in the absence of exercise training. Three studies show that the odds of being at work at 6 months after MI or coronary artery bypass graft is significantly increased by relaxation therapy. These effects were not demonstrated in abbreviated relaxation therapy, but there was no difference between full or expanded relaxation therapy.
(Waddell & Burton 2004) Evidence synthesis	**Concepts of rehabilitation for the management of common health problems** [Report commissioned by UK Department for Work and Pensions] 24 reviews on cardiac rehabilitation (7 systematic) showed that. • In principle, the provision of vocational advice is recognised as a fundamental aspect of cardiac rehabilitation, along with lifestyle/psychological interventions and educational advice. Employers should be involved early in the rehabilitation process in order to avoid prolonged inactivity, and there is a need for greater collaboration between cardiac rehabilitation and occupational health medicine to ensure optimum and effective return to work. However, there is little evidence this has been implemented in practice. • Return to work following a major cardiac event is a major milestone in the rehabilitation process. However, it is a complex issue that involves the patient and the employer as well as clinical decision-makers. Once the decision is made (which should be as early as possible) communication and contact are paramount, both within and outwith the rehabilitation team, in order to identify and modify obstacles to return to work. • Good communication between medical staff and those providing vocational counselling in respect of medical status, exercise tolerance, and psychological factors are essential for successful return to work. • n 2004, any impact on return to work was unclear, firstly because of the limited evidence available and secondly because of the many factors influencing return to work after a major cardiac event. *(This extract is limited to the evidence on cardiac rehabilitation after MI).*

TABLE 5a: CARDIAC/CARDIOVASCULAR CONDITIONS

(Waddell & Burton 2006)	**Is work good for your health and well-being?**
	[Report commissioned by UK Department for Work and Pensions]
Evidence synthesis	Returning workers with cardiovascular and respiratory conditions to work is a generally accepted goal that is incorporated into clinical guidance.
	There is strong evidence that many workers with cardiovascular conditions do manage to return to work, but the rates vary and return to work may not be sustained.
	The return to work process for workers with cardio-respiratory conditions is generally considered to require a combination of both clinical management and occupational risk control.
	There is limited evidence that rehabilitation and return to work for workers with cardio-respiratory conditions can be beneficial for general health and well-being and quality of life.
	Risk factors for return to work:
	• Return to work is contingent on many social and policy issues.
	• (*Several reviews conclude that functional capacity is poorly correlated with return to work*). Coronary risk status is much more important than functional capacity in determining RTW.
	• Although more severe infarctions reduce the chance of return to work, psychosocial factors appear to have a greater impact. Return to work is less likely in women, blue-collar workers particularly with physically strenuous jobs, and patients with emotional problems.
	• Resumption of work is largely determined by factors that cardiac rehab cannot influence – age, severity of disease, educational level, and adequacy of pension and retirement benefits
	Specific suggestions for facilitating RTW were involvement early in the worker's recuperative period, including early contact with the worker, offering support and encouragement by telephoning/visiting, maintaining links to the workplace, encouraging co-workers, supervisors, and/or subordinates to maintain contact with the worker.
	(*This review focused on the health benefits of work and provided little direct evidence on the effectiveness of vocational rehabilitation interventions. However, the overall conclusion was that*: The impact of rehabilitation on vocational outcomes is difficult to evaluate because return to work depends on many complex factors.

[CHD = coronary heart disease; MI = myocardial infarction; RCT = randomised controlled trial; RTW = return to work]

Table 5b: Respiratory conditions

TABLE 5b: RESPIRATORY CONDITIONS	
Authors	**Key features** (*Reviewers' comments in italic*)
(Ameille & Descatha 2005) Narrative review	**Outcome of occupational asthma** Most studies show that patients with occupational asthma continue to deteriorate of they continue in the same job. Therefore there is general consensus that complete and definitive removal from exposure is the key to treatment of occupational asthma. Complete avoidance of exposure is associated with improvement in asthma symptoms and functional parameters, though symptoms and non-specific bronchial hyper-responsiveness (NSBH) persist in approximately 70% of cases. Several studies show that improvement in symptoms and NSBH can continue over several years after cessation of exposure. However, it is not always possible for affected individuals to find alternative employment. Furthermore, patients with occupational asthma become unusually sensitive to non-specific stimuli such as cold air, dust or other irritants often present in the workplace. Inadequate compensation in many countries may also contribute to the decision of workers to continue the in the same employment after diagnosis. Reduction of exposure, which can be achieved by relocation to a less exposed job, improvement in workplace hygiene, use of modified material, and use of personal protective devices, is therefore an alternative worth considering. Quotes Vandenplas 2003 analysis of 6 studies to show that reducing exposure is more frequently associated with persistent asthma symptoms and NSBH and with worsening of asthma compared with complete removal, though this may vary with different causative agents.
(Antó et al. 2001) Narrative review	**Epidemiology of chronic obstructive airways disease** Chronic obstructive pulmonary disease (COPD) is a leading cause of mortality and disability worldwide, affecting ~5-15% of adults in industrialised countries. COPD has a chronic long-lasting course characterized by irreversible decline of forced expiratory volume in one second (FEV1), increasing presence of dyspnoea and other respiratory symptoms, and progressive deterioration of health status. After diagnosis the 10-yr survival rate is ~50% with more than one-third of patients dying due to respiratory insufficiency. (*No data on occupational impact*).
(Banks & Jalloul 2007) Narrative review	**Occupational asthma, work-related asthma and reactive airways dysfunction syndrome** Over the past 20 years, it has become recognised that work related asthma includes three entities, all of which can adversely affect workers' health and, in many instances, require the worker to leave the job: Occupational asthma (allergic or irritant): Most is known about the natural history of occupational asthma. It is generally agreed that workers must leave the workplace where exposure occurs when this diagnosis is made. Work-aggravated asthma: This remains the least well described, and has only been accepted as part of work-related asthma in the last few years. There is some evidence that reducing exposure to respiratory irritants and optimising asthma therapy may allow some patients to continue in the same job. However, this has not yet been confirmed by clinical trials and the most appropriate management is still not agreed. Reactive airways disease syndrome: This is not well understood. It is generally a severe medical illness, usually occurring after an acute exposure, and usually leads to persisting respiratory problems.

TABLE 5b: RESPIRATORY CONDITIONS

Reference	Content
(Beach et al. 2005) Report	**Diagnosis and management of work-related asthma** [US Agency for Health Care Policy & Research: evidence review and Health Technology Assessment] 5-15% of adult onset asthma is thought to be occupational. Included 124 diagnostic studies and 64 management studies, including both removal from the workplace and reduced exposure at the workplace. Standard treatments for asthma appear to be effective in occupational asthma; however, there is limited research. Occupational asthma appears to be slow to resolve, and may worsen over time irrespective of subsequent exposure status. Patients who are removed from *(continued exposure at)* the workplace show improved lung function and decreased non-specific bronchial responsiveness at follow-up, but rarely experience complete resolution, experience continued airflow limitation and may require continued medication. Approximately one third of workers are unemployed 6 years after initial confirmed diagnosis. Most workers who are diagnosed appear to have reduced earnings over time (greater if removed from the workplace, but even if managed by reduced exposure in the same workplace).
(Bradley et al. 2002) Cochrane review	**Physical training for bronchiectasis** Only included two studies, which showed that inspiratory muscle training improved endurance exercise capacity and health-related quality of life (HRQoL), compared to sham or no training. *(HRQoL was based on subjective measures, related to symptoms. No occupational outcomes).*
(British Thoracic Society & SIGN 2007) Clinical guideline	**British guideline on the management of asthma** [British Thoracic Society and Scottish Intercollegiate Guidelines Network] *(Mainly concerned with clinical management of asthma in general. No information on vocational rehabilitation or occupational outcomes for non-occupational asthma).* Section 8.4 on occupational asthma: The aim of management is to identify the cause, remove the worker from exposure, and for the worker to have worthwhile employment. Relocation away from exposure or substitution of the hazard should occur as soon as diagnosis is confirmed, and ideally within 12 months of the first work-related symptoms of asthma. Workers who remain in the same job and continue exposure are unlikely to improve and symptoms may worsen. Complete avoidance of exposure may or may not improve symptoms and bronchial hyper-responsiveness. There is consistent evidence from clinical and workplace studies that about one third of workers are unemployed up to 6 years after diagnosis, though it is unclear if this is any different from non-occupational asthma.
(Cambach et al. 1999) Systematic review & meta-analysis	**The long-term effects of pulmonary rehabilitation in patients with asthma and chronic obstructive pulmonary disease** *(A critical review and meta-analysis of articles published since the 1950s).* Patients with asthma and chronic obstructive pulmonary disease benefit from pulmonary rehabilitation. Significant summary effect sizes were found for maximal exercise capacity, endurance time and walking distance, and for health-related quality of life (dyspnoea, fatigue, emotion and mastery). *(Interventions varied. No occupational outcomes).* *(This review pre-dates 2000, but was retained because it provides a good summary of the evidence from the previous 50 years).*
(Camp et al. 2004) Narrative review	**Women and occupational lung disease: sex differences and gender influences on research and disease outcomes** It is unclear how sex differences in lung anatomy and physiology may influence the development of lung disease. Research into women's health and occupational lung disease must consider possible sex differences in susceptibility to various exposures and development of occupational lung disease, as well as likely gender differences in their occupations, occupational environment and exposures. In some countries, the prevalence of occupational asthma is higher in men, but in others, the rates seem to be similar. In the United Kingdom, surveillance data suggests higher rates in men than women; however, when occupation is taken into consideration the rates are similar in both sexes. Gender differences have been identified in studies of respiratory signs and symptoms in various occupational settings, but there is no consistent pattern. *(Nothing on vocational rehabilitation or occupational outcomes).*

TABLE 5b: RESPIRATORY CONDITIONS

(Datta & ZuWallack 2004)
Narrative review

High vs. low intensity exercise training in pulmonary rehabilitation: is more better?

Exercise training is considered a necessary part of respiratory rehabilitation but there is no consensus on the best exercise strategy. As in healthy individuals, the effect of exercise training on patients with chronic lung disease is dose dependent, with higher intensities resulting in greater physiological adaptations and greater exercise performance. However, it is not clear that this translates into reduced symptoms or better quality of life. (No occupational outcomes).

(Effing et al. 2007)
Cochrane review

Self-management education programmes for chronic obstructive pulmonary disease

Included 14 trials of various kinds of education programmes in self-management with variable duration of follow-up. There were small and variably significant reductions in symptoms and improvements in health-related quality of life, but these were not clinically meaningful. There was conflicting evidence on numbers of exacerbations but a significant reduction in hospitalisations (OR 0.64; 95% CI (0.47 to 0.89). No significant effects were found on lung function, exercise capacity, and days lost from work.

(Gibson et al. 2002)
Cochrane review

Self-management education and regular practitioner review for adults with asthma

Self-management education programmes made no difference to pulmonary function, but significantly improved health-related quality of life and significantly reduced health care use. 16 studies reported the impact on days off work or school, with significant improvement. Economic analysis showed increased direct (health care) costs, significant reduction in indirect (social) costs, and non-significant reduction in total costs. (No update since 2002).

(Goetzel et al. 2005)
Narrative reaview

Return on investment in disease management

12 studies of asthma were included, 7 of which were RCTs. Per-patient costs averaged $269 and savings $729. An overall Return on investment (ROI) of $2.72 was calculated for studies providing both cost and benefit data. Of the seven RCTs examined, six produced savings in medical costs, but only two had savings that were high enough to result in a positive ROI, and those two studies had very few cases. (This review only covered direct medical costs and there were no data on indirect costs such as sickness absence. Generic material in Table 7).

(Henneberger 2007)
Systematic review

Work-exacerbated asthma

6 recent epidemiological studies suggest that work-exacerbated asthma accounts for 26% of working adults with asthma and 45% of all work-related asthma. Work-exacerbated asthma can result from a variety of occupational triggers including physical factors (e.g. extreme temperatures, exercise), behavioural states (e.g. strong emotions, stress), odours (e.g. perfume), general irritants and dust, and second hand cigarette smoke. Demographic and clinical features are similar to adult asthma and occupational asthma.

More severe cases may require a change of job, while other cases may be able to remain at work if exposures are lowered and asthma medication optimised. Exposures should be lowered by engineering controls (e.g. improved ventilation) when possible, with reliance on personal respirators only for short-term special situations. Since work exacerbated asthma can result in job loss or change largely unwanted by the patient, it is important that the patient receives appropriate social service support.

(HSE 2007b)
Statistics

Occupational asthma - statistics

The 2006/07 Self-reported Work-related Illness survey estimated that there were 142 000 people in UK with 'breathing or lung problems' which they believed to be 'work-related'. In 2006, there were 592 new cases – an incidence rate of about 20 per million workers per year – recorded by respiratory and occupational physicians reporting to The Health and Occupation Reporting (THOR) network. This is probably a substantial under-estimate. It compares with an incidence of 160 new cases of occupational asthma assessed for disablement benefit under the Industrial Injuries Disablement (IIDB) scheme.

The most common age groups for new cases of occupational asthma were 35–44 and 45–54 years – each accounting for around one-quarter of the total. 72% of males and 77% of females were aged <55 years. (THOR data) www.hse.gov.uk/statistics/causdis/asthma/index.htm (accessed 20 November 2007).

TABLE 5b: RESPIRATORY CONDITIONS

| (HSE 2007a)

Guidance | **Asthma - guidance**

[UK Guidance]

Occupational asthma is the most frequently reported occupational respiratory disease in Great Britain; work-related asthma (asthma made worse by work) is substantially more common. Key elements of management:

- Risk assessment and control of substances injurious to health is a legal requirement on employers
- Importance of health surveillance and early detection
- The fundamental principle of clinical and occupational management and vocational rehabilitation is to stop or control exposure combined with routine clinical management of asthma

(There is no suggestion that people with asthma should not work, or that work is detrimental (provided appropriate risk assessment & control). No evidence on effectiveness or occupational outcomes).

www.hse.gov.uk/asthma *(accessed 20 November 2007)* |

| (Iqbal et al. 2002)

Systematic review | **Worldwide guidelines for chronic obstructive pulmonary disease: A comparison of diagnosis and treatment recommendations**

41 clinical practice guidelines showed similar approaches to diagnosis and management of COPD, but the detail and clarity of the recommendations varied. Key differences included the lung function parameters that define a diagnosis and severity assignment of COPD. The use of anticholinergics, alone or in combination, was listed as a consideration for first-line therapy for persistent COPD in all 41 guidelines. There was consensus regarding reserving corticosteroids for selected patients. *(This review focused entirely on clinical diagnosis and management, with no mention of vocational rehabilitation or occupational outcomes).* |

| (Jeebhay & Quirce 2007)

Narrative review | **Occupational asthma in the developing and industrialised world**

The proportion of adult asthma cases attributable to work is similar in industrialised countries and developing countries undergoing rapid industrialisation (3-15%), but lower in less industrialised developing countries (6%).

Primary and secondary prevention strategies should be directed at controlling workplace exposures, accompanied by educational and managerial improvements. Appropriate treatment remains early removal from exposure to the causal agent, and to minimise the consequences to the worker. This includes providing health care and rehabilitation, as well as assisting the worker to obtain adequate compensation and preservation of income. Systems that incorporate retraining, such as the Quebec system, may be more effective than those that do not. However, many workers with occupational asthma continue to remain exposed to the causal agent, and up to one third suffer prolonged work disruption, discrimination and long-term unemployment. Unfortunately, occupational asthma remains under-recognised, poorly managed and inadequately compensated, especially in developing countries. |

TABLE 5b: RESPIRATORY CONDITIONS

(Lacasse et al. 2006) Cochrane review	**Pulmonary rehabilitation for chronic obstructive pulmonary disease** Included 31 RCTs. Rehabilitation was defined as exercise training for at least four weeks with or without education and/or psychological support. There was modest improvement in respiratory function and exercise capacity (6 or 12 minute walking tests), and statistically and clinically significant improvement in health-related quality of life (Chronic Respiratory Questionnaire scores for Dyspnoea, Fatigue, Emotional function and Mastery). *(No occupational outcomes).*
(Malo 2005) Narrative review	**Future advances in work-related asthma and the impact on occupational health** Asthma is one of the most common occupational respiratory disease; 10% of people with adult onset asthma say that their symptoms are aggravated by work. More is known about allergic and, to a lesser extent, irritant induced occupational asthma but much more research is needed on work-aggravated asthma. Further research is required on the genetic basis and cellular mechanisms of asthma. The best method to characterize exposure is still open to debate. For irritant-induced occupational asthma, measures should be directed to reducing the likelihood of accidental inhalational episodes. For allergic occupational asthma, the efficacy of primary prevention surveillance programmes may be greatly hampered by psychological and cultural factors. For secondary prevention of allergic occupational asthma, cases have to be identified early, as the earlier the worker is removed from exposure the more likely he/she is to be cured. Better field means should be developed by molecular biologists for the early identification of cases of sensitization to occupational agents. Occupational asthma too often remains undiagnosed and incorrectly or insufficiently investigated by clinical and functional means. Diagnosis of occupational asthma is based on a stepwise approach: questionnaire, immunological assessment (when relevant and feasible), lung function and inflammatory tests and specific inhalation challenges. Further evidence is required on the validity of some of these steps. Although occupational asthma is a prescribed disease in many jurisdictions, the protection offered to workers is generally inadequate. Diagnostic services for occupational asthma are often unsatisfactory and take time. Affected workers frequently continue to be exposed or, if not, encounter serious socio-economic losses. Yet occupational asthma is a condition that can be cured if the diagnosis is made rapidly. It can have minimal impact on one's health and life if adequate re-adaptation is proposed. Moreover, occupational asthma usually affects young people, so efforts to cure it have a long-term benefit. Once the diagnosis is made, the worker should be assessed and a suitable re-adaptation programme offered. In young individuals, this might mean returning to further education, training and professional development programmes in which, ideally, they are no longer exposed to the causal agent. If this is done, it has been estimated that the quality of life of workers with occupational asthma will be satisfactory, and at an acceptable socioeconomic cost. More cost-benefit data on the socio-economic impact of occupational asthma and various aspects of its management should be gathered worldwide.
(Mannino & Braman 2007; Mannino & Buist 2007) Narrative reviews	**The epidemiology and economics of chronic obstructive pulmonary disease** *(US epidemiology and costs).* COPD is "a disease state characterized by airflow limitation that is not fully reversible. The airflow limitation is usually both progressive and associated with an abnormal inflammatory response of the lungs to noxious particles or gases". COPD is a preventable and treatable disease responsible for a large human and economic burden around the world. During 2000, COPD in the United States was responsible for: • 8 million physician office and hospital outpatient visits • 1.5 million emergency department visits • 726,000 hospitalizations • 119,000 deaths

TABLE 5b: RESPIRATORY CONDITIONS

Cigarette smoking is the main risk factor for COPD in the developed world, although other important risk factors include occupational exposures, air pollution, airway hyper-responsiveness, asthma, and genetic predisposition. One report estimated that 19% of COPD cases in the USA were attributable to work exposures, with this proportion being 31% in never-smokers. In most of the world, COPD prevalence and mortality continue to rise in response to increases in smoking, particularly by women and adolescents. COPD is also an important cause of disability, and is linked to co-morbid diseases, such as depression and cardiovascular disease, which increase the costs. COPD is a very costly disease in the United States, with estimated direct medical costs in 1993 of $14.7 billion (69). The estimated indirect costs related to morbidity (loss of work time and productivity) and premature mortality is an additional $9.2 billion, for a total of $23.9 billion. By 2002 this cost was estimated at $32.1 billion. The annual societal costs of COPD per patient in the United States are estimated to be $5,646, ranging from $2,000 among patients with mild COPD to $16,000 among patients with severe COPD. Additional estimates of the costs associated with COPD have noted a significantly higher burden of disability (22.8 vs. 7.3%) in the population aged 40–63 years, with a higher cost ($8,559 vs. $5,443).

(Mapp et al. 2005)
Narrative review

Occupational asthma

Occupational asthma has become one of the most common forms of occupational lung disease in many industrialized countries, and has been implicated in 9–15% of adult asthma. Occupational asthma is defined as a disease characterized by variable airflow limitation and/or airway hyper-responsiveness due to causes and conditions attributable to a particular occupational environment and not to stimuli encountered outside the workplace. Work-related asthma includes (1) immunologic occupational asthma, characterized by a latency period before the onset of symptoms (about 90% of cases); (2) non-immunologic occupational asthma, which occurs after single or multiple exposures to high concentrations of irritant materials (about 7% of cases); (3) work-aggravated asthma, which is pre-existing or concurrent asthma exacerbated by workplace exposures; and (4) variant syndromes. Assessment of the work environment has improved, making it possible to measure concentrations of several high- and low-molecular-weight agents in the workplace. The identification of host factors, polymorphisms, and candidate genes associated with occupational asthma is in progress and may improve our understanding of mechanisms involved in occupational asthma. A reliable diagnosis of occupational asthma should be confirmed by objective testing early after its onset. Removal of the worker from exposure to the causal agent and treatment with inhaled glucocorticoids lead to a better outcome. Finally, strategies for preventing occupational asthma should be implemented and their cost-effectiveness examined.

Management:

When asthma is induced by a workplace sensitizer, strict exposure control is needed. For employees sensitized to low molecular weight agents (e.g., isocyanates), complete cessation of exposure is the most desirable intervention.

For patients with occupational asthma induced by an acute exposure to an irritant at work, steps should be taken to prevent further exposure to high concentrations of the irritant.

Patients with pre-existing asthma that is aggravated at work should limit exposure to irritants, tobacco smoke, and relevant environmental allergens. If asthma is mild, the employee can stay in the same job, provided that exposure to non-specific triggers is reduced (e.g., by moving to a different work area, improving ventilation, or using a respirator for short-term exposures to irritants). In addition to these types of changes, the physician may recommend periodic monitoring of symptoms and objective criteria of lung function. By contrast, if the disease is severe, a job change may be necessary.

TABLE 5b: RESPIRATORY CONDITIONS

	Early removal of the employee from exposure to the offending agent, although associated with a better medical outcome, has the worst socioeconomic outcome, unless compensation programs are satisfactory and offer adequate financial coverage. *(This is one of the most comprehensive reviews of occupational asthma, with 443 references).*
(Moscato & Rampulla 2003) Narrative review	**Costs of occupational asthma and of occupational chronic obstructive pulmonary disease** *(US costs).* Estimates were based on 15% of adult asthma, 15% of chronic bronchitis and 18% of COPD attributable to work. Total annual costs in the United States in 1996 were estimated to be $1.6 billion for occupational asthma and $5 billion for occupational COPD. The ratio of direct to indirect costs was higher for asthma (74% : 24%) than for COPD (56% : 44%). In view of the rising prevalence of occupational asthma and occupational COPD, these costs are likely to rise. A patient with confirmed occupational asthma should be considered 100% incapacitated on a permanent basis for the job that caused the disease and any other jobs involving exposure to the same agent. Studies show that cessation of exposure to the causal agent results in decrease of asthma severity and medical costs, but is associated with adverse economic and employment consequences for the individual (professional downgrading, loss of income, and 30% long-term unemployment).
(Namath & Kuschmer 2006) Narrative review	**Work-related airways disease** *(Most of this paper reviews the epidemiology, pathogenesis and classification of work-related asthma and COPD but it also deals specifically with economic and medicolegal issues for each disease from a US perspective).* Occupational asthma has a significant economic impact on workers who develop the disease and become disabled. Although symptomatic improvement can occur for up to 5 years, symptoms persisting beyond 2 years after last exposure may be considered 'permanent' impairment. The negative impact of unemployment on the individual and the community may be offset by retraining programmes, allowing workers impaired by occupational asthma to continue gainful employment, sometimes in alternative employment with the same employer. The diagnosis of occupational COPD is often made around retirement age, so costs relate mainly to (slightly early) retirement.
(Newman Taylor et al. 2004) Report	**Guidelines for the prevention, identification & management of occupational asthma: evidence review & recommendations** [British Occupational Health Research Foundation Report] Asthma is 'work-related' when there is an *association* between symptoms and work. The different types of *work-related asthma* should be distinguished, since the implications to the worker and the occupational health management of the disease differ. *Work-related asthma* includes two distinct categories: • *work aggravated asthma,* i.e. pre-existing or coincidental new onset adult asthma which is made worse by non-specific factors in the workplace, and • *occupational asthma i.e. adult asthma caused by workplace exposure and not by factors outside of the workplace. Occupational asthma can occur in workers with or without prior asthma.* *Occupational asthma can be subdivided into:* • *allergic occupational asthma characterised by a latency period between first exposure to a respiratory sensitiser at work and the development of symptoms, and* • *irritant-induced occupational asthma that occurs typically within a few hours of a high concentration exposure to an irritant gas, fume or vapour at work.*

TABLE 5b: RESPIRATORY CONDITIONS

Occupational factors account for 9-15% of cases of asthma in adults of working age. Almost 90% of cases of occupational asthma are of the allergic type.

Occupational asthma is unique in that it is the only type of asthma that is readily preventable. Prevention depends on the effective control of exposure to respiratory sensitisers in the workplace. Occupational asthma has important long-term adverse health and economic consequences. Although symptoms may resolve completely with early diagnosis and early removal from exposure, many patients fail to recover even when completely removed from exposure.

*** The symptoms and functional impairment of occupational asthma caused by various agents may persist for many years after avoidance of further exposure to the causative agent.

*** The likelihood of improvement or resolution of symptoms or of preventing deterioration is greater in workers who have no further exposure to the causative agent.

** The likelihood of improvement or resolution of symptoms or of preventing deterioration is greater in workers who have relatively short duration of symptoms, relatively normal lung function. Ideally, complete and permanent avoidance of exposure is the mainstay of management. In practice, workers may reject this advice for social or financial reasons. If it is possible to relocate the worker to low or occasional exposure work areas, he or she should remain under increased medical surveillance.

* Redeployment to a low exposure area may lead to improvement or resolution of symptoms or prevent deterioration in some workers, but is not always effective.

There is consistent evidence derived from clinical and workforce case series in a limited number of countries that about one third of workers with occupational asthma are unemployed after diagnosis. The risk of unemployment may fall with increasing time after diagnosis. There is consistent evidence that loss of employment following a diagnosis of occupational asthma is associated with loss of income.

** Approximately one third of workers with occupational asthma are unemployed up to 6 years after diagnosis.

** Workers with occupational asthma suffer financially.

What is the effectiveness of compensation being directed towards rehabilitation? There are no studies that have made direct comparisons between different systems of rehabilitation either under different jurisdictions or within the same jurisdiction at different times. Systems that incorporate retraining may be more effective than those that do not.

These guidelines do not override legal obligations.

(NICE 2004b)	**Managing stable chronic obstructive pulmonary disease** [UK National Institute for Clinical Excellence]
Guideline	*(Brief summary of physiotherapy and clinical rehabilitation recommendations but nothing on vocational rehabilitation interventions, effectiveness or occupational outcomes).*

TABLE 5b: RESPIRATORY CONDITIONS

(Nicholson et al. 2005) Systematic review & UK guidelines	**Evidence-based guidelines for the prevention, identification, and management of occupational asthma** Occupational factors are estimated to account for 9–15% of cases of asthma in adults of working age, including new onset or recurrent disease. Management of the worker with occupational asthma: Health surveillance can detect occupational asthma at an earlier stage of the disease and improve outcomes. Outcome is better in workers who have shorter duration of symptoms prior to diagnosis, relatively normal lung function at diagnosis, and no further exposure to the causative agent after diagnosis. Measures should be taken to ensure that workers diagnosed as having of occupational asthma avoid further exposure to its cause in the workplace. Studies investigating the effectiveness of respiratory protective equipment in those with occupational asthma are limited to small studies in provocation chambers or limited case reports. The outcome of interventions following a confirmed diagnosis of occupational asthma may depend on several factors, including the worker's age and the causative agent. Approximately one third of workers with occupational asthma are unemployed up to six years after diagnosis. It is suggested that systems that incorporate retraining may be more effective than those that do not. *(No direct evidence on further vocational rehabilitation interventions, effectiveness or cost-effectiveness).*
(Ofman et al. 2004) Systematic review	**Does disease management improve clinical and economic outcomes in patients with chronic diseases?** 9 studies of asthma were included: 9 out of 36 comparisons (25%) showed significant effects for the Disease Management intervention in terms of symptoms, health related quality of life and direct health care costs*(though it was not specified which effects were significant).* 6 studies of chronic obstructive airways disease were included: only 2 out of 22 comparisons showed a significant benefit for the Disease Management intervention. *(No occupational outcomes or indirect costs. Further extract in Table 6c).*
(Peters et al. 2007) Systematic review	**Predictors of delayed return to work or job loss with respiratory ill-health** Included 5 studies on asthma, occupationally induced or not, and 2 studies also covering COPD or rhinitis, of variable methodological quality. In the single study of a general working population, blue collar workers with either asthma or COPD, were 2-6X less likely to return to work within 6 months compared with office workers. In those with occupational asthma, job loss was also more likely if working in smaller companies and being less well educated. Overall, the risk of becoming unemployed was high, and three times higher in those with all forms of asthma compared with rhinitis.
(Rachiotis et al. 2007) Systematic review	**Outcome of occupational asthma after cessation of exposure** 39 studies reported wide variation in rates of symptomatic recovery, with an average of 32%: 28 studies showed that 73% of patients had some degree of persistent non-specific bronchial hyper-responsiveness. Recovery was higher with shorter duration of symptoms, and lower with increasing age and in series from specialist clinics (probably a case selection effect). *(No data on occupational outcomes).*
(Ram et al. 2005) Cochrane review	**Physical training for asthma** 13 studies included. Physical training programs have been designed to improve physical fitness, muscle coordination and confidence. Physical training improves cardiopulmonary fitness as measured by an increase in maximum oxygen uptake and maximum expiratory ventilation. It has no effect on resting lung function or the number of days of wheeze (but, importantly, does not make them any worse). Three studies were reported to show a significant improvement in 'work capacity' but that appears to have been a measure of physical exertion and the studies were in children. *(No occupational outcomes).*

TABLE 5b: RESPIRATORY CONDITIONS

(Smidt et al. 2005) Systematic review	**Effectiveness of exercise therapy: a best-evidence summary of systematic reviews** Asthma: 4 systematic reviews provided insufficient evidence to support or refute the effectiveness of exercise therapy for adults (or children) with asthma, compared to no treatment or other conservative treatments. Bronchiectasis: There is only one systematic review which includes two RCTs. There is insufficient evidence to support or refute the effectiveness of exercise therapy for patients with bronchiectasis. Chronic obstructive pulmonary disease: 11 systematic reviews from 1992-2002 showed that exercise therapy is effective for patients with COPD, compared to no treatment. Exercise therapy consisted of (treadmill) training in walking, and lower limb strengthening exercises (e.g. stair climbing). The patients were encouraged to continue with daily walking exercises at home until they felt moderate pain. No conclusions can be drawn with regard to the effectiveness of a specific type of exercise therapy. *(No evidence on occupational outcomes. Other extracts in Tables 3 and 5a).*
(Smith et al. 2005) Systematic review	**The impact of psycho-educational interventions on health outcomes and costs in adults and children with difficult asthma** [UK Health Technology Assessment] 8 RCTs and 1 controlled clinical trial reported school or work time lost *(though data was not reported separately for work loss).* Overall, there was no clear evidence of any significant effect on short, medium or long-term work loss.
(Talmage & Melhorn 2005) (Hyman 2005) Physician guidance	**A physician's guide to return to work: working with common cardiopulmonary problems** [American Medical Association] *(Guidance book for primary care physicians and care providers to assist navigation of return to work issues, supported by science and consensus).* The potential risk of working with lung disease relates to work exposure to a chemical or substance that caused or aggravates the disease: hence the importance of risk assessment and control. If there is no causal or aggravating exposure, risk is not an issue. Capacity for work can be judged by pulmonary function. Cardiopulmonary conditions are common, and the physician should think through the issues of risk, capacity and tolerance. As a general principle, any known risk factors that may have contributed to the disease formation should be assessed and modified (in addition to rehabilitation and return-to-work support). As with other body system problems, patients with cardiopulmonary disease are rarely harmed by return-to-work recommendation. The considerable benefits of returning to work usually outweigh the risk. *(Provides a reasoned case for promoting and assessing capacity for return to work with cardiac conditions. No further information on vocational rehabilitation interventions, effectiveness or occupational outcomes). (Entries on working with musculoskeletal conditions are in Table 3).*
(Taylor et al. 2005) Systematic review	**Effectiveness of innovations in nurse led chronic disease management for patients with COPD** Included 9 RCTs, all variations on a case management approach. Two studies of brief interventions did not show any benefit. Seven longer-term interventions did not show any influence on mortality at 9-12 months, and did not improve patients' health related quality of life, psychological wellbeing, disability, or pulmonary function. One study showed an equivocal improvement in readmission rates. Authors' conclusion: There is little evidence to date to support the widespread implementation of nurse led management interventions for COPD. *(No occupational outcomes).*
(Toelle & Ram 2004) Cochrane review	**Written individualised management plans for asthma in children and adults** Included 7 small trials. Overall, there was no consistent evidence that written plans produced better patient outcomes than no written plan. 3 studies that reported data on days lost from work or school *(data were not reported separately)* showed no significant effect.

TABLE 5b: RESPIRATORY CONDITIONS

(Trikalinos et al. 2006) Health technology assessment	**Pulmonary rehabilitation for COPD and other lung diseases** [US Agency for Health Care Policy & Research, Health Technology Assessment] Based on 70 RCTs, almost all on COPD. Pulmonary rehabilitation was defined as a multidisciplinary and comprehensive intervention, including an exercise-training component of at least 2 weeks' duration, with or without one or more non-exercise components: educational, psychosocial support, breathing exercises, respiratory muscle training, or nutritional interventions. Overall, exercise-based pulmonary rehabilitation is effective in improving patients' disease-specific health-related quality of life (dyspnoea, mastery, fatigue and emotions), as well as their functional and maximal exercise capacity, compared with usual care. Especially in the short term, the improvements are significantly larger than the minimal clinically meaningful improvement. *(No evidence on occupational outcomes).*
(Turnock et al. 2005) Cochrane review	**Action plans for chronic obstructive pulmonary disease** Included 3 RCTs. Action plans are designed to help an individual recognise a deterioration in their symptoms and initiate changes to treatment early and so reduce the impact of the exacerbation. Action plans had a significant positive effect on self-management knowledge, resulting in an increased ability to recognise and react appropriately to an exacerbation by individuals. Unfortunately there was no evidence these behavioural changes altered health-care utilization, health-related quality of life, lung function, functional capacity, symptom scores, mortality, anxiety, or depression. The review looked for days lost from work but none of the studies reported this outcome.
(Van Weel et al. 2006) Narrative review	**Occupational Health and general practice: from opportunities lost to opportunities capitalized?** *(Perspective was General Practice in The Netherlands. This paper covered chronic diseases like cardiovascular disease, diabetes, COPD and asthma, but the main emphasis was on chronic respiratory diseases. Generic material in Table 7).* Cardiovascular disease, COPD and asthma all have high prevalence and consultation rates, indicating a high level of GP involvement in diagnosis and management. A majority of patient with heart disease and COPD were over age 65, though the majority of patients with asthma were under retirement age. Only the guideline on asthma provided *(minimal)* advice about work. However, analysis of work-related functioning in chronic respiratory disease highlighted that work-related factors and circumstances played an important role in patients' coping strategies. Patients tended to ignore negative effects of their workplace on their physical condition and as a consequence adopted inefficient coping strategies and suffered undue limitations. Several studies have shown that work status and the prediction of future sickness absence is related to chronic respiratory symptoms rather than to objective pulmonary function. In one study, patients with COPD who remained in paid employment reported a higher quality of life than those who left work, even though their objective pulmonary function was comparable. *(Though it is unclear if this was cause and effect or selection bias).* In another study, guided self-management of asthma resulted in a substantial and lasting reduction of days with respiratory-related socio-economic limitations (OR=0.49) compared with usual GP supervised care.
(Vandenplas et al. 2003) Narrative review	**Health and socioeconomic impact of work-related asthma** Follow-up studies of workers with immunological occupational asthma have shown that avoidance of exposure to the causative agent results in a significant improvement in asthma symptoms, airway obstruction, and nonspecific bronchial hyper-responsiveness (NSBH). Nonetheless, removal from exposure does not necessarily lead to complete recovery from asthma. Approximately 70% of affected workers still experience asthma symptoms and retain NSBH several years after cessation of the offending exposure. NSBH can, however, further improve >5 yrs after exposure cessation. Persistence of asthma has been consistently associated with a longer duration of work-related symptoms before removal and with a more severe asthma at the time of diagnosis. Atopy and tobacco smoking have not been identified as significant determinants of outcomes in occupational asthma. The long-term health effects of reducing rather than eliminating exposure to the agent causing occupational asthma remain uncertain. Reducing exposure is more frequently associated with persistence of asthma symptoms (93%) and NSBH (95%), and with worsening of asthma (28%) than complete removal (61%, 75%, and 12%, respectively). Available studies suggest that the pattern of functional changes in irritant-induced occupational asthma may be remarkably similar to what has been described in subjects with immunological occupational asthma after cessation of exposure to causative sensitising agent, as NSBH can continue to improve for up to 3 yrs following an inhalation accident.

TABLE 5b: RESPIRATORY CONDITIONS

The negative socio-economic impact of asthma can take many forms, including reduced workforce participation and employment rates, changes in employment or job duties as an adjustment to the asthmatic condition, asthma-related lost work days, and impaired work effectiveness while on the job. Partial work disability, defined as any change in job duties or reduction in work hours due to asthma, has been described in 5% to 20% of adult asthmatics attending specialist clinics. The work impact appears to be even more dramatic among the subset of adults with occupational asthma. Multiple studies conducted in various countries have shown that immunological occupational asthma is associated with considerable professional and financial consequences: 25–38% of subjects with occupational asthma suffer prolonged work disruption and 42–78% report a substantial loss of income. A number of vocational and sociodemographic factors adversely affect employment and socioeconomic status in workers with occupational asthma; these include unskilled jobs, lower levels of education, older age or younger age, a lower number of economically-dependent subjects and being employed in small-sized firms. Interestingly, the clinical severity of asthma does not appear to be an important determinant of employment status in subjects with occupational asthma. In the only available study that compared immunological occupational asthma with non-work-related asthma, the rate of unemployment was similar in the two groups, whereas a reduction of income was more frequently reported by subjects with occupational asthma (62%) as compared with those with asthma unrelated to work (38%). The socioeconomic impact of work-aggravated asthma symptoms has received relatively little attention given the potential magnitude of the problem. The results of the few available studies show that, even in the absence of occupational asthma or irritant-induced asthma, work-aggravated asthma is associated with a considerable socioeconomic impact.

Available information indicates that financial compensation for occupational asthma is currently inadequate in European countries, since about one third of subjects with occupational asthma remain exposed to the agent causing their asthma in order to avoid or minimise the adverse financial effects that would result from complete avoidance of exposure. It appears that the rate of unemployment is lower among subjects with occupational asthma in Quebec (25%) than in other countries despite removal from exposure of all affected workers. This lower rate of unemployment is coincident with a higher proportion of workers who benefit from professional retraining programs (22%) and/or find another job with the same employer (31% versus 15–21%). Extrapolating from this limited information, compensation schemes might be more effective to the extent that they can be redirected toward facilitating relocation into non-exposed jobs in the same company or retraining for other jobs rather than providing inadequate financial compensation. Furthermore, to be more equitable, compensation should ensure more appropriate income replacement when relocation or professional rehabilitation brings about a loss of earnings.

Concepts of rehabilitation for the management of common health problems
[Report commissioned by UK Department for Work and Pensions]

Exercise training should be included in the management of patients with chronic obstructive pulmonary disease.

Asthma is the most prevalent cause of respiratory ill health during working life but most of the literature on asthma is about primary or secondary prevention by controlling exposure or medical treatment. There is no clear evidence on the efficacy of breathing exercises for the rehabilitation of asthma or other respiratory disorders, but general pulmonary rehabilitation can improve exercise capacity and quality of life, and education in asthma self-management coupled with regular medical review can improve health outcomes, including days off work. *(No further information on the effectiveness or cost-effectiveness of vocational rehabilitation interventions)*.

(Waddell & Burton 2004)

Evidence synthesis

TABLE 5b: RESPIRATORY CONDITIONS

(Waddell & Burton 2006) Evidence synthesis	**Is work good for your health and well-being?** [Report commissioned by UK Department for Work and Pensions] There is strong evidence that many workers with respiratory conditions do manage to (return to) work. There is general clinical consensus that return to (suitably controlled) work is an appropriate and desirable goal for many people with respiratory conditions. There is strong evidence that prevention of further exposure is fundamental to the clinical management and vocational rehabilitation of occupational asthma. *(No further information on the effectiveness or cost-effectiveness of vocational rehabilitation interventions).*
(Yorke et al. 2006) Cochrane review	**Psychological interventions for adults with asthma** Included 15 studies (687 patients) though studies were generally small and of poor quality and only a few studies looked at any particular intervention and outcome. Interventions included cognitive behavioural therapy (CBT), relaxation therapy and biofeedback therapy. CBT improved health-related quality of life. Relaxation therapy made no significant difference to Peak expiratory flow or FEV1, reduced medication use, but made no difference o depression scores. Biofeedback therapy reduced peak expiratory flow. All other findings were conflicting. Overall, the reviewers concluded that there is insufficient evidence to determine whether psychological interventions for adults with asthma help to improve symptoms and mental health. Two small studies reported school/work absenteeism but showed no significant effect on this outcome.

[COPD = chronic obstructive pulmonary disease; RCT = randomised controlled trial]

TABLE 6: REVIEWS AND REPORTS ON DELIVERY

Table 6a: Primary health care

TABLE 6a: PRIMARY HEALTH CARE	
Authors	**Key features** *(Reviewers' comments in italic)*
(Black et al. 2000) Physician guidance	**Injury/illness and return to work/function: a practical guide for physicians** Prepared by the Physician Education Project in Workplace Health of the Ontario, Canada Workplace Safety and Insurance Board. This guide highlights the key role of treating physicians and the importance of collaboration and coordination of management with other key stakeholders, e.g. in the workplace. The physician has a responsibility to understand the patient's role in the workplace and to support safe and timely return to work as the desired outcome. This includes responsibility to: assess; diagnose; treat; develop a return-to-work plan; monitor progress; provide reports; communicate with the patient, other health professionals, relevant authorities and employer; and prevent recurrence. *(Builds upon and complements Kazimirski 1997 (Table 6a). No direct evidence on effectiveness).*
(Breen et al. 2006) Workshop report	**Mono-disciplinary or multidisciplinary back pain guidelines? How can we achieve a common message in primary care?** Developed from a workshop held at the Fifth International Forum on Low Back Pain in Primary Care in 2002. Despite a considerable degree of acceptance of current evidence-based guidelines, in practice, primary health care providers still do not share a common message. Participants in this workshop contributed to an open discussion on 'how and why' evidence-based guidelines about back pain do or do not work in practice. How to share the evidence and make it meaningful to practice stakeholders is the main challenge of guideline implementation. Guidelines should be developed and monitored by a multidisciplinary team, but may be transferred to practice by mono-disciplinary messengers. Despite general agreement that multi-faceted interventions are most effective for implementing guidelines, the feasibility of doing this in busy clinical settings is questioned. Research is needed from local implementation pilots and quality monitoring studies to understand how to develop and deliver the contextual understanding required. This relates to processes of care as well as outcomes, and to social factors and policymaking as well as health care interventions.
(Crawford & Laiou 2005) Report + survey	**Effective management of upper limb disorders by general practitioners and trainee occupational physicians** Aimed to identify best practice in the clinical management of work related upper limb disorders by reviewing the literature and contacting relevant institutions and associations *(the review data are in Table 3)*. To determine the nature of teaching on this subject in the training of Occupational Physicians and GPs To gather information via focus groups and questionnaire survey to identify perceived difficulties in the management of upper limb disorders and identify training needs. The majority of universities surveyed covered musculoskeletal issues, however, not every course could identify what they covered for work related musculoskeletal disorders. The focus groups and questionnaire identified that the majority of training in musculoskeletal disorders was during the registrar years by Continuous Medical Education. When comparing management with the evidence reviewed, good practice was identified in a number of disorders but this was not always consistent. With regard to diagnosis, diffuse non-specific upper limb disorders were as an issue. The areas identified as being problematic in managing were psychosocial factors, recurrent symptoms, chronicity and the patient's high expectations compared to other issues. A key recommendation was that there is a need to ensure that the patient is as well informed as possible about the possible duration of symptoms. Furthermore, research is vital with regard to psychosocial issues and their impact on musculoskeletal disorders as is improving the time taken to see other specialists. Where training is concerned, this needs to be accessible hands-on training but investigation should also be made of the usefulness of electronic media including CD-ROMs and accredited websites. *(This report highlights some UK training and professional education issues that may impact on delivery of effective rehabilitation).*

TABLE 6a: PRIMARY HEALTH CARE

Doctors.net 2007 – unpublished data Survey	**Health, work and well-being survey of general practitioners** *(Survey of UK GPs, prepared for the Department for Work and Pensions).* • 79% of GPs agree that return to work is an important outcome measure of successful clinical management in people of working age. • 78% of GPs agree that, for most jobs, work is beneficial for physical health, and 90% for mental health. • 62% of GPs agree and 24% are undecided (only 14% disagree) that they have a key role in helping people with a health problem or disability to retain their jobs, though they are not convinced that they have a key role in helping these people to obtain employment. • 49% of GPs 'somewhat agree' that they are confident dealing with patient issues around return to work. • 84% of GPs feel they could provide more advice and support to return to work if there were more services to support patients to remain in or return to work. • The main suggestions for additional support were more occupational health facilities and more (GP) training. *(Other parts of the survey dealt with issues around sick certification).*
(Foreman et al. 2006) Report	**Barriers and facilitators to return to work: a literature review** [Report prepared for the South Australian WorkCover Corporation] An overall summary of the literature in terms of its implication for service delivery is that: • Effective management of return-to-work requires addressing individual psychological characteristics (particularly cognitions and expectations about the condition and return-to-work, and negative emotions) and workplace factors (particularly job design and workplace support) in addition to appropriate clinical management. • A coordinated approach between all stakeholders is essential (particularly important is linking the clinician/treating practitioner with those rehabilitation and workplace personnel who are involved with the injured worker). • There is an increasing body of research on best practice clinical management of various work related conditions that should be incorporated into practice guidelines for clinicians working with workers compensation clients. • Return-to-work interventions may need to differ in emphasis and content depending on time since injury.
(Frank & Sawney 2003) Editorial	**Vocational rehabilitation** Referring to a review from the Organisation for Co-operation and Economic Development was mainly about 'top down' policy approaches but these cannot succeed without 'bottom up' approaches by health professionals and employers. For health professionals, the most vital message of the report concerns early intervention—the most effective measure against long-term ill health and consequent dependence on social security benefits. In this respect the strategy usually pursued in the UK, whereby the patient's possible return to work is considered only after completion of medical care, has come in for strong criticism. There is a window of opportunity: at first patients see themselves as 'sick' but with the prospect of returning to work; later they see themselves as 'disabled' and consequently unable to do so. The first phase is thought to last 2-4 months and is the time at which vocational rehabilitation is most likely to be effective through psychological and multidisciplinary management. All health professionals should seek to give positive advice about return to work before negative attitudes are formed.

TABLE 6a: PRIMARY HEALTH CARE

What does bottom-up rehabilitation demand of health professionals? First, all health professionals must recognize a responsibility to assist ill or disabled people back into work where practicable - a culture largely lacking in the NHS. Secondly, general practitioners and the primary health care team are pivotal through their clinical management and their provision of sick notes which trigger or perpetuate absence from work. Where available, occupational health practitioners can give much assistance through job modification in arranging a phased return to work and support after return to work. Good communication is crucial—particularly between general practitioners and occupational health physicians. Poor communication often results from a lack of clear rehabilitation goals from the outset. This in turn derives from the fact that, in many countries the world over, the management of work disability has not been viewed as an important part of medical practice outside the specialties of rehabilitation and occupational medicine.

(FOM 2005) Physician guidance	**The health and work handbook: patient care and occupational health: a partnership guide for primary care and occupational health teams** [Faculty of Occupational Medicine/Royal College of General Practice/Society of Occupational Medicine, UK] Starts from the standpoint that work is important for people. Helping patients to stay in work, or return to work, after absence due to illness or injury, is an important part of the therapeutic process, improves health outcomes in the long-term, is essential to restoring quality of life, and is an indicator of successful outcome of treatment. Primary care teams and occupational health professionals have a central role to play in return to work. GPs are well placed to offer simple fitness for work advice to their patients and to provide the focused support necessary to assist their recovery and retention in work. Occupational health professionals can provide more specialist advice and support in developing return to work programmes which will ensure that workers can return to work and that such return can be sustained. Close working and effective communication between primary care and occupational health professionals is essential.
(Garg et al. 2005) Systematic review	**Effects of computerized clinical decision support systems on practitioner performance and patient outcomes** Included 100 studies of diagnostic, reminder, disease management, and drug prescribing systems. Many systems improved practitioner performance, but the effects on patient outcomes remain under-studied and, when studied, inconsistent. *(No occupational outcomes).*
(Goldfarb et al. 2004) Narrative review	**Impact of appropriate pharmaceutical therapy for chronic conditions on direct medical costs and workplace productivity** Pharmaceutical management is a cornerstone of chronic disease management. Four chronic conditions – asthma, migraine, diabetes and heart failure - were reviewed, based on their prevalence, costs and relevance to employers. The review found that the large majority of published evidence makes a compelling case that appropriate drug therapy improves the health status and quality of life of individuals with chronic illness while reducing health care consumption and costs. Much research remains to be done to better establish the link between pharmacotherapy and workplace productivity, but early evidence identified in this review suggests that workers whose chronic conditions are effectively controlled with medications are more productive. For employers, the evidence translates into potential direct and indirect cost savings.
(Grimshaw et al. 2001) Review of systematic reviews	**Changing provider behavior: an overview of systematic reviews of interventions** An overview of 41 systematic reviews of professional behaviour change interventions published between 1966 and 1998. In general, passive approaches are generally ineffective and unlikely to result in behaviour change. Most other interventions are effective under some circumstances; none are effective under all circumstances. Promising approaches include educational outreach (for prescribing) and reminders. A consistent finding is that multifaceted interventions targeting different barriers to change are more likely to be effective than single interventions. However, it is difficult to disentangle which components of multifaceted interventions are likely to be effective and complementary under different settings.

TABLE 6a: PRIMARY HEALTH CARE

(Grimshaw et al. 2004) Systematic review	**Effectiveness and efficiency of guideline dissemination and implementation strategies** Systematic review of the effectiveness and costs of different guideline development, dissemination and implementation strategies. To estimate the resource implications of these strategies. To develop a framework for deciding when it is efficient to develop and introduce clinical guidelines. There is an imperfect evidence base to support decisions about which guideline dissemination and implementation strategies are likely to be efficient under different circumstances. Decision makers need to use considerable judgement about how best to use the limited resources they have for clinical governance and related activities to maximise population benefits. They need to consider the potential clinical areas for clinical effectiveness activities, the likely benefits and costs as a result of any changes in provider behaviour. Further research is required to: develop and validate a coherent theoretical framework of health professional and organisational behaviour and behaviour change to inform better the choice of interventions in research and service settings, and to estimate the efficiency of dissemination and implementation strategies in the presence of different barriers and effect modifiers. *(Highlights the difficulties of implementation of novel clinical guidelines – it may be expected that implementation of novel non-clinical interventions will require similar efforts).*
(Grimshaw et al. 2005) Cochrane review	**Interventions to improve outpatient referrals from primary care to secondary care** Included 17 studies, 14 of which evaluated professional educational interventions. Generally effective strategies included dissemination of guidelines with structured referral sheets (four out of five studies) and involvement of consultants in educational activities (two out of three studies). Three studies evaluated organisational interventions (patient management by family physicians compared to general internists, attachment of a physiotherapist to general practices and requiring a second 'in-house' opinion prior to referral), all of which were effective. Ineffective strategies included: passive dissemination of local referral guidelines (two studies), feedback of referral rates (one study) and discussion with an independent medical adviser (one study). Five studies evaluated financial interventions, with variable effects. *(No data on occupational outcomes).*
(HTA 2008) Report	**Service delivery organisation for acute low back pain** [Health Technology Assessment] The main conclusions and suggestions *(not 'recommendations' because these have a legal status in an HTA)* were: • In planning services for LBP, NHS Boards should take account of existing evidence based guidelines for the management of low back pain. • Services are used appropriately and that patients with non-specific LBP should be streamed to physiotherapy services and not onto orthopaedic waiting lists. • The balance of evidence suggests that triage by a specialist gatekeeper, whether a physiotherapist, nurse or other clinician, results in shorter orthopaedic appointment times and higher conversion to surgery rates. Estimates typically exceed 80% for the proportion of patients managed entirely by physiotherapy, advice and/or exercise. If orthopaedic departments have their referrals triaged their time will be freed up for patients requiring surgery, who will get faster access to the surgeon. Patients not needing surgery will be managed more appropriately and quickly. • The available evidence (despite its limitations) indicates that patients who self-refer to physiotherapy have shorter waiting times than those who are referred by a GP. • Many of these studies show increased levels of patient satisfaction. • As NHS boards develop back pain services, staff will need appropriate training for new and extended roles. Structured, evidence-based training for physiotherapy staff who triage and manage patients with LBP is paramount in delivering quality services. • Any redesign of physiotherapy services for LBP should include evaluation of clinical outcomes, effectiveness and cost-effectiveness. *(The available evidence was mainly about process measures and patient satisfaction, but no evidence was found on clinical or occupational outcomes).*

TABLE 6a: PRIMARY HEALTH CARE

(Jamtvedt et al. 2006) Cochrane review	**Audit and feedback: effects on professional practice and health care outcomes** Providing healthcare professionals with data about their performance (audit and feedback) can be effective in improving professional practice, but the effects are generally small to moderate. Effectiveness is likely to be greater when baseline adherence to recommended practice is low and when feedback is delivered more intensively. The results of this review do not support mandatory or unevaluated use of audit and feedback as an intervention to change practice.
(Kazimirski 1997) Policy document	**The physician's role in helping patients return to work after an injury or illness** [Canadian Medical Association Policy Document] Addresses the role of attending physicians in assisting their patients to return to work after an illness or injury. The physician's role is to diagnose and treat the illness or injury, to advise and support the patient, to provide and communicate appropriate information to the patient and employer and to work closely with other involved healthcare professionals to facilitate the patient's save and timely return to the most productive employment possible. Carrying out this role requires the physician to understand the patient's roles in the family and workplace. It requires physicians to recognise and support the employee-employer relationship and the primary importance of this relationship in the return to work. Finally, it requires physicians to have a good understanding to the potential roles of other health care professionals and employment personnel in assisting and promoting the return to work. • The physician should help the patient to develop a return to work plan. • Early in the course of treatment, the physician should discuss with the patient expected healing and recovery times as well as the importance of an early graduated increase in healing for physical and psychological recovery. • The physician should encourage communication between patient and employer early in treatment and rehabilitation. • The physician should, as early as possible, identify and address potential obstacles to recovery of function and return to work. • The physician should be knowledgeable about and should refer to, communicate with and coordinate management with occupational health, a multidisciplinary rehabilitation team or other appropriate health professionals, as and when required. *(Evidence based but essentially a consensus document with no evidence linking or direct evidence on effectiveness).*
(Moffett & McLean 2006) Narrative review	**The role of physiotherapy in the management of non-specific back pain and neck pain** This paper provides an overview of best practice for the role of physiotherapy in managing back pain and neck pain, based mainly on evidence-based guidelines and systematic reviews. More up-to-date relevant primary research is also highlighted. A stepped approach is recommended in which the physiotherapist initially takes a history and carries out a physical examination to exclude any potentially serious pathology and identify any particular functional deficits. Initially, the term 'brief intervention' generally refers to any minimal intervention usually of one or two sessions only. Advice providing simple messages of explanation and reassurance will form the basis of a patient education package. Self-management is emphasized throughout and a return to normal activities is encouraged. Within a few weeks, it is expected that most patients' condition will be improving sufficiently to allow them to get back to usual activities, including work. For the patient who is not recovering after a few weeks, a short course of physiotherapy may be offered. This should be based on an active management approach, such as exercise therapy. Manual therapy should also be considered. Any passive modalities of treatment should only be used if required to relieve pain and assist in helping the patient get moving. Barriers to recovery need to be explored. Those few patients who have persistent pain and disability that interferes with their daily lives and work need more intensive treatment or a different approach. There is strong evidence that intensive multidisciplinary biopsychosocial rehabilitation with a functional restoration approach is effective, although it is not widely available. Liaison with the workplace and/or social services may be important. Getting all players on side is crucial, especially at this stage.

TABLE 6a: PRIMARY HEALTH CARE

(Mowlam & Lewis 2005) Report	**Exploring how General Practitioners work with patients on sick leave** [UK Department for Work and Pensions research report] In-depth interviews with 24 GPs. Dealing with sickness absence was a daily issue for GPs. Most absences were short; longer and more problematic absence was particularly associated with back pain, depression, stress and anxiety. Most GPs believed that sickness absence is almost always genuine. However, patients' behaviour and motivation was said to be influenced by issues such as subjective reactions to the experience of illness, organisational culture and financial circumstances. There was a widespread view among GPs that work can be of therapeutic benefit for a range of physical and psycho-social reasons. This view was qualified, however, where patients worked in low-paid jobs of low social status, and where the job itself was believed to cause or exacerbate a physical or psychological condition. Four key factors were identified as constraints on GPs' involvement in return to work issues. The importance of preserving the doctor-patient relationship, based on mutual trust and an assumption that the doctor is acting in the patient's best interests, was stressed. GPs sometimes perceived a conflict between their obligations to patients and either the benefits system or employers. Shortage of time and lack of occupational expertise also made it difficult for GPs to address work issues. These considerations underpinned different views about the extent to which vocational rehabilitation is part of the GP's role. At one end of the spectrum were GPs who took a holistic viewpoint, seeing work as an important element of health and return to work as an integral part of medical rehabilitation. At the other end of the spectrum were GPs who felt their role was to focus on medical treatment and recovery; although this might lead to return to work, work issues were not in themselves part of the GP remit.
(Sainsbury 2008) Report	**Employment Advisers in GP surgeries** [UK Department for Work and Pensions report] Key Findings: • The 'gateway' model was practicable as a means of connecting people with employment and other support services. • GPs in the study were enthusiastic and positive about the *Pathways to Work* Advisory Service. Having direct and easy access to an employment and social security expert allowed them to support their patients in newer and more constructive ways than previously. • Physically locating advisers in GP surgeries was highly valued and considered essential by GPs. • There was evidence from the survey and qualitative components of the study that the intervention of the adviser was an essential catalyst for some people in moving them towards or into work. • Advisers dealt with a wide range of people beyond the main target population of Statutory Sick Pay (SSP) and long-term Incapacity Benefit recipients, and provided help and support beyond employment advice. • There is scope for increasing the numbers of people meeting an adviser by increasing GPs' awareness of what advisers can offer, and by publicising the service more widely.
(Seddon et al. 2001) Systematic review	**Systematic review of studies of quality of clinical care in general practice in the UK, Australia and New Zealand** Included 90 studies of quality of care for chronic conditions such as cardiovascular disease, hypertension, diabetes and asthma. Most of the studies were from UK. In almost all the studies the processes of care did not attain the standards set out in national guidelines or by the researchers themselves. The review helps to identify deficiencies in the research, quality and policy agenda in a part of the health care system where quality of care has been largely ignored. Further work is required to evaluate quality of care in a representative sample of the population, to identify reasons for sub-standard care, and to develop and test strategies to improve clinical care in general practice. (*This review focussed on the process of care, which has potential implications for clinical and occupational outcomes, but no direct evidence provided of the impact on outcomes*).

TABLE 6a: PRIMARY HEALTH CARE

(Van Weel et al. 2006) Narrative review	**Occupational health and general practice: from opportunities lost to opportunities capitalized?** *(Perspective was General Practice in The Netherlands. This paper covered chronic diseases like cardiovascular disease, diabetes, COPD and asthma, with a major emphasis on chronic respiratory diseases – separate data in Table 5b).* An increasing proportion of the population are living with chronic disease, where the main principles of management are: • Ongoing health care aimed at minimizing symptoms, preventing complications and optimizing life expectancy and quality of life. • Shifting from 'treatment' to supporting and coaching patients in self management to meet the needs and demands of their individual life circumstances. • Self-management programmes emphasise continuous adjustment of treatment as patients' condition and life circumstances change. Most patients with chronic conditions are treated by GPs in primary care. There are guidelines for the management of the common chronic conditions in this setting. Work is in principle an important part of activities of daily living in patients with chronic diseases who are of working age. However, advice and support about work is uncommon in primary care: GPs ask about work in <¼ - ½ of consultations. There is also a lack of communication between primary care and occupational health. This paper analyses the importance of advice about work and the potential benefits for patients. It suggests that clinical practice guidelines should incorporate advice about work; in view of the limited research evidence in this area, it may be necessary to rely on 'common sense consensus'.
(Verbeek et al. 2002) Narrative review	**Evidence-based medicine for occupational health** *(Despite the title, this review seems more relevant to primary care).* One reason patients perceive a lack of advice and support about 'return-to-work issues' might be that most doctors feel unsure *how* they could be involved. This review therefore considers the most important theories involved in return to work and the evidence on the effectiveness of interventions that improve a patient's functioning, including return to work after an episode of illness. Opportunities for intervention are considered within the framework of the WHO International Classification of Functioning, supplemented by psychosocial theories of illness and illness behaviour. A systematic literature search found evidence of effective interventions for heart disease, rheumatoid arthritis, back pain and common mental health disorders *(though only brief findings were given from selected studies and reviews. There was no systematic report of the findings).* The author concluded that all doctors should ask patients if they work and if they have reported sick. Possible hindrances for return to work such as failure to make special arrangements in the workplace or misconceptions about disability should be explored. These issues can then be addressed by referring patients to an occupational health professional or by using cognitive-behavioural techniques. To facilitate implementation of these measures in practice, clinical guidelines should include guidance on return-to-work interventions.
(Verbeek 2006) Narrative review	**How can doctors help their patients return to work?** Author considered that the implication of the evidence reviewed is firstly that all doctors should ask patients if they work and if they have reported sick. General practitioners (with appropriate training) can carry out psychological (cognitive behavioural) interventions. Possible hindrances for return to work such as a failure to make special arrangements in the workplace or misconceptions of disability should be explored. These issues can subsequently be addressed by referring patients to an occupational health professional or by directly using the cognitive-behavioural techniques. To facilitate the implementation of these measures in practice, clinical guidelines should include guidance on return-to-work interventions.

TABLE 6a: PRIMARY HEALTH CARE

(Weevers et al. 2005) Systematic review	**Work-related disease in general practice: a systematic review** Objective was to determine the prevalence of potentially work-related diseases in the general practice population and the incidence of consulting a GP. Included 24 studies. The authors defined 'work-related diseases' as 'multi-factorial diseases among a working population, which are partly caused by work, and/or aggravated, accelerated or exacerbated by occupational exposures, and/or the cause of impaired work capacity'. *(This definition is rather imprecise and confounds symptoms with disease).* Based on this *(probably over-inclusive)* definition, they found a high prevalence and incidence of 'work-related' musculoskeletal conditions *(back, neck and shoulder pain)* among GP consulters. The authors argue that GPs have an important role in identifying and managing work-related diseases. They suggest that, frequently, GPs do not recognize the work-relatedness of diseases, which may lead to more serious health problems or unnecessary (long) absenteeism from work; conversely, if GPs were more able to recognize the work-relatedness of a disease, there is a potential for more adequate prevention and less absenteeism from work. *(Whilst these latter interpretations are theoretically plausible, no evidence is presented to support them. The authors' discussion of 'work-related' implies that these conditions are* **caused** *by work, but that is not supported by the cited evidence - a point acknowledged by the authors' comment that 'GPs should consider the work factor because patients often link their work with their illness'. The issue of work as the primary cause becomes important when considering how GPs should address 'the work factor': inappropriate assumptions about the causal role of work can lead to advice that might actually have a negative or iatrogenic effect).* The authors conclude that 'Training of GPs in occupational medicine and proper communications with their patients on this topic can improve managing work-related health problems in primary care' *(though no evidence is presented on whether GP attention to these issues actually improves occupational outcomes).*

Table 6b: Workplace interventions (including occupational health)

TABLE 6b: WORKPLACE (INCLUDING OCCUPATIONAL HEALTH)

Authors	Key features *(Reviewers' comments in italic)*
(ACOEM 2006) Guideline	**Preventing needless work disability by helping people stay employed** [American College of Occupational and Environmental Medicine] Although most injured or ill people can cope with their problem and make either temporary or permanent life and work adjustments, a large minority cannot. This minority does not recover successfully, adopts disabled self-concept, and experiences either needlessly prolonged absence or permanent withdrawal from work in problematic situations, the stay-at-work/return-to-work (SAW/RTW) process is usually inadequate and ill-suited to detect and effectively address the most important issues related to the outcome. Because this minority accounts for such large portion of all disability program costs, 1% reduction in cases with prolonged disability should generate substantially larger reduction in overall system cost. Therefore, the focus of the SAW/RTW process should shift away from 'managing' or 'evaluating' disability to preventing it. The fundamental reason for most lost workdays/lost jobs is not medical necessity, but the non-medical decision making and poor functioning of the SAW/RTW process. Employers, insurance carriers, and government agencies currently burdened by the costs of preventable disability, and worried about the future implications of the aging workforce, should consider underwriting efforts to more effectively prevent disability. Recommendations to improve the SAW/RTW process will require: • A sense of urgency; • Attention and priority; • Research; • Experimentation with new methods and interventions; • Infrastructure development; • Policy revision; • Methodological improvement and dissemination; • Education and training; • Incentive alignment; and • Funding. Avoiding the unfortunate outcome of iatrogenic or system-induced disability is worthwhile. Improving the appropriateness and usefulness of services available to people coping with illness and injury is also of value. It also is sensible, if not urgent, to curtail needlessly using resources and losing personal and industrial productivity.

TABLE 6b: WORKPLACE (INCLUDING OCCUPATIONAL HEALTH)

(Boardman & Lyon 2006) Research report	**Defining best practice in corporate occupational health and safety governance** Evidence suggests that in many sectors there is still a lack of engagement at the highest levels in UK organisations – and that directors are still unclear as to their role in occupational health and safety leadership and in ensuring that risks to health and safety within their business are properly controlled. Develops the argument and provides best practice guidance for directors and boards to take a leading role in occupational health and safety.
(BOMEL Ltd 2005) Research report	**Occupational health and safety support systems for small and medium sized enterprises: a literature review** The aim of this literature review was to identify and review occupational health (OH) support models and programmes for small and medium size enterprises. There is little evidence in the occupational health literature, but internet searches and personal contacts identified a total of almost 40 projects / programmes from the UK, from Europe and the rest of the world. Most reports lacked quantitative information or only measured process rather than occupational health outcomes. A number of qualitative benefits of OH models were identified, including: opportunities for employees to develop and learn new skills; reductions in staff turnover and absences; rehabilitation services for workers who have been away from work for long periods of time; the provision of a community service with regional OH models; and lower insurance premiums for the employer as a result of participating in the OH models. However, the lack of evaluation data precluded quantitative appraisal of the benefits. The authors found a general lack of cost-effectiveness data.
(Brewer et al. 2007) Systematic review	**A systematic review of injury/illness prevention and loss control programs (IPCs)** Systematic review of 53 high or medium quality studies to determine whether injury/illness prevention and loss control programs are effective in reducing workplace injury/illnesses and/or workers' compensation claims. Across all studies, the results suggest a mixed level of evidence for the effect of injury/illness prevention and loss control programs. However, when the 'prevention' interventions were separated from the 'loss control' programs the results took on a different appearance. The prevention programs still provide a mixed level of evidence. The loss control programs – those focusing on reducing the duration of injuries, amount of time off work, associated injury costs and insurance costs – show a strong level of evidence for positive effects on both the duration and costs of injuries/illnesses. The studies variously examined graded activity, rehabilitation, therapy, early intervention, disability case management and RTW policies. In summary: (1) there is strong evidence supporting the effectiveness of multicomponent disability management programs, using an approach that involves the healthcare provider, company supervisors and workers, and workers' compensation carriers; (2) there is moderate level of evidence that supervisor practices, workstation adjustments, and exercise have a positive effect on reducing injuries/illnesses. Workstation adjustment or ergonomic training alone has no effect on reducing injuries/illnesses.
(Butterfield & Ramseur 2004) Systematic review	**Research and case study findings in the area of workplace accommodations including provisions for assistive technology** Included 30 papers (11 studies and 19 case studies). The most common accommodations were workplace provisions for computer technologies, environmental access, tool operations, and seating & positioning. All but one study were for people with musculoskeletal or visual limitations. No evidence was found or presented for the effectiveness of these workplace accommodations.

TABLE 6b: WORKPLACE (INCLUDING OCCUPATIONAL HEALTH)

(CBI 2000)	**Their health in your hands: focus on occupational health partnerships**
Report	[Confederation of British Industry] Business recognises the importance of health and fitness at work, as well as the need to manage occupational risks to health. There is scope for improvement in UK occupational health management. Businesses are often not as systematic in their approach to occupational health as they are to safety management. Best practice needs to be shared and encouraged, including policies to manage long-term sickness absence. Health professionals (particularly GPs) need greater awareness, education and training in occupational health issues so that they can provide better advice about health and work issues. Employee involvement at all levels is essential to identify and manage workplace health, and this role is valued by employers. The key to sustainable improvement in occupational health is a partnership between business, government, trade unions and employees in the workplace.
(CBI/AXA 2007)	**Attending to absence: CBI/AXA absence and labour turnover survey 2007: a summary**
UK Survey	[Confederation of British Industry/ AXA UK] In 2006 sickness absence rose slightly to an average of 7 days per employee (3.3% of working days), though this ranged from 2.7-12 days in the best and worst performing organisations. Public sector absence averaged 9 days compared with 6.3 days in the private sector. Across the UK economy, a total of 127 million days were lost. The direct costs – based on salary costs of absent employees, replacement costs and lost productivity – was £537 per employee and totally £13.4 billion. Long-term absence (20 days or more) accounted for 43% of costs. Few organisations were able to quantify indirect costs. *(Note that (Bevan & Hayday 2001) concluded that such surveys seriously under-estimate the true costs of sickness absence, possibly be a factor of three or more).* The key to good absence management is commitment from senior management and having the right policies in place. Where senior managers had primary responsibility for absence management, absence rates averaged nearly a day lower. They were also lower where Human Resources managers had primary responsibility. However, in 71% of organisations line managers have day to day responsibility for absence management. Employers typically take action after 10 days or three spells of sickness absence, but the best performing organisation trigger their absence management policies earlier.
(CIPD 2007)	**Absence management**
UK Survey	[Chartered Institute of Personnel and Development] The 2006 CIPD survey showed that sickness absence fell slightly (from 3.7 to 3.5% of working days) to an average of 8 days per employee (9.9 days in the public sector). The average cost was £598 per employee per annum. Almost 60% of absence was short term (up to 7 days). Minor illness was the most significant cause of short-term absence for both manual and non-manual employees. For manual workers, back pain (responsible for 19% of absences), musculoskeletal injuries (17%), and acute medical conditions (15%) were the top three causes of long-term absence. For non-manual workers, stress (33%), acute medical conditions (19%) and mental ill health (13%) came top 46%) of employers reported an increase in stress-related absence compared with a year earlier. 42% of organisations have a target for reducing employee absence, while 37% benchmark their absence rates against comparable employers. 90% have a written sickness absence or attendance management policy and 70% reported that their organisation has made changes in the last two years to how sickness absence is managed. More than 70% of employers provide information on levels of absence to line managers as a means of helping to manage short-term absence and around half train managers in absence management. 72% of respondents considered return-to-work interviews the most effective method of managing short-term absence. 38% of respondents considered the involvement of occupational health professionals the most effective means of managing long-term absence (though only 62% of organisations use them for this purpose), compared with 19% rehabilitation programmes and 15% changes to working patterns.

TABLE 6b: WORKPLACE (INCLUDING OCCUPATIONAL HEALTH)

(Curtis & Scott 2004) Narrative review	**Integrating disability management into strategic plans: creating healthy organizations** *(Provides an overview of initiatives that integrate return to work management into the company's everyday functioning, with a focus on the employer's role).* The cost of people off work relates not only to direct costs, such as wages, WorkCover premiums, and medical costs. The impact on the organisation is through loss of staff, turnover, reduced productivity, and impact on the company's product, or relationships with customers. The smaller the organisation the larger the impact on staff turnover, and the increased likelihood of impact on customers. When employees become ill or injured they have reduced productivity levels, or may be unavailable for work. Employees who have positive experiences with their employer remain engaged, and more likely to be productive, provide customer care, and contribute to the organisation.
	• Employee engagement is important enough for the company to develop a strategic plan for disability management. Disability management has been shown to result in 10% to 50% savings in the costs associated with time off work. Senior management involvement is necessary for any disability management program, and must be incorporated into strategic planning.
	• Intervention undertaken early in the case is associated with improved results. Absences exceeding three to five days need proactive management. Maintaining work connection is a key factor in reducing lost time. Even casual contact with the employee has been shown to reduce time off work by 30%. Supporting the individual to get appropriate medical care, and avoid delays. They may need someone to advocate on their behalf, if they are in difficult circumstances.
	• A return to work model should be articulated and clear to all members of the company. Effective programs require clear goals, available modified and meaningful duties, and a co-ordinated approach with treating practitioners. Targets are best set before the program is initiated, and a review of results conducted annually by senior management.
	Integrating disability management into the company's strategic plan is a solid and cost-effective way of improving the corporate culture and productivity, reducing staff turnover, and improving the company's profitability.
(EEF 2004) Employer guide	**Fit for work: the complete guide to managing sickness absence and rehabilitation** Comprehensive guide from EEF (Engineering Employers Federation) addressing attendance management. The approach intends to foster a climate of good attendance and a strong rehabilitation and health and safety culture. The guide is primarily concerned with getting those who are already in employment back to work or, if still at work, working more efficiently; managing both short-term and long-term sickness absence is considered. A six-step strategy is set out:
	• Clearly defined roles within the company
	• Identify priorities for action
	• Inform and involve the workforce
	• Establish ready access to occupational health support
	• Focus on rehabilitation
	• Tackle frequent short-term absence
	Typical rehabilitation measures: keep in touch; phased return to work; alter pattern of work, tasks/work content, workplace, pace of work, tools/ equipment; training and information; mobility/transport. *(Vocational rehabilitation seems to be seen largely as health care and work adaptation).* Return-to-work interviews encapsulate key elements of good strategy for maximizing attendance: they encourage communication and action with shared responsibilities. *(Comes, understandably, from an employers' perspective, dealing with legal requirements as well as the 'business case', but recognizes workers' needs and concerns. Guidance based more on experience and common sense than scientific evidence, but represents a modern approach encouraging getting all players onside. Linked to HSE 2004).*

TABLE 6b: WORKPLACE (INCLUDING OCCUPATIONAL HEALTH)

(Employers' Forum on Disability 2008) Employer guide	**Attendance management and disability: line managers guide** Line managers have a vital role in managing attendance and performance. This guide aims to help line managers: • spot the signs that someone might have a disability • recognise when absence might be disability related • learn how to manage different types of absence • treat disabled colleagues fairly • identify how work can be done differently to maximise the performance of disabled staff • decide if an adjustment is reasonable • make sure not to break the law • know where to go for more help and advice Reasonable adjustments: The law requires employers to make 'reasonable adjustments' for disabled employees. This means removing barriers wherever possible that get in the way of a disabled person doing their job. This can mean changing where they work, the way in which they do their job or providing equipment to help them.
(Franche et al. 2005b) Systematic review	**Workplace-based return-to-work interventions: a systematic review of the quantitative literature** Included 10 studies published from 1990-2003. There was strong evidence that work disability duration is significantly reduced by work accommodation offers and contact between healthcare provider and workplace; and moderate evidence that it is reduced by interventions which include early contact with worker by workplace, ergonomic work site visits, and presence of a RTW coordinator. For these five intervention components, there was moderate evidence that they reduce costs associated with work disability duration. Evidence for sustainability of these effects was insufficient or limited. Evidence regarding the impact of supernumerary replacements was insufficient. Evidence levels regarding the impact of the intervention components on quality-of-life was insufficient or mixed. Authors' conclusions: Our systematic review provides the evidence base supporting that workplace-based RTW interventions can reduce work disability duration and associated costs; however, the evidence regarding their impact on quality-of-life outcomes was much weaker.
(Greenstreet Berman Ltd 2004) Report	**Costs and benefits of return to work and vocational rehabilitation in the UK** (See entry in Table 1 for distinction between 'return to work' and 'rehabilitation' interventions). Return to work and vocational rehabilitation are essential aspects of improving the health and well-being of staff and reducing the cost of work related injury and ill-health. Early intervention can prevent: minor injury becoming serious; acute injury becoming chronic; and serious injury becoming disabling. Genuine attempts to restore an injured employee's well being can mean that employees are less likely to feel aggrieved and less likely to seek 'justice' through a compensation claim. This can result in: • Fewer employers' liability claims • Less staff absence incurred by employers • Reduced or contained employers liability costs, and • Fewer injuries reportable to the Health and Safety Executive or local authority under the RIDDOR regulations

TABLE 6b: WORKPLACE (INCLUDING OCCUPATIONAL HEALTH)

Studies show there are significant benefits to employers, employees and insurers when RTW and rehabilitation are implemented effectively. A previous review of the impact of such schemes on compensation costs concluded that they can lead to 10% to 40% reduction in compensation costs. Since employers derive additional benefits such as reduced absence and improved workplace productivity, the ratio of benefit to cost is greater for employers than insurers. However, these studies also suggest that there is significant scope for improvement in the UK in the provision and hence the impact of vocational rehabilitation.

Examples of effective low to no-cost options include:

- Offering reduced hours
- Offering light or transitional duties
- Carrying out return to work interviews
- Modifying the workplace, such as reducing the height of shelves etc, and

Additional effective options include:

- Setting up 'on demand' or insurance-provided rehabilitation services e.g. through NHS Plus or private health care services
- A general absence management scheme is more cost-effective.

Key factors in making return to work and rehabilitation include:

1. Ensuring early intervention following injury or absence - necessary to prevent deterioration of the condition and the employee becoming distanced from work: mainly dependent on the employer and the employee.
2. Ensuring health care is directed to the goal of returning the individual to work: dependent on health care professionals, employee and employer
3. Employee motivation to return to work - central to a successful outcome: can be influenced by the employer.

(Hanson et al. 2007) Pilot study	**Evaluation of OHSxtra, a pilot occupational health case management programme within NHS Fife and NHS Lanarkshire** [Occupational Health and Safety Extra: an NHS service] A pilot study of occupational health services provided for NHS Scotland staff who were 'struggling' at work or off sick. Used a case management model of fast-track referral to physiotherapy, occupational therapy, counselling or CBT treatment, as appropriate. - Significant improvement in subjective performance ratings at work activities and WorkAbility Index. - 97% of clients had a positive overall impression of the service. - 95% of employers had positive overall impression of the service. - 98 of line managers felt it improved service delivery. - 72% of sick absent clients returned to work (but no control group); 99% of those 'struggling' did not go absent. - Estimated that every £1 spent saved £1.66 in absence costs *(These results provide evidence about a service delivery model; there was no control group so it is not evidence on effectiveness. The intervention described seems to be more a model for delivering early access to health care, rather than an example of vocational case management (Hanson et al 2006 – Table 6c).*

TABLE 6b: WORKPLACE (INCLUDING OCCUPATIONAL HEALTH)

| (Hill et al. 2007)

Research report | **What works at work?**

Report by Institute for Employment Studies, commissioned by UK Department for Work and Pensions: reviews the effectiveness of workplace interventions to prevent and manage common health problems

The research question was: 'What workplace practices and interventions have been shown to be effective in reducing health related negative work outcomes? Key findings:

Consistent with the biopsychosocial model, the health condition of the employee is only one of a number of factors in their rehabilitation. One of the key themes to emerge from this research is the importance of addressing multiple barriers in ill-health prevention, management of health problems, and promotion of recovery from ill-health.

Interventions which included some form of employer/employee partnership, and/or consultation, demonstrated improved results (compared to those which did not).

It is not only the employee's health condition that is important to consider, but also their attitudes and beliefs. Cognitive behavioural approaches are one way of effectively addressing this aspect of health and recovery.

Interventions should be comprehensive, addressing both individual- and organisational-level factors. Specific interventions have also been shown to be effective if, for example, organisational interventions are combined with a complementary individual intervention.

Improved communication, co-operation and common agreed goals between employers, employees, occupational health providers and primary care professionals can result in faster recovery, less re-occurrence of ill-health, and less time out of work overall.

Common mental health problems have been addressed in the workplace using a wide range of intervention types; however, there is only a limited amount of good quality evaluation evidence on the effectiveness of these interventions. The available evidence also mainly relates to individual level intervention types, showing that cognitive behavioural approaches in general, and CBT in particular, can be effective in reducing ill-health and absenteeism. There were contradictory results for organisational-level interventions, although this is largely influenced by the sparseness of good quality data.

There was evidence that educational interventions for back pain and musculoskeletal disorders, designed to address an individual's beliefs and attitudes about that pain, were effective. Interventions should also address employees' attitudes and beliefs, as well as. Evidence was also found to suggest the importance of organisational policies and practices, and of employed tackling potential organisational barriers to promoting and maintaining health at work, and promoting recovery through work. The timely provision of modified duties was found to be effective in managing back pain at work and in helping those with back pain to return to work.

This review identified very little evidence in relation to the management or rehabilitation of workers with cardio-respiratory health problems in the workplace. (*However, a large part of the review concerned health promotion, and it argued that improved health outcomes might in principle lead to improved occupational outcomes in the medium to long-term. The conclusions of this review focus on broad principles, similar to Waddell & Burton 2004. The review provides limited hard evidence on clinical or occupational interventions or their effectiveness for occupational outcomes*). |

TABLE 6b: WORKPLACE (INCLUDING OCCUPATIONAL HEALTH)

(HSE 2004c)	**Managing sickness and return to work: an employers and managers guide**
Employer guide	[UK Health & Safety Executive]
	Document covers a wide range of areas:
	• Importance and understanding of the issues
	• Legal obligations and responsibilities
	• Managing recovery at work
	• Recording sickness absence
	• Keeping in contact
	• Return to work interview
	• Planning workplace adjustments
	• Making use of professional and other advice and treatment
	• Agreeing and reviewing a return to work plan
	• Coordinating the return to work process
	• Developing and implementing a sickness absence and return to work policy.
	(A major Health and Safety Executive guidance document on sickness absence management. Notes that contacting sick-listed workers or helping them return to work is not a legal requirement; but rather a duty of care (though there is legislation covering protection after return to work). Importantly, there is a focus on recovery of 'health at work' and comprehensive guidance showing a mix of evidence-based and consensus-based best practice).
(HSE 2004b)	**Managing sickness absence in the public sector**
Report	[Health & Safety Executive/Ministerial Task Force for Health, Safety and Productivity, and the Cabinet Office]
	Case studies and interviews with practitioners and stakeholders show that managing sickness absence is not 'rocket science'. Concluded that three key fundamental systems changes are needed:
	• Boards of departments and agencies should take responsibility for absence management, set up and oversee attendance management strategies for their departments, and report regularly on performance.
	• Management information systems need to provide for real time recording and audit. This will give managers and HR departments more timely data so that they can monitor absence, take action and initiate support at agreed trigger points, and ensure that well established procedures are adhered to in practice.
	• As departments install new HR management systems, managers should receive formal training in both the systems and procedures and the skills they need to deal with case management, referral and return to work discussions. This should be complemented by central HR support to enable departments to move towards integrating absence and performance management.

TABLE 6b: WORKPLACE (INCLUDING OCCUPATIONAL HEALTH)

IIAC 2007 – personal communication Compilation of material from various sources	**The effectiveness of vocational rehabilitation** [UK Industrial Injuries Advisory Council] *(Provides examples of UK best practice)* In British Telecom, Health and Safety is within the HR section and is covered by the BT People Strategy of 'creating a healthy environment where excellence prospers'. There are three steps to the consideration of health and safety – primary engagement, secondary intervention (formerly prevention) and tertiary restitution (formerly rehabilitation). Most workers who are sick or injured require simple and temporary measures to help them to return to work and avoid long term sickness absence. Line managers are key to tertiary restitution in keeping in regular contact with workers on sickness absence to remind them they are part of the work community. Contact is usually by telephone, but may also be face-to-face at the workers home. Line managers can arrange practical interventions to support return to work (e.g. flexibility for home working, funding transport to work). BT has an external provider for occupational health services and other outside providers are also used when required. However, in the majority of cases the problems are relatively simple and BT actively discourages abrogation of responsibility to experts. Line managers have the levers, support and guidance they need. In 5 years, the scheme has reduced sickness absence by about 1/3. Most of that has been produced by reducing long-term absence of more than 6 months stood at 33%, but this has now risen to 75% (and to the same job). The largest drop has been in absence due to musculoskeletal conditions, which was previously the largest cause. The highest proportion of absence is now due to mental health problems. Employer liability litigation has dropped. Transport for London has had high sickness absence rates (particularly high in London underground with 12 days per employee per annum). A business case was made to improve occupational health provisions, focusing on two main areas i) musculoskeletal disorders, primarily back pain and ii) stress, anxiety and depression. Guidance on managing and preventing back pain was incorporated into basic training for managers and employees. A physiotherapy service was introduced for those with back pain and voluntary back fitness classes. Stress reduction workshops consist of 2 hour sessions for 6 weeks are provided for closed groups of workers who may self-refer or be referred by their line manager. There are specific services for workers who are assaulted or exposed to stressful incidents. Transport for London are also piloting a programme which funds rehabilitation for a minority of people due to the length of NHS waiting times. This is extremely difficult to manage and has had variable results, because return to work is much more about the psychosocial rather than the biological aspects of a person's illness. Royal Mail was the first large public business to directly employ occupational therapists in the mid 90s. Initially, an occupational health nurse makes an assessment to determine whether the worker should be referred to an OT or physiotherapist. If these procedures are unsuccessful, the worker is assessed for referral to a specialist rehabilitation programme, which is contracted out to an independent company. This was piloted 4 years ago on 'tough' cases of chronic back pain who had little hope of improvement: 44 were on long term sickness absence (averaging 31 weeks); 42 were on extended periods of modified duties (averaging < 50% productivity for > 1 year); 22 had had episodic absences (averaging 7 weeks). The programme was very successful, with 80% clinical improvement and 69% return to work rate: 75 workers returned to full duties, and a further 8 to full-time modified work; many remain at work 2 years later. The success of the scheme shows the need for a multiplicity of approaches. Looking at the results, vocational rehabilitation was considered not a simple single intervention issue. The location of the rehabilitation programmes on site, at the workplace, was crucial to success. Whilst there was a significant cost in setting up the scheme, there was a high return on the investment (> 5:1). This equated to a £700,000 saving at one site in terms of days lost, anticipated terminations of employment and legal issues and long term pension contributions.

TABLE 6b: WORKPLACE (INCLUDING OCCUPATIONAL HEALTH)

An earlier controlled longitudinal study of 'Royal Mail's early intervention programme following psychological trauma' (Rick et al. 2006) concluded that there was robust evidence from an organisational perspective that:

- the trauma management procedures used at RMG are a safe response to trauma;

- the 'support post trauma' protocol is effective in relaying information to employees about symptoms and further sources of support within the organisation;

- organisational activity which enhances an employee's feeling of support post-trauma (particularly practical support) is associated with lower symptoms at 3 months and lower absence at 12 months.

Rolls-Royce implemented a company-wide absence management policy and developed an effective sickness absence management programme (HSE 2005). Trade union representatives from a number of different unions were consulted over the proposed procedures at the planning stage. All staff were trained on the new policies & procedures, explaining the responsibilities of managers, human resources and occupational health advisors. An IT programme was introduced that monitors employee absence, records the reasons for the absence and calculates costs. Early rehabilitation is provided to anyone who is absent for 4+ weeks, including an action plan and physiotherapy services (for both work and non-work related injuries).

The Health & Safety benefits include:

- The ability to analyse the causes of staff absence accurately. For example, Rolls-Royce has recorded a drop in the proportion of staff absence due to stress from 20% to 16%

- Fewer staff days absence due to illness

The business benefits include:

- A reduction in staff absence from an average of 2.9%(1999) to 2.4%(2002) of the workforce, saving around £11m

- The average number of days lost per employee per year has fallen to 4.2 (compared with a national average of 6.8)

- Consequently, more staff contribute to Rolls-Royce's business activities at any one time

- Employees feel managers are positively interested in their prompt return to work

- As employees return to work more quickly, management time spent on each absence is more effective

- By reducing absence by about 15%, the company has saved approximately £11 million

TABLE 6b: WORKPLACE (INCLUDING OCCUPATIONAL HEALTH)

(ILO 2002) Code of practice	**Managing disability in the workplace: ILO code of practice** [International Labour Organization] *(Broad policy approach to disability issues and employment, and responsibilities of key stakeholders including employers and workers' representatives. It includes 'job retention by employees who acquire a disability'. Importantly, it emphasises that vocational rehabilitation is one aspect of comprehensive occupational health and disability management policies).* The disability management strategy should be linked to a workplace-level policy on promoting a safe and healthy workplace, including provision for occupational safety and health measures, risk analysis of any adaptation adjustment or accommodation, early intervention and referral to treatment and rehabilitation of those who acquire a disability while in employment, and a mentoring system to ensure that integration of disabled employees is fostered. The importance of involving workers' representatives, employee awareness and communication is emphasised. Where existing employees acquire a disability while in employment, employers can continue to benefit from their accumulated expertise and experience by taking steps to enable them to retain their employment, including: (a) early intervention and referral to appropriate services; (b) measures for a gradual resumption of work; (c) opportunities for workers with disabilities to test work or obtain experience in an alternative job if they are unable to resume their previous jobs; (d) the use of support and technical advice to identify any opportunities and adjustments which might be required. The competent authorities should promote the availability of opportunities for workers who become disabled, experience work-related injuries, or develop occupational diseases in the course of their working life to remain economically active through: (a) vocational retraining opportunities including those suited to a variety of sectors on the open labour market; (b) the promotion and support of information and advisory services relating to job retention and return to work; (c) the development of materials, if possible in the form of an electronic database, illustrating examples of successful job-retention practices and experiences suited to women and to men, to older and younger workers and to urban and rural areas, and appropriate to national conditions; (d) active programmes to facilitate the integration or reintegration of persons with disabilities into the labour market; (e) monitoring the compatibility of social security systems supporting workers with disabilities with the goals of job retention and return to work.
(IWH 2007) Guidance	**Seven 'principles' for successful return to work** [Institute for Work and Health] These principles were developed from a systematic review of the literature completed in 2004, which included both quantitative studies and qualitative studies, and from other current research on return to work. The review focused on three outcomes: duration of work disability, costs of work disability, and quality of life of workers. Overall, the review found that workplace-based return-to-work interventions have positive impacts on duration and costs of work disability. However, only weak evidence was found to support that these interventions had a positive impact on workers' quality of life, suggesting the need for more research in this area. The seven principles are based on what is known to date and may change as new research evidence becomes available. 1. The workplace has a strong commitment to health and safety which is demonstrated by the behaviours of the workplace parties. 2. The employer makes an offer of modified work (also known as work accommodation) to injured/ill workers so they can return early and safely to work activities suitable to their abilities.

TABLE 6b: WORKPLACE (INCLUDING OCCUPATIONAL HEALTH)

	3. Return to work planners ensure that the plan supports the returning worker without disadvantaging co-workers and supervisors. 4. Supervisors are trained in work disability prevention and included in return to work planning. 5. The employer makes an early and considerate contact with injured/ill workers. 6. Someone has the responsibility to coordinate return to work. 7. Employers and health care providers communicate with each other about the workplace demands as needed, and with the worker's consent.
(James et al. 2002) Narrative review	**Absence management and the issues of job retention and return to work** A large proportion of working days lost through sickness absence stem from relatively long spells of absence. A proactive approach to supporting the return to work of ill and injured workers can have beneficial consequences. However, few UK organizations have comprehensive arrangements in place to handle cases of long-term absence. • In most companies, line managers have the primary responsibility for maintaining contact with absent employees and exploring whether anything can be done to facilitate their return to work. • Workplace adjustments: two thirds report that changes to working hours are considered as an option. Changes in job content (e.g. lighter duties) are also common. However, operational factors may limit the extent to which these are possible. • A few companies support faster access to medical advice and treatment. However, most rely on the National Health Service, with some comment on delays for appointments or treatment. *(The authors highlight key aspects of sickness absence management, but also identify significant difficulties).*
(James et al. 2003) Research report	**Job retention and vocational rehabilitation: the development and evaluation of a conceptual framework** Theoretical framework, evidence review and stakeholder consensus on the main processes and practices that are considered to contribute to effective rehabilitation activity on the part of the employer: • Early and timely identification of vulnerable workers through surveillance: recruitment and selection procedures, health checks and medicals, staff appraisals, absence statistics, regular contact with absent workers, return to work interviews, and fitness for work assessments; • Provision of rehabilitation support in the form of health care *(again the assumption seems to be that health care is one of the main forms of rehabilitation),* and the provision of various 'vocational services' such as functional evaluations, training, 'social support' and workplace adjustments; • Co-ordination of the rehabilitation process by the creation of systems that facilitate sufficient communication, discussion and 'joined-up' action between all potentially relevant actors: human resource staff, safety practitioners, occupational physicians and nurses, psychologists, disability advisers, equal opportunities personnel, trade union and other workplace representatives, and external medical personnel; • Involvement of worker representation to facilitate an environment of openness and trust; • Establishment of policy frameworks that clearly detail support structures, and clarify responsibilities and accountability; • Systematic action, including the provision of required training, to ensure proper implementation of policy frameworks; • Adoption of feedback/reassessment frameworks to identify (and address) any weaknesses in the content and operation of established policy frameworks. *(Delivery of all the elements may be difficult – especially in small and medium sized enterprises – but the <u>principles can be incorporated into locally developed implementations</u>).*

TABLE 6b: WORKPLACE (INCLUDING OCCUPATIONAL HEALTH)

(Kumar 2001) Narrative review	**Disability, injury and ergonomics intervention** The estimated prevalence of disability varies from 0.2 – 20.9%, depending on the definition of disability and the method of measurement. The major categories of disability were described as cardiovascular conditions, respiratory conditions and joint diseases. There is a major association with aging, and demographic trends make this important. Disability has a significant socioeconomic impact with differential employment rates for disabled and non-disabled workers. Using a functional classification and developing functional profiles of people with disability may allow ergonomists to develop generic as well as specific solutions to successfully intervene in many cases and improve their functional capacity.
(Marsden et al. 2004) Research Report	**The development of case studies that demonstrate the business benefit of effective management of occupational health and safety** This study reviewed specific business cases for health and safety in a range of UK organisations. It provides material that a range of stakeholders can use to engage with decision-makers to persuade them of the business case for improved health and safety. The key finding was that in each of the cases described, whatever the original motivation, organisations believed that improving health and safety was integral to business risk management. The organisations decided to improve aspects of health and safety because their business cases showed the benefits to the organisation. These benefits included a mix of both tangible and intangible benefits, such as maintenance of brand and reputation, client requirements, and staff morale, as well as health and safety. In these cases the organisations considered their own business cases so compelling that they did not need a fully quantified cost benefit analysis. However, it was also found that organisations rarely systematically or comprehensively track the costs and benefits of undertaking a particular initiative, particularly where health and safety is integral to management. Example headline savings: • £11 million saved due to absence management (Rolls Royce); • Costs of flu vaccination recouped in one month (Barts and The London NHS Trust); • Manual handling injuries eliminated and lost hours reduced to zero (MFI); • £12 saved for every £1 spent on manual handling improvements (British Polythene Industries); • Almost 70% reduction in staff absence rates (Port of London Authority).
(Nice & Thornton 2004) Research report	**JRRP: Employers' management of long-term sickness absence** *(Employers survey as part of the background to the UK Job Retention and Rehabilitation Pilots (JRRP)).* Employers perceive sickness absence to be a problem because of: difficulties in providing cover for absences; stress and overload on staff; costs; effects on productivity and profitability; and effects on customer service. Among managers there was some lack of sympathy towards days off for 'minor' complaints and suspicions that short-term absences were not always 'genuine'; this created some tensions with HR staff who wanted to avoid a disciplinary approach. In practice, the approach to managing short-term absence was typically non-interventionist. While it was widespread practice for the employee to make contact on the first day of absence, only one employer in the study was proactive at this point in that they offered occupational health advice for selected conditions. There was rather little evidence of active management of sickness absence in the first two to three weeks. Return to work interviews, or less formal discussions, were almost universal, but sometimes cursory. Although it was sometimes recognised that repeated short spells of absence, like occasional days off, could be the precursor to prolonged sickness absence, there as a tendency for them to be seen as suspect.

TABLE 6b: WORKPLACE (INCLUDING OCCUPATIONAL HEALTH)

	There was a widespread desire to retain staff absent with long-term sickness in order to keep specialist skills, maximise investment in training, avoid costs of recruiting and training new staff, circumvent the shortage of new recruits and to give the wider message to staff and job applicants that they are valued. Almost all organisations defined when continued absence became regarded as long-term, usually 4 or 3 weeks. The earliest thresholds, from ten days, had been chosen as the most appropriate at which to intervene with rehabilitation efforts. Prior to that point, the line manager was usually the main actor. After that point, there were 5 main models: • prime responsibility with departmental or line managers, common in public sector organisations; • shared between line managers and human resources (HR); • led by HR; • led by the occupational health department, in one organisation; • shared by HR, occupational health nurse and line managers. Some problems were associated with leaving responsibility to managers: other pressures on their time, limited knowledge or skills, and inconsistent treatment. Back up from human resources included more proactive advice, and, in large companies, central telephone-based help teams. There was difficulty dealing with uncertain duration of absence, particularly for mental health conditions, and managers had some scepticism about 'stress-related' conditions. In general, employers were willing to consider and make adjustments or adaptations to employees' working conditions and the workplace. A wide variety of modifications were reported including phased returns, altering or reducing hours worked and tasks undertaken, adapting equipment and the place of work, and temporary or permanent redeployment. The survey gave a strong impression that sickness absence policies and procedures were evolving rapidly *(in 2003–04)*.
(NIDMAR 2000) Code of practice	**Canadian National Institute of Disability Management and Research: code of practice for disability management** Provides a framework within which employers, unions, legislators, insurers and providers can work together to support return to work for workers with disabilities. Identifies best management practices and policies for sound workplace programmes in disability management. The main 'values' are: • Safe and productive employment of workers with disabilities. • Safe and healthy working • Reduced occurrence and impact of illness and injury due to work • Consensus among government, labour and management on the achievement of these values Disability management requires the coordination of health care and support services, protection of confidentiality and informed consent, return to work planning, coordination of financial resources and information, occupational health and safety, dispute resolution procedures, education of all parties. Central to the approach is to remove obstacles within the workplace, workplace programmes, policy and regulations. Lays out the responsibilities of the key participants in disability management, including a return to work coordinator/disability management professional.
(Norwich Union Healthcare 2006) UK Survey	**Health of the workplace report** Only 6% of GPs in UK feel that employers are doing enough to stop workers going on to long-term sickness or to help rehabilitate them to return to work sooner. Employers believe that GPs are not playing as effective a role as they could *(in rehabilitation)*. 85% of employers believe GPs are too quick to sign sick notes.

TABLE 6b: WORKPLACE (INCLUDING OCCUPATIONAL HEALTH)

(Ruotsalainen et al. 2006) Narrative review	**Evidence on the effectiveness of occupational health interventions** Aimed to provide an overview of the range of evidence currently available regarding the effectiveness of occupational health interventions. 148 occupational health intervention articles published in 2000 and 2001 were examined. In 21% of the studies the study design was a randomized controlled trial, in 28% it was a controlled trial, an interrupted time-series in 7% and a different design in 44%. The occupational health outcome was exposure in 27% of the studies, worker behaviour in 12%, disease symptoms in 30%, disability or sickness absence in 24%, injuries in 4%, and quality of care in 3%. Concluded that high quality evaluation studies are conducted in all areas of occupational health; however, it is clear that more are needed and the methodology could be improved. *(This is a review of the kinds and methodology of evidence available and does not give any findings).*
SIGN 2007 – unpublished data Summary paper	**Short-life working group on occupational health** [Scottish Inter-collegiate Guideline Network] Paper agreed at Scottish Inter-collegiate Guideline Network council 7 November 2007. The aim is to strengthen occupational and vocational rehabilitation and increase awareness that maximising functional capacity and addressing a return to work will achieve the best outcome for an individual's health and wellbeing. It was agreed that every guideline development group or review group should be asked to identify whether there may be any occupational health issues within their area of work.
(Stephens et al. 2004) Narrative review	**Occupational health and SMEs: focused intervention strategies** SMEs are very diverse but, in general, they do not invest much resources or money in occupational health. SMEs have 'gatekeepers' who provide, or more often withhold, resources that would improve occupational health. Gatekeepers are key stakeholders within an SME with access to resources. The gatekeeper is often the owner, 'boss' or, in larger SMEs, a senior manager with assigned OH responsibilities. Effective occupational health interventions need to target the gatekeeper with the aim of persuading them to adopt improved practices and propagate them throughout their organisation. 'Persuasion' may be in the form of incentives that promote the value of good practice or, provide a threat of negative repercussions if good practice is not followed. However, SME gatekeepers are often resistant to making changes to occupational health practices. The strengths and weakness of any proposed intervention depend on a set of attributes: task influences; incentives; targeting; medium; and route. Taking the notions of the gatekeeper and interventions together, the authors concluded that an effective intervention strategy is one that will consist of complementary interventions, which compensate for each others respective weaknesses. Furthermore, to maximise the impact of the intervention strategy, there should be interventions aimed at the workforce and separate interventions aimed at the 'gatekeepers'. In this way a 'pincer' effect is created, with pressures on the gatekeeper coming from outside the SME and from within via a more OH aware workforce.

(The Work Foundation 2006)
 	
Toolkit
	The well managed organisation: diagnostic tools for handling sickness absence
	
	The Work Foundation was invited by the Ministerial Task Force (2004) to produce, with Government, a clear profile for the well managed organisation. A diagnostic toolkit covers:
	
	• Management skills and training needs:- monitoring, measuring and understanding absence information
	   o managing sickness absence when it happens
	• Promoting a healthy environment *(with a particular focus on HSE Stress Management Guidelines):*
	   o tackling the underlying causes of absence (work organization and job design)
	   o promoting a culture that encourages attendance
	• Involving the workforce and their representatives in creating a healthier workplace
	
	Linked publications consider the roles and responsibilities of Boards and of Directors, with a strong emphasis on the importance of their involvement in sickness absence management issues

TABLE 6b: WORKPLACE (INCLUDING OCCUPATIONAL HEALTH)

(Thornbory 2008) Report	**Occupational health 2008: making the business case**

(*Special report by the Workplace Law Group, aimed at the legal and allied professions*). Provides a comprehensive description of the legal framework, modern concepts of occupational health and occupational health services. Considers the legal, financial, cost-benefit analysis and moral reasons that support the business case for occupational health. Summarises the principles of managing absence, disability and rehabilitation (*consistent with other recent UK publications in this Table*).

(TUC 2002) Report	**Rehabilitation and retention: what works is what matters**

[UK Trades Union Congress]

There is growing acceptance that greater effort is needed to retain employees who have been affected by poor health, injury, or disability, in paid employment. Employers have a key role in this, and new research reveals that it can best be achieved where they:

- Make rehabilitation a policy goal
- Invest in employee health, providing access to good occupational health facilities and workplace health initiatives
- Respond to absence: monitoring health, keeping in touch with sick employees, responding early with referral for medical checks, being alert to disability issues, and applying practical rehabilitation measures
- Do not make health a disciplinary matter
- Assume in the first instance that sickness absence is due to work-related causes which should be investigated
- Involve all levels of management in rehabilitation, including line managers, personnel/human resources (HR) managers, occupational health (OH), and senior managers
- Work with unions and their members, being open on health and absence issues, and involving them fully in the development of relevant policies.

(*These principles are consistent with all of the other evidence and views on sickness absence management, with the exception of the assumption in the first instance that sickness absence is due to work-related causes. For discussion, see Evidence findings and Table 2 in present report*).

(Tyers et al. 2007) Report	**Workplace Health Connect – January 2007 progress report**

[UK Health & Safety Executive report]

Workplace Health Connect was a 2-year pilot initiative, launched in February 2006. It was a free, no-obligation service providing small and medium enterprises (SMEs) with advice on workplace health and safety: a telephone advice line for employers and employees; problem solving visits; signposting to approved local specialists. As of November 2006, fewer than 4,000 calls had been received by the advice line (reflecting lack of advertising), but 1,130 adviser visits had been conducted (reflecting a high rate of referral from the advice line). A survey of SME employer attitudes towards occupational health, showed that they tended to:

- agree that health issues are important to them
- strongly agree that it isn't always clear what employer responsibilities are in the area of employee health
- feel that it can be difficult to get employees to take their own health seriously
- feel that some health and safety procedures are not practical.

The overall levels of satisfaction with the services offered were extremely high. SMEs that received a visit found it useful: 87% said the recommendations were useful, 70% had already made changes and 22% planned to. The most common changes already made were updating health and safety policies or conducting a risk assessment. Only a minority of companies had a specific interest in sickness absence or return to work issues, but those who did had been helped by Workplace Health Connect to resolve any issues. Further evaluation is expected.

TABLE 6b: WORKPLACE (INCLUDING OCCUPATIONAL HEALTH)

(Waterman 2007) Narrative Review	**The future for occupational health in the United Kingdom**

Since the 1970s, the UK Health and Safety strategy has reduced the number of work accidents, but the huge costs and personal suffering associated with health issues has lagged far behind. UK does not have a single, coherent approach to occupational health services: there is no statutory provision, and occupational health (OH) is not part of the NHS. Instead, OH is a patchwork of public and private providers, mainly in large companies and generally limited in small and medium enterprises (SME): there are various estimates that only about a third of employees have access to OH, though many of these are far from comprehensive.

Outlines a fundamental debate in UK, Europe and worldwide a) between those who argue for a comprehensive OH *service* which is available to everyone, stands outside the normal day-to-day running of enterprises, and possibly integrated into the NHS, and b) OH *support* for the key relationship between workers and employers; the challenge being to get employers and workers to take responsibility for work-related health standards and to initiate seeking support Argues that, at present in the UK, the balance of opinion is for the *support model.* Describes various pilot studies of this approach. Workplace Health Connect is one example for SMEs in England:

- a confidential service designed to give free, practical advice on workplace health, safety and return to work issues
- an Adviceline and supporting website giving tailored, practical advice to managers and workers
- aims to transfer knowledge and skills directly to managers and workers, enabling them to tackle workplace health issues themselves.
- working in partnership with the Health & Safety Executive and based around an Adviceline/website and local problem-solving services.

(An evaluation of Workplace Health Connect is due to be published within the next year).

(WHO 1995) Strategy document	**Global strategy on occupational health for all**

Health at work and healthy work environments are among the most valuable assets of individuals, communities and countries. Occupational health is an important strategy not only to ensure the health of workers, but also to contribute positively to productivity, quality of products, work motivation, job satisfaction and thereby to the overall quality of life of individuals and society.

The 10 priority objectives proposed by the strategy were:

- Strengthening of international and national policies for health at work and developing the necessary policy tools
- Development of healthy work environment
- Development of healthy work practices and promotion of health at work
- Strengthening of occupational health services
- Establishment of support services for occupational health
- Development of occupational health standards based on scientific risk assessment
- Development of human resources for occupational health
- Establishment of registration and data systems, development of information services for experts, effective transmission of data and raising of public awareness through public information
- Strengthening of research
- Development of collaboration in occupational health and with other activities and services

[GP = General Practitioner; OH = occupational health; RTW = return to work; SAW = stay at work; SME = small and medium enterprises]

Table 6c: 'Structured' vocational rehabilitation interventions

Authors	Key features (*Reviewers' comments in italic*)
TABLE 6c: 'STRUCTURED' VOCATIONAL REHABILITATION	
(BSRM 2000) (BSRM 2003) Working Party Report	**Vocational rehabilitation: the way forward** [British Society of Rehabilitation Medicine] Reviews deficiencies within vocational rehabilitation in UK and makes recommendations. A survey of 30 non-governmental organisations found that they considered: • Waiting times for National Health Service (NHS) services unacceptable • Services inflexible • Lack of understanding about the impact of disease and disability on work • Lack of awareness of options to prevent work loss • Notable lack of inter-agency working In particular, in the NHS, there was: • Loss of the culture of facilitating employment as a key element of effective health care. • Ignorance of means of re-integrating individuals into employment • VR usually only considered **after** completion of 'treatment' • Little designated responsibility to facilitate inter-agency working • Poor recognition of the value of Occupational Health in facilitating vocational rehabilitation. General practitioners have a pivotal role to play in vocational rehabilitation. Because they have responsibility for sick certification they are in a key position to provide advise about work and to trigger vocational rehabilitation. However, lack of time, resources and interest generally precludes this. Recommended that the NHS and Employment Services should recognise formally that early, professional and accessible vocational rehabilitation: • Should be equitably available early following illness or injury. • Requires a multi-disciplinary team spanning the health and employment services to support patients and employers at a district level • Requires one member of the district rehabilitation services to have responsibility and skills to lead vocational rehabilitation in the health service and liaise with the District Employment Adviser • Requires close liaison with occupational health services • Requires an enhanced role for the District Employment Adviser (DEA) who needs access to district rehabilitation services.

TABLE 6c: 'STRUCTURED' VOCATIONAL REHABILITATION

The precise relationship between these services and NHSPlus needs further investigation.

Case management should be adopted formally as the means to assist individuals with complex disabilities back into work.

A National Service Framework for vocational rehabilitation would ensure national standards across the UK and should be developed by Department of Health.

Undergraduate and post-graduate training programmes and accreditation should be developed for health professionals, DEAs and case managers.

(CSAG 1994) Report	**Back pain**

[Clinical Standards Advisory Group]

This report on UK services for back pain developed the first UK clinical guidelines for the management of acute low back pain and made recommendations on early intervention and the management of non-specific LBP in primary care. *(These were similar to and superseded by more recent guidelines, e.g. COST B13 Working Group 2004)*. In addition, it recognised that, no matter how good the service, a small minority of patients would require further, more specialised treatment. It therefore recommended that each District should have a dedicated back pain rehabilitation service, led by a consultant, and including facilities for psychological support, advice about work, and communication with the workplace to facilitate return to work.

(DH 2004) Guidance note	**Improving chronic disease management**

[UK Department of Health]

Disease management is generally provided by multidisciplinary teams providing high-quality, evidence-based care, including the use of pathways and protocols. There is growing evidence, from service improvements, initiatives already in place and the experience of other countries, that the essential components of good chronic disease management include:

- Use of information systems to access key data on individuals and populations
- Identifying patients with chronic disease
- Stratifying patients by risk
- Supporting patients to take an active role in managing their own condition: self-care and self-management
- Coordinating care (using case-managers)
- Using multidisciplinary teams
- Integrating specialist and generalist expertise
- Integrating care across organizational boundaries
- Aiming to minimise unnecessary visits and admissions
- Providing care in the least intensive setting

(See also Table 7a)

TABLE 6c: 'STRUCTURED' VOCATIONAL REHABILITATION

(Dunstan & Covic 2006) Narrative review	**Compensable work disability management: a literature review of biopsychosocial perspectives** Minimising work disability and facilitating work participation are a major focus of occupational therapy, and the specific brief of therapists working as case managers in the occupational injury arena. This paper reviews and discusses the empirically supported critical factors in the development, maintenance and management of work disability, and outlines the essential components of multidisciplinary biopsychosocial rehabilitation. By implementing the biopsychosocial model and time off work as the framework in which work disability is conceptualised and occupational rehabilitation plans are developed, case managers can play a key role in promoting evidence-linked practice to reduce the cost and suffering associated with long-term work disability.
(Epping-Jordan et al. 2004) Narrative review	**Improving the quality of health care for chronic conditions** Non-communicable conditions and mental disorders accounted for 47% of the global burden of disease in 2002 and this is projected to increase to 60% by 2020. At the same time many people with chronic conditions are failing to receive appropriate care. Managing the quality of health services for chronic conditions is a seemingly daunting challenge. To meet this challenge, the World Health Organisation has adapted the Chronic Care Model to produce the Innovative Care for Chronic Conditions. This expands community and policy aspects and concludes complements at the micro (patient and family), meso (healthcare organisation and community) and macro (policy) levels. The framework provides a flexible but comprehensive base on which to build or redesign health systems in accordance with local resources and demands.
(Frank & Thurgood 2006) Editorial	**Vocational rehabilitation in the UK: opportunities for health-care professionals** In view of demographic changes, increasing emphasis on preserving an active and healthy workforce, and the goal of increasing employment rates including for people with ill health or disabilities, all health professionals caring for people of working age will increasingly need to provide advice about health and work. Yet many therapists (*and other health professionals*) have little training in vocational rehabilitation. There is now widespread agreement that maintaining an active and healthy workforce needs close collaboration between the employment and health sectors, and that a cohort of trained health professionals is required to cross this divide, There is, however, increasing concern that there are inadequate numbers of appropriately trained health professionals to fill such roles. There are likely to be increasing openings for therapists with interests in this area.
(Gobelet et al. 2007a) Narrative review	**Vocational rehabilitation: a multidisciplinary intervention** Vocational rehabilitation is by definition a multidisciplinary intervention in a process linked to the facilitation of return to work or to the prevention of loss of the work. Clinical staff in contact with a person who has lost his job (general practitioner, specialized physician) must promote vocational rehabilitation. Medical rehabilitation for those with disabilities, whether new or old, has to be followed without delay by vocational rehabilitation. These two intertwined processes (medical and vocational rehabilitation) are overlapping. The vocational aspect of the rehabilitation should be introduced as soon as possible in the course of the medical rehabilitation programme. If help is to be provided early for the person who is going off work and in danger of losing their job, the effective and knowledgeable intervention of the line manager at the workplace is crucial, as is that of the counsellor at the workplace or the occupational health professional. They involve many professionals including physiotherapists, occupational therapists, psychologists, vocational trainers, job counsellors, teachers, case-managers, job placement agencies. Vocational rehabilitation has a financial cost, borne by many state organizations (security, social system, social affairs) as well as by employers and private insurances, which are in case of accident, concerned by this process. However, the evidence suggests that these costs are recouped 2- to 10-fold (*this figure appears to be based entirely on reference to BSRM 2000 – Table 6c*).

TABLE 6c: 'STRUCTURED' VOCATIONAL REHABILITATION

(Goetzel et al. 2005) Narrative review	**Return on investment in disease management** Disease Management is a multi-disciplinary, coordinated, continuum- based approach to healthcare delivery and communications for populations with, or at risk for, established medical conditions. Effective Disease Management programs should contain the following eight elements: (1) an identified population with specific health and disease conditions; (2) the application of evidence-based practice guidelines to treat those patients; (3) a process that encourages collaboration among physicians and other providers; (4) risk stratification, matching interventions with need; (5) patient self-management education (that may include primary prevention, behaviour modification programs, and compliance/surveillance); (6) process and outcomes measurement, evaluation, and management; (7) routine reporting and feedback loops that include communication with the patient, physician, health plan, and ancillary providers; and (8) appropriate use of information technology. A positive ROI was found for programs directed at CHF and multiple disease conditions. Some evidence suggests that diabetes programs may save more than they cost, but additional studies are needed. Results are mixed for asthma management programs. Depression management programs cost more than they save in medical expenses, but may save money when considering productivity outcomes. *(This review only covered direct medical costs and there were no data on indirect costs such as sickness absence. Separate entries in Cardiac, respiratory and mental health Tables).*
(Green-McKenzie et al. 2004) Narrative review	**Managing workers' compensation costs: success of initiatives to change outcomes** General overview of workers compensation health care costs and 9 US examples of system interventions which improved outcomes. A general thread of the successful programmes was integrated management of delivery of health care to the injured worker, which emphasised a gatekeeper approach and improved communication among the main stakeholders. Case management often played a useful role and could be pivotal in helping to improve communication. Modified duties were common, allowing workers to return to work in a safe and productive capacity, and reducing the likelihood of re-injury. Some of these programmes were integrated with injury prevention. *(Despite the emphasis on controlling costs, many of the findings and conclusions were actually about improved occupational outcomes).*
(Hanson et al. 2006) Narrative review	**The costs and benefits of active case management and rehabilitation for musculoskeletal disorders** Case management is a collaborative process which assesses, plans, implements, coordinates, monitors and evaluates the options and services required to meet an individual's health care, educational and employment needs, using communication and available resources to promote quality, cost-effective outcomes. (Case Management Society UK www.cmsuk.org) This project aimed to review evidence on the costs and benefits of active case management and rehabilitation programmes for musculoskeletal disorder; to identify potential incentives, and obstacles to, the adoption of these programmes; and, to describe a model programme based on the evidence and assess its acceptability to stakeholders. The authors concluded there is moderate evidence that case management approaches are effective and can yield a variety of benefits that are cost effective. The benefits observed include reduced healthcare costs, reduced treatment duration, reduced sick-leave and time off work, improved worker productivity, reduced compensation claims and litigation, reduced claim duration and more rapid claim closure. An outline of the key components of successful and cost-effective case management was provided. (See also Table 2).
(Isernhagen 2006) Narrative review	**Job matching and return to work: occupational rehabilitation as the link** Caring physicians generally do not know enough about their patients' job demands to advise about work. Patients themselves tend to provide the lowest estimate of their job capabilities. Physician recommendations of restrictions may be counter-productive and act as a barrier to RTW: because of their lack of job knowledge, physicians often 'play safe' and are too conservative; employers often find the recommended restrictions impractical. Functional capacity evaluation is reliable but its predictive value for return to work is low to moderate. A reliable method that matches objective FCE to objective job specific information may produce a stronger match. The authors propose a new model of job function matching, based on research and the skills of occupational rehabilitation professionals, to bridge the gap between the medical community, employers and workers. *(No evidence is presented on the effectiveness of this approach).*

TABLE 6c: 'STRUCTURED' VOCATIONAL REHABILITATION

(IUA/ABI 2007) Industry guidance	**The rehabilitation code** [International Underwriting Association / Association of British Insurers] Targeted at insurers and solicitors with the aim of promoting rehabilitation and early intervention in the compensation process. It shall be the duty of every claimant's solicitor to consider, from the earliest practicable stage, and in consultation with the claimant and where appropriate the claimant's treating physician(s), whether it is likely or possible that early intervention, rehabilitation or medical treatment would improve their present and/or long term physical and mental well being. It shall be the duty of the insurer, from the earliest practicable stage in any appropriate case, to consider whether it is likely that the claimant will benefit in the immediate, medium or longer term from further medical treatment, rehabilitation or early intervention. Unless the need for intervention, rehabilitation or treatment has already been identified by medical reports obtained and disclosed by either side, the need for and extent of such intervention, rehabilitation or treatment will be considered by means of an assessment by an appropriately qualified person. The assessment report will be disclosed to both sides. The insurer will be under a duty to consider the recommendations and to consider funding them.
(Kenyon 2003) Report	**Cost benefit analysis of rehabilitation services provided by CRS Australia** [Institute for Research into International Competitiveness for Commonwealth Rehabilitation Service Australia] Analysed 16,348 clients who received vocational rehabilitation over 18 months to December 2002. The average client had approx 30 hours contact with CRS Australia, of which 4.5 hours were spent in pre-programme activities including referral and initial assessment, and 26 hours in a rehabilitation programme. The average cost of delivering the programme was $4,397 and the Total Social Benefit $133,389, with a Net Social Benefit of $128,991 and benefit to cost ratio of 30.
(MBWDC 2000) Report	**Report of the task force on vocational rehabilitation in workers compensation** [Michigan Bureau of Workers' Disability Compensation] From 1965, the Michigan Workers Disability Compensation Act made vocational rehabilitation a benefit to injured workers. In the late 1990s there was concern about abuses, including delayed referrals, under-qualified providers, inadequate evaluations, unrealistic demands for immediate job placement with high pressure tactics and little or no concern about wage recovery, and injured workers who did not cooperate with vocational rehabilitation. The Task Force recognized the accepted principle that rehabilitation is an inherent part of the workers compensation system, while acknowledging the difficulty in translating that principle into cost-effective programs that serve the needs of both injured employees and employers. It proposed a definition of vocational rehabilitation (See Table 1) to eliminate confusion over this important area of professional practice. It recommended enhanced qualifications for providers, requiring Bureau approval at the individual provider level to provide vocational rehabilitation services, and upgraded service delivery standards to improve the quality and appropriate use of vocational rehabilitation. The recommendations call for the Bureau to strengthen enforcement of vocational rehabilitation practice standards for all the parties, to encourage early intervention, and to develop and emphasise continuing education for all participants with assistance from appropriate educational partners. It also recommended better data recording of vocational rehabilitation and further consideration of the role of case management.

TABLE 6c: 'STRUCTURED' VOCATIONAL REHABILITATION

(Ofman et al. 2004) Systematic review	**Does disease management improve clinical and economic outcomes in patients with chronic diseases?** Overall (in 102 studies of 11 chronic conditions: depression, diabetes, rheumatoid arthritis, chronic pain, coronary artery disease, asthma, heart failure, back pain, chronic obstructive pulmonary disease, hypertension, and hyperlipidemia) patient satisfaction with treatment had the highest percentage of statistically significant comparisons favouring the treatment group (71%), followed by patient adherence to treatment recommendations (47%), measures of disease control (45%), and provider adherence to guidelines (40%). Utilization and cost-related outcomes showed benefit in relatively few studies, as evidenced by the following: other utilization (e.g., provider visits) (16%), cost (14%), emergency department visits (11%), and hospitalizations (11%). *(No occupational outcomes or indirect costs. Separate data in cardiac, respiratory and mental health Tables).*
(Price Waterhouse Coopers LLP 2008) Report	**Building the case for wellness** The objective was to build the wider business case for workplace wellness programmes and then specifically the economic case for UK employers, based on a review of relevant UK case studies, supplemented by a review of the published literature. *(The literature included in PWC 2008 was mainly on health promotion, which is excluded from the present review).* Some employers have identified clear demographic, societal and economic realities that have led to their implementing wellness programmes. Others have instituted programmes for specific reasons such as improved retention, recruitment and company image. The wellness programmes generally included a) health and safety, b) prevention and health promotion, and c) managing ill health (occupational health, absence management and disability management). The report evaluated the evidence from 55 organisations in the UK that had implemented a variety of wellness programmes and initiatives in recent years. Overall, in most cases reviewed, an improvement in key intermediate performance measures could be seen and in a number of cases the organisations linked these improvements through to an estimation of the financial benefits. The improvement in intermediate and financial benefits was observed in various different types of organisations, across different sectors and firm sizes, and for various types of interventions. . 45 out of 55 cases reported a reduction in days lost through sickness absence as a consequence of wellness interventions. The reductions in lost days vary enormously, ranging from 10% to 97% over the evaluation period, with the reported average around 30-40%. Seven case studies with detailed economic analysis reported a return on investment in terms of a benefit-cost ratio ranging from 1-34. The magnitude of the benefits varied significantly, depending not only on what type of organisation and programme involved, but also on the way in which the programme was planned and executed. Overall, the authors concluded that successful wellness programmes were those that were specifically designed to meet employee needs. As there is no 'one-size fits all' offering, there is a need for a framework that offers a practical approach to implementation which focuses on employee need and value *(No separate analysis presented on the effectiveness of specific vocational rehabilitation interventions).*
(Shaw et al. 2007) Systematic review	**A literature review describing the role of return-to-work coordinators in trial programs and interventions designed to prevent workplace disability** Included 22 studies (40 articles), mainly of musculoskeletal conditions or work injuries. The primary aim of the review was to analyse the activities of RTW coordinators and the necessary competences. The focus was RTW coordinators providing direct, on-site workplace liaison to reduce work absences associated with physical health ailments. 29 RTW coordinator activities were identified, but there was variation in the training background, workplace activities, and contextual setting of RTW coordinators. Based on these activities, six preliminary competency domains were identified: (1) ergonomic and workplace assessment; (2) clinical interviewing; (3) social problem solving; (4) workplace mediation; (5) knowledge of business and legal aspects; and (6) knowledge of medical conditions. The principal activities of RTW coordination involve workplace assessment, planning for transitional duty, and facilitating communication and agreement among stakeholders. It was concluded that successful RTW coordination may depend more on competences in ergonomic job accommodation, communication, and conflict resolution than on medical training.

TABLE 6c: 'STRUCTURED' VOCATIONAL REHABILITATION

In the majority of studies, RTW coordination was only one of several elements included within a larger intervention. Other elements included medical case management, multidisciplinary rehabilitation, physiotherapy, early medical management by a rehabilitation specialist, physician recommendations to stay active, improvements in employer safety practices, adoption of a managed care approach to medical care, and improved database tracking of claims costs and lost time claims. Thus, benefits of RTW coordination were difficult to distinguish from other program benefits. In two studies where workplace intervention was assessed independently from a clinical intervention, the workplace intervention appeared to have the greater benefit. In terms of the overall intervention programs, most studies reported either improvements in aggregated disability costs or lost-time claims (range of 20–60%). When the relative odds of returning to work was the principal outcome, most studies reported at least a two-fold increase. One study assessing cost–benefit found a net savings of CAN$16,000 per case, while another showed improved outcomes with no significant increase in overall treatment cost. Only 2 of the 22 studies reported no improvement in disability outcomes after intervention.

| (VRA 2007)

Professional standards | **Vocational rehabilitation standards of practice**

[Vocational Rehabilitation Association]

Provides a professional definition of vocational rehabilitation (*see Table 1*), identifies the disciplines and process that define the field and how it differs from other forms of professional practice, and describes the knowledge, skills and training required by VR professionals to provide an effective service.

(Focused on professional standards and process rather than outcomes or effectiveness). |
| (Von Korff et al. 2002)

Narrative review | **Organising care for chronic illness**

[BMJ Series – ABC of psychological medicine]

(This is the only review found which is about the management of chronic illness (directly concerning common health problems) as opposed to chronic disease). Details will vary with the chronic illness in question, but there are common principles for the management of all chronic conditions. Common elements include:

- Collaboration between service providers and patients
- A personalised written care plan
- Tailored education in self management
- Planned follow up
- Monitoring of outcome and adherence to treatment
- Targeted use of specialist consultation and referral
- Protocols for stepped care (*See also Table 7a).* |

TABLE 6c: 'STRUCTURED' VOCATIONAL REHABILITATION

(WAG 2006) Report	**Improving health and the management of chronic conditions in Wales. Self management and independence: a report by the Task and Finish Group** [Welsh Assembly Government]

The Cochrane database of systematic reviews was searched using the MeSH term 'self care' (14 reviews), text terms 'self management' (45 reviews) and 'education' (145 reviews). Abstracts of these reviews were searched to determine their applicability, and the findings were summarized. Distillation of the material provided in the systematic reviews yielded valuable information, based largely on the strength of evidence, that permitted categorisation of the nature and modes of intervention.

<u>Outcomes are improved by:</u>

- Interventions which are based on models of increasing self empowerment.
- Exercise training.
- Models based on regular interaction with health professionals focused on proactive recall and review of patients, particularly if patient oriented.
- Use of patient specific materials such as written action plans especially when supplemented by verbal information for asthma, or practical skills in medication management.
- Combining all of these approaches appears to provide optimal outcomes
- Interactive computer based programmes which provide feedback, behaviour change support and peer support as well as information

<u>Less successful models:</u>

- Models based solely on education, provision of written materials or encouraging adherence to treatment are less successful

<u>Models where these reviews did not yet provide evidence of effectiveness:</u>

- The effectiveness of lay-led self management programmes. A Cochrane review of evidence in this area is expected shortly.
- The value of training health care providers to be more 'patient centred' in clinical consultations.

Some of the reviews point to problems with literacy levels, or difficulties in improving outcomes in marginalised populations, but no reviews provided evidence of how to overcome these problems; more research is needed in this area.

(Weingarten et al. 2002) Meta-analysis	**Interventions used in disease management programmes for patients with chronic illness - which ones work?**

Included 102 studies of 118 disease management programmes. Patient education was the most commonly used intervention (92 programmes), followed by education of healthcare providers (47) and provider feedback (32). Most programmes (70/118) used more than one intervention. Provider education (effect size 0.44 95% CI 0.19 - 0.68), feedback (0.61, 0.28 - 0.93), and reminders (0.52, 0.35 - 0.69) were associated with significant improvements in provider adherence to guidelines, and with significant improvements in patient disease control (effect sizes 0.35 (0.19 to 0.51), 0.17 (0.10 to 0.25), and 0.22 (0.1 to 0.37) respectively). Patient education, reminders, and financial incentives were all associated with improvements in patient disease control (effect sizes 0.24 (0.07 to 0.40), 0.27 (0.17 to 0.36), and 0.40 (0.26 to 0.54) respectively). Measures of provider adherence to guidelines were used as key processes of care and measures of disease control as key outcomes of care (*but no clinical or occupational outcomes*).

[RTW = return to work]

Table 6d: Social security and policy interventions

TABLE 6d: SOCIAL SECURITY AND POLICY	
Authors	**Key features** (*Reviewers' comments in italic*)
(Bambra et al. 2005) Systematic review	**Does 'welfare-to-work' work? - a systematic review of the effectiveness of the UK's welfare-to-work programmes for people with a disability or chronic illness** Included 16 studies. There were five main welfare-to-work strategies operating in the 1990s: Three of the strategies focused on individuals with a disability or chronic illness—by aiming to raise their education and vocational skills levels; providing support and advice in locating and obtaining work; or overcoming financial concerns about the benefits-to-work transition. The other two strategies concentrate on the work environment: by providing incentives to employers to employ people with a chronic illness or a disability, and by improving the physical accessibility of the workplace environment. Overall, each of these strategies helped people with disabilities into work, who were previously on benefits. The proportion of participants gaining employment after involvement ranged from 11% to 50%, dependent on characteristics of participants, such as 'job-readiness', as well as wider labour market context. The evidence tentatively suggests that some types of welfare-to-work— most notably education, training and work placement, and vocational advice and support services—are more soundly based than others. However, no single UK welfare-to-work approach stands out as by far the best way of solving the twin policy problems of low employment rates amongst people with a disability or chronic illness, and rising numbers of incapacity benefit claimants. As most studies were uncontrolled, it was difficult to determine if the improved employment chances were due to the effectiveness of the welfare-to-work interventions themselves or to external factors. Wider impact, such as uptake of schemes as a proportion of the total target population, was weak. The qualitative components identified barriers and facilitators concerned with effective implementation, to aid design of future initiatives.
(Corden & Thornton 2002) Research report	**Employment programmes for disabled people: lessons from research evaluations** [UK Department for Work and Pensions research report] Reviewed 6 international examples of employment programmes for disabled people: • New Deal for Disabled People Personal Adviser Service – UK • Project NetWork - USA • National Vocational Rehabilitation Programme - Canada • Intensive Assistance - Australia • Case Based Funding Trial for Disability Employment Assistance - Australia • Arbeitsassistenz - Austria The following findings emerged from the review of the six programmes: • There was general support among clients for the personal case management approach (even when clients were critical of actual services provided). • Quality of services offered can be highly variable, and there is need for firm quality control.

TABLE 6d: SOCIAL SECURITY AND POLICY

	• Different kinds of organisations and service models were able to recruit people receiving disability-related benefits for **voluntary** participation in vocational rehabilitation.
	• The rate at which those recruited completed the agreed programmes and subsequently moved into work varied and was hard to compare across programmes. What evidence there was suggested that programme impacts in terms of moves into work or increased earnings may be relatively modest
	• Conclusive evidence on relative impacts of different models of case management and service delivery is difficult to achieve.
	Evidence from these six programmes was supplemented by the wider research literature on case-managed employment services for disabled people, which provides support for holistic and individualised approaches. There is rather little evidence of the service process affecting placement outcomes, but assistance with job search appears to be effective.
(DWP 2004) Government report	**Building capacity for work: a UK framework for vocational rehabilitation** [UK Department for Work and Pensions] In promoting work as the best form of welfare for people of working age while protecting those in the greatest need, the UK Government would like to enable more people who have health conditions, impairments or injuries to access, remain in, or return to work. The Government also recognises that absence management is an important issue for many businesses and that more could also be done to minimise the effects of illness caused or made worse by work activities. This Framework was a first step to collecting stakeholders' views and case examples, considering the issues, producing a working description of vocational rehabilitation and developing a common agenda.
DWP-1	**Job Retention and Rehabilitation Pilot (JRRP)** [UK Department for Work and Pensions] The JRRP was designed to help people who had been off work 6-26 weeks but who were still employed, with the goal of preventing long-term incapacity. It was budgeted at £17.75 This was a randomised controlled trial comparing a health care and a workplace intervention, separately and in combination, against 'usual care', and using several delivery models. Participants were randomised to: • a workplace intervention, aimed at achieving a return-to-work by addressing issues in the workplace; • a health intervention, aimed at achieving a return-to-work by addressing the health issues of the individual; and • a combined intervention, this being a mix of the above two interventions (the appropriate mix per individual being left to the judgment of the intervention provider). • a control group of 'usual care'. 2845 subjects were recruited in six areas of the country between April 2003 and December 2004, which was considerably short of the planned 5,400. The context of the JRRPs is described in two research reports on employers' (Nice & Thornton 2004 - See Table 5a) and GPs' (Mowlam & Lewis 2005 – see Table 5c) management of sickness absence.

TABLE 6d: SOCIAL SECURITY AND POLICY

DWP-1 contd	
(Farrell et al. 2006) Research report	**Experiences of the Job Retention and Rehabilitation Pilot** A qualitative study of the experience of participants and staff providing the JRRP services. Participants were generally positive about the staff they met, the premises and the pace at which help was provided, and could be particularly impressed by how it compared with routine NHS provision. Particularly well received were psychological therapies, physical therapies, help with NHS case management, complementary therapies, support in negotiations with employers, and workstation or functional capacity assessments and advice. The case manager role emerged as an important element of the service. In general, the emotional and practical help provided by case managers was highly valued, though contact was not always maintained. Returns to original jobs were the most common route back to work for those who went back to work, and these were aided by the availability of light duties and phased returns. Overall, improvements to health were what allowed people to go back to work and this is where they felt that JRRP had the most impact. Persistent health problems and difficulties in finding suitable work were the main barriers to returning to work among those who did not return to work. People felt unfit to work because their health conditions had not seen a significant improvement. Not having suitable work to go back to was a barrier to returning to work both for those who did feel fit enough to work and those who did not. The reactions of those assigned to the control group varied considerably from mild disappointment to strongly expressed frustration. Staff considered that 'what works' in delivering a job retention service included a number of approaches in working with clients, services, key actors and working relationships were identified by staff as important. Above all else, staff felt it was important to be responsive to individual clients' needs. In addition, important elements in the way they worked with clients were the capacity to intervene early, focusing on the client at all times, taking an holistic approach and trying to tackle a range of problems in a coordinated fashion, tailoring packages of support for individuals, being readily available to talk to clients, having the flexibility to spend money as required, and providing quick access to intensive and focused interventions. Effective health interventions included psychological therapies, physiotherapy, access to specialist medical help, complementary therapies and exercise programmes and facilities. The case management model was popular. Other stakeholders helpful at times were employers, GPs, other NHS workers, family and friends, Jobcentre Plus advisers and trades unions representatives. Helpful employers were willing to help employees return to work, willing to work with JRRP, open to new ideas for rehabilitation, and had effective occupational health services and supportive sick pay schemes. Some GPs aided client progress by encouraging people to think positively about work and to proceed with JRRP rehabilitation plans. They also provided useful background information for provider staff and made helpful suggestions for referrals.
(Purdon et al. 2006) Research report	**Impacts of the Job Retention and Rehabilitation Pilot** The primary outcome measure for the trial was sustained return to work for 13 weeks or more and, given the power of the trial, a difference of 6% between any of the intervention groups and the control group would have been significant. There was a high drop-out rate of 30% (45% for the workplace intervention): 5% withdrew between randomization and interview with the provider, a further 10% between interview and receiving the intervention, and a further 15% did not formally drop out but claimed they never received the intervention. Another 12% refused particular interventions offered - most commonly counselling and CBT, contact with the employer, and complementary therapies. The cross-over rate was low at 5-7%. There were almost identical return-to-work rates for each of the four groups: 44% for the health intervention; 45% for the workplace intervention; 44% for the combined intervention; and 45% for the control group. No benefits were found in other work-elated outcomes, including weeks in work, weeks out of work and receipt of Incapacity Benefits. None of the interventions had any statistically significant or clinically meaningful effect on return to work.

TABLE 6d: SOCIAL SECURITY AND POLICY

DWP-1 contd (Taylor & Lewis 2008) Working Paper	**Understanding the impact of JRRP for people with mental health conditions** JRRP interventions were found to have a negative impact on people with mental health conditions, i.e. those who took part in JRRP had a lower rate of return to work than those who did not use the service. Nine possible hypotheses wire explored. The analysis concluded that it was probably not due to design-related issues. The most plausible explanations were that: • Returns to work appear to have been delayed because of: 1) focus on the same employer where it may have been more productive to seek a new job; 2) waiting for a more complete health recovery, and 3) dependency on the Provider. • There appeared to be less scope to boost NHS provision for mental health conditions compared to other conditions. • There was some evidence of employer behaviours that were more supportive (or less obviously obstructive) of a return to work which meant less scope to improve the workplace context for mental health.
(Stratford et al. 2005) Research report	**The Job Retention and Rehabilitation Pilot: reflections on running a randomised controlled trial** This report was based on data collected by three 'research advisers' who conducted site visits to providers and the Contact Centre to monitor the trial throughout its operation, as well as data from two surveys of participants and the screening instrument. It identified major problems with the running of the trial: • Poor recruitment, lack of awareness of the trial, marketing • the screening process for entry criteria (one third of potential recruits were ineligible) and to eliminate 'deadweight (40–45%) • problems with the control group, • low intensity of contact, lack of engagement and delay in receiving interventions • the high drop-out rate • lack of engagement of GPs and employers, affecting recruitment; and acting as barriers to service providers • lack of standardization and control of the **content** of the interventions, both in health care and particularly in the workplace • although there was little cross-over, the presence of JRRP in an area may have had a wider influence on patients, GPs and employers (hence affecting the controls) The organisation and management of the trial was extremely complex. *(It was originally conceived by the Department for Employment and HM Treasury, and then inherited by DWP, none of whom had any experience of running such a randomised trial (M Aylward 2008, Personal communication)).* The DWP project management team was split into two discrete parts: Disability and Work Division (DWD), in London, had responsibility for the evaluation, and the contract management group within Jobcentre Plus in Sheffield, had responsibility for service delivery. The National Centre for Social Research helped to design and monitored trial procedures and acted as an intermediary. There was a central Contact Centre in Glasgow. The interventions were actually provided by 6 groups of Providers in six parts of UK, each group consisting of widely disparate health and other professionals who were not accustomed to working together as a team. Other stakeholders offer different explanations why JRRP failed. One provider suggested that intervention was too late (about half the interventions did not start till >12 weeks sickness absence, and that the screening process selected people who were in situations where the help available would not be effective (Pickvance 2006). On the other hand, Margaret Hodge, then DWP minister for employment and welfare reform and involved in setting up the JRRP, believed that the intervention was 'probably a little too soon' and 'not sufficiently targeted to those who really need help.' This reflected the Treasury view that it is mainly a matter of 'deadweight' (Ballard 2006). *(However, in the event, 55% of participants failed to return to sustained work, which shows they very clearly needed and were candidates for help. Moreover, the belief that intervention was 'too soon' is completely contrary to the scientific evidence throughout the present review).*

TABLE 6d: SOCIAL SECURITY AND POLICY

DWP-2 (Stafford 2007) (Orr et al. 2007) (Greenberg & Davis 2007) Research reports	**New Deal for Disabled People (NDDP)** [UK Department for Work and Pensions] **New Deal for Disabled People: Third synthesis report – key findings from the evaluation** **Long-term impacts of the New Deal for Disabled People** **Evaluation of the New Deal for Disabled People: the cost and cost-benefit analyses** NDDP is the major national employment programme available to people claiming Incapacity Benefit (IB) and other disability-related benefits in UK, and it is an important part of the Government's welfare to work strategy. NDDP is a voluntary programme that provides a national network of Job Brokers to help people with health conditions and disabilities move into sustained employment. This synthesis report highlights key findings from a large-scale, comprehensive and multi-method evaluation of NDDP, the period July 2001 to November 2006. Overall, the take-up rate was variously estimated o be 2-3.1% of those eligible. 43% of participants entered work, but only 57% of those remained in work for 13 weeks. NDDP increased employment for all 21 subgroups of existing recipients and new claimants. The share working two years after entering the programme rose 4-16% because of the intervention, depending on the subgroup. The average cost to Job Brokers of delivering NDDP programme services to a typical registrant was between £600 and £900. Including both costs incurred by Job Brokers and the central administrative costs incurred by Jobcentre Plus, the cost per client who entered work was £2 - 3,000 and the cost per client who retained a job for at least 6 months was £4 – 5000. NDDP's **net** benefits (i.e. its benefits less its cost) were: • For each pound expended on NDDP, the Government saved between £3.41 and £4.50 for continuing claimants and between £1.71 and £2.26 for new claimants in benefit payments and administrative expenditures. • There is considerable uncertainty about the extent to which NDDP is cost-beneficial from the perspective of NDDP registrants, especially for continuing claimants, because of difficulty estimating costs and benefits in economic terms. • The net benefits of NDDP to society as a whole are £2,915 to £3,163 for typical continuing claimants and £613 to £861 for average new claimants or about £4 or £5 for each pound the Government expended on continuing claimants and around £2 for each pound expended on new claimants.
DWP-3	**Pathways to Work** [UK Department for Work and Pensions] *'Pathways to work'* is an integrated package of support designed to help Incapacity Benefit (IB) recipients to manage their health problems and get back to work. The initial pilots started in October 2003, initially for new claimants (inflow) with existing recipients (stock) able to participate on a voluntary basis. Since then it has been progressively rolled out to cover the whole country by April 2008. Two models of *Pathways* are now being delivered – JCP *Pathways* is already available across 40% of the county, provider-led *Pathways* (private or voluntary sector led) will cover the other 60%. *Pathways* to Work is particularly appropriate for those with common health problems, e.g. mild/moderate mental illness or musculoskeletal pain, and targets a number of the health-related, personal and occupational barriers to return to work. It is the first large-scale example of joint working between the Department of Health and the Department for Work and Pensions, delivered by the NHS and Jobcentre Plus employment support. *Pathways* has four main elements: • Claimants are required to attend a series of mandatory Work Focused Interviews (WFIs). • Condition Management Programmes are a new and innovative NHS service to help people to manage their health condition (voluntary).

TABLE 6d: SOCIAL SECURITY AND POLICY

DWP-3 contd

- Existing services such as the New Deal for Disabled People (NDDP), Work-Based Learning for Adults (WBLA), Training for Work (TfW) and Programme Centres have been brought together into a coherent 'Choices package' that provides systematic work-focused support (voluntary).

- Participants can also be eligible for increased financial and other support which aims to encourage a move into paid employment (Return to Work Credit).

(For more detailed descriptions of these elements see Waddell & Aylward 2005 – see entry below).

Anon 2008

DWP Administrative data

Pathways to Work Performance Summary: March 2008

This summary is based on administrative data up to October 2007 and some more recent but provisional data. In total, there have been:

- 733,740 starts to *Pathways to Work*, for 564,570 individuals (i.e. some repeated).
- 289,740 mandatory initial WFIs and 276,270 mandatory repeat WFIs.
- 96,530 starts to Choices programmes, for 79,730 individuals, including: 50,610 NDDP starts, 36,220 Condition Management Programme Referrals and 9,700 other programme starts.
- 83,770 job entries for 64,240 individuals (to April 2007) and 75,760 RTWC awards for 49,950 individuals (to October 2007).

(Corden & Nice 2006)

Research report

Pathways to Work: Findings from the final cohort in a qualitative longitudinal panel of incapacity benefits recipients

Qualitative research showed evidence of satisfaction with what had been offered. There was general support for the principles of *Pathways*, but strong emphasis on the importance of the intervention coming at the right time and the support offered suiting the circumstances of individual people. Understanding the effects of a range of conditions and being able to tailor information giving, and timely and appropriate support requires considerable skill and training among Personal Advisers. The first Work Focused Interview was important in clarifying the purpose in meetings, establishing trust and rapport and reducing anxieties, and the adviser's personal approach was critical. Information about financial aspects was understood and remembered, and practical help with applications for in-work financial support was appreciated. There was limited use of services within the Choices package: those who did were already focused on working or who saw some possibility of working in the future. Despite considerable interest in the Condition Management Programme, few people went on to use it. In retrospect, the most important influence for many was their perception of their health. Few people felt that taking part in *Pathways* had made a major difference in their views about work or their behaviour in relation to work.

(Bailey et al. 2007)

Research report

Pathways to work: customer experience and outcomes

These results were based on interviews of 3,507 new or repeat clients in the first seven *Pathways to Work* pilot areas, an average of 14 months after taking part.

- Customers were generally positive about their experience of the Work Focused Interviews.
- 23% of participants took up one or more of the Choices package of services: most commonly NDDP job brokers (9%), or work-related training (8%).
- Only 4% took part in a Condition Management Programme.
- 35% of participants were in paid work around 14 months later and a further 20% were actively looking for work or waiting to start a job. However, 45% were not seeking work, and a majority of this group did not expect to look for work within the next year.

TABLE 6d: SOCIAL SECURITY AND POLICY

DWP-3 contd

(Bewley et al. 2007)

Research report

The impact of Pathways to Work

The evaluation compared changes in the outcomes among a sample of individuals in the pilot areas with corresponding changes in individuals in a set of similar looking comparison areas. The main results are based on the April 2004 pilot areas.

1. *Pathways* had no significant effect on the probability of individuals stating that they had a health condition or disability that limited their ability to carry out their everyday activities. (*Though that was based on a crude population questionnaire, not clinical data*).

2. *Pathways* significantly increased the probability of being employed after 18 months by 7.4 percentage points. This employment effect was quite stable over the latest six or so months observable.

3. The impact of *Pathways* on the probability of receipt of IB after 18 months was small and non-significant.

Findings 2 and 3 appear contradictory. Basically, it is because not working and receipt of Incapacity Benefit are not entirely congruent. Further analysis showed that *Pathways* increased the probability of working and not receiving incapacity benefits a year and a half after the enquiry by 8.7 percentage points. This was mostly accounted for by a decrease of 6.9 percentage points in the probability of not working and not receiving incapacity benefits. (*However, this whole analysis was extremely complex and difficult for a non-statistician to understand*).

4. *Pathways* appeared to have stronger employment effects on women than men, on those aged under 50, and on those with musculoskeletal conditions. It had no effect on those with mental health conditions.

A cost-benefit analysis of Pathways to Work for new and repeat incapacity benefits claimants

The financial benefits of *Pathways to Work* were estimated to significantly exceed the estimated financial costs, with net measured benefits both to *Pathways* participants and the Exchequer. The average net cost of *Pathways* for individuals who made an incapacity benefits enquiry was £340. *Pathways* increased the likelihood that these individuals would be in paid work 18 months later. If it was conservatively assumed that *Pathways'* effects continued for 70 weeks, the measured benefits were estimated to be £1,041 per person, with £526 of this amount accounted for by increases in the disposable incomes of the individuals and £515 accruing to the Exchequer. If, instead, it was more optimistically assumed that programme effects persist for 150 weeks, *Pathways'* benefits were estimated to total £2,023, with £935 accruing to individuals and £1,088 to the Exchequer. Despite the considerable uncertainty that surrounded these estimates, the authors concluded that *Pathways* had positive net measured benefits. This corresponded to a return to the Exchequer of £1.51 (£515/£340) for each pound invested in *Pathways* if programme effects lasted for 70 weeks or £3.20 (£1,088/£340) per pound invested if the effects of *Pathways to Work* effects lasted for 150 weeks.

(Adam et al. 2008)

Research report

TABLE 6d: SOCIAL SECURITY AND POLICY

DWP-3 contd	
(Waddell & Aylward 2005) Narrative review	**Future challenges to Pathways** 1. Evaluation of *Pathways* is ongoing. 2. *Pathways* is resource and staff intensive and requires a high level of staff skills and competencies, both for Personal Advisers and the Condition Management Programmes. This has implications for training and staffing of national roll-out. 3. There are still questions about the effectiveness and cost-effectiveness of the different elements of *Pathways*, the Condition Management Programmes and different service delivery models which require continuing research and evaluation. 4. There is mixed evidence about the impact of *Pathways* on claimants with mental health conditions, and limited evidence about the impact on claimants over age 50 and existing (long-term) clients. Further research is required to develop and evaluate effective interventions for these groups. 5. A large minority of claimants regard themselves as 'too ill to work' and/or are regarded by Personal Advisers as 'hard to help': Personal Advisers may waive WFIs for these reasons. (It is not clear if these are the same groups, or how far they overlap with 4.) 6. The success of *Pathways* will depend, to at least some extent, on the success of broader policies including IB Reform, the *Health, Work and Well-Being Strategy* and employment policy. Though, conversely, the demonstrable success of *Pathways* may contribute to these broader policies.
(GAO 2007) US Government report	**Vocational rehabilitation: report to congressional requesters** [US Government Accounting Office Report to Congressional Requesters] A study of the long-term outcomes for over 303,500 Social Security Administration beneficiaries (Disability Insurance and Supplemental Security Income) who participated in vocational rehabilitation (VR) in 1000-03. Approximately 40% increased their earnings in the year following VR compared to the year prior to VR services, while 32% did not have any earnings and another 28% had fewer earnings. More Supplemental Security Income beneficiaries (42%) than Disability Insurance beneficiaries (36%) increased their earnings. However, 88% had annual earnings below the threshold for 'substantial gainful employment' and remained on Social Security Administration disability benefits.
(Gründemann 1997) Summary Report	**Preventing absenteeism in the workplace: research summary** [European Foundation for the Improvement of Work and Living conditions] This is a summary report of a European project on 'Ill-health and workplace absenteeism: initiatives for prevention' which aimed to document and assess organizational, health, rehabilitation and other initiatives designed to improve workers' health and attendance at work. Recommended: • Higher priority and better statistics on absenteeism and its causes. • Governments, employers' organisations and unions together should establish national action programmes to address absenteeism and ill health. • Employers and employees require information about the possibilities (methodologies, tools and practical experiences) to reduce absenteeism related to ill health by preventive activities and reintegration of long term absentees. • Education and training on health, work and absenteeism for health professionals. • Support and encouragement for small and medium size enterprises to address work and health and absenteeism. (*Although described as a 'research summary' this paper did not present evidence on occupational outcomes, effectiveness or cost-effectiveness*).

TABLE 6d: SOCIAL SECURITY AND POLICY	
(Hasluck & Green 2007) Research report	**What works for whom?** [UK Department for Work and Pensions report] Overview of the effectiveness of DWP interventions to get all categories of beneficiaries off social security benefits. For disabled people and people with health problems, there is a need to distinguish between 'what works' at programme level and 'what works' for individuals: both should be taken into account. Across a number of programmes, individual beliefs, attitudes and intentions are important factors in determining 'what works'. Those most motivated to return to work are likely to be more successful (holding other factors constant). In contrast, financial incentives and other interventions have less impact on those who are not ready or willing to consider receiving help or support to overcome barriers and move towards work. There are issues concerning the type of work entered and the profile of employers recruiting disabled people and those with health conditions. Employers' perceptions and attitudes matter for the employment prospects of people with disabilities and health conditions. Disability is not static: there is a need for responsiveness and flexibility in meeting individual customer needs. For some people with disabilities, policy interventions alone might be insufficient in moving towards or entering work; rather, an underlying improvement in health may be the key change in moving towards work, while deterioration in health can make entry to work less likely or lead to a premature exit from the labour market, so trajectories of health and perceptions of health are crucial. *(New Deal for Disabled People and Pathways to work are summarised elsewhere in this Table. This report does not provide any quantitative evidence of effectiveness).*
(Hogelund 2001) Narrative review	**Work incapacity and reintegration** An overview of selected studies from the clinical, economic and public policy literature. In sum, clinical studies suggested that psychological variables may affect the likelihood of work resumption whereas socio-demographic, medical, job related and lifestyle factors seem to be of no, or only very limited, importance in the return to work of long-term incapacitated persons. However, non-clinical studies find socio-demographic variables (i.e. age) to be of importance. There is only modest evidence *(up to 1997)* that clinical interventions have any impact on the rate of return to work. The economic literature reviewed provided no clear evidence on whether vocational rehabilitation has a positive effect on work resumptions. The social policy literature showed that legal-formal characteristics of sickness benefit and disability benefit schemes and how they are administered influence how the schemes are used, which may in turn affect return to work. There was relatively clear evidence that benefit levels and some aspects of eligibility criteria have an effect. It seemed likely that financial and organisational conditions are very important, but their possible effects are difficult to measure. The sociological literature provided some evidence that labour market conditions and working conditions have a significant effect on the rate of return to work. Surprisingly, there was more uncertainty about whether unemployment conditions are of any importance. These various factors may interact and the combined effect on return to work may be greater than any one factor.

TABLE 6d: SOCIAL SECURITY AND POLICY

(HSA 2008)	**Workplace health and well-being strategy**
	[Irish Health and Safety Authority]
Policy Paper	The primary objective of the national Strategy for workplace health and wellbeing is to create a workplace culture and environment that will promote health and well being, prevent ill health and support the rehabilitation back to the workplace of those who are out of work through ill health or disability. This will be achieved through the implementation of a set of separate but complementary and pragmatic recommendations that will address the current issues and shortcomings in relation to health and wellbeing in Irish workplaces. The case for action is based on:
	• the ever increasing costs of ill health which impact at an individual, enterprise and societal level
	• the demographics of an aging workforce
	• sickness absence
	• the challenges of providing equal access to OH in SMEs
	Makes a large number of recommendations, the most important of which include:
	• Develop a service model to support SMEs
	• Research into early retirement and support to continue working beyond retirement age.
	• An awareness campaign for both employers and employees on the role and responsibilities of each in relation to workplace health.
	• Different government departments, agencies and non government organisations must work more in partnership on workplace health issues.
	• Ensure that all workers have access to competent occupational health advice.
	• Develop a model which links primary care to occupational health services.
	• Embark on a collaborative initiative with GPs which builds on the positive aspects of early return to work and the consequent need to modify the management and certification of sickness absence.
	• Develop better vocational rehabilitation and return to work infrastructure
	• Develop better information, reporting and analysis systems on workplace health
	(Recommendations on musculoskeletal conditions were mainly around manual handling, and on mental health conditions around stress and bullying. Further recommendations on noise and vibration, and on asthma, dermatitis, etc.)
	To implement this:
	1. a relevant Government Department should take overall leadership for the implementation of the Strategy;
	2. this lead Department should establish a National Implementation Group, consist of representatives of all the key stakeholders;
	3. a full-time National Coordinator should be appointed;
	4. a detailed Action Plan should be prepared that will set out in the form of detailed projects and programmes how the specific recommendations contained in the Strategy will be implemented.
	Concludes that 'The implementation of this Strategy will be challenging. However, the benefits at an individual and a national level are clear and achievable. What is required are the resources and structures and the combined efforts of all the key organisations to ensure that the challenge is successfully met and the benefts fully realised.'

TABLE 6d: SOCIAL SECURITY AND POLICY

(Kornfeld & Rupp 2000)	**The net effects of the Project NetWork return-to-work case management experiment on participant earnings, benefit receipt, and other outcomes**
Research report	[US Social Security Administration (SSA)] This randomised controlled trial started in 1991 in 8 demonstration sites, and tested a case management approach to promoting employment for people with disabilities. The intervention consisted of intensive outreach, work-incentive waivers and case management/referral services. Participation was voluntary, and 8248 applicants and recipients of SSA benefits took part – most of the sites easily reached their enrolment targets. Administrative data showed that Project Network produced a significant increase in net earnings over the first two years of \$200 or 11%. However, this declined to zero in the third year. There was no significant reduction in reliance on SSA benefits, Authors' conclusion: Project Network produced modest net benefits to people with disabilities and net costs to taxpayers. Combining case management services with other initiatives such as benefit changes or support into work could produce different results. These effects could also be sensitive to economic, labour market and local conditions.
(Leigh-Doyle & Mulvihill 2004)	**Illness and employment: retaining the link to work**
Policy paper	[European Foundation for the Improvement of Work and Living conditions] *(Policy paper, based on an EFILWC conference)* Retention and reintegration strategies: There is general agreement that, while there is a great potential for retaining in work people who develop a chronic illness, this is not generally realised. Job retention or reintegration is often impeded by a lack of coherence and coordination between systems, particularly social security and employment services. At the workplace level, different strategies must concentrate on prevention, retention and reintegration. People who experience severe mental health difficulties during their working life must be re-empowered and assisted to reintegrate. The three approaches – occupational health and safety, workplace health promotion, and rehabilitation/reintegration – should be developed and strengthened within companies. A more pro-active role is required, which may involve a modernised role for occupational health and safety, and its integration with human resources and other departments in companies. There is a lack of knowledge of what constitutes best practice, and empirical research is required to demonstrate the most effective measures. Social partner roles and responsibilities: The social partners are major actors in maintaining, retaining or reintegrating people with a chronic illness or disability in employment. Strategies for maintaining people at work must be multi-faceted but coordinated – involving the employer, social security systems, the individual concerned and his/her family. Employers, unions and work colleagues all have a role in ensuring a supportive work environment. Employers should address the integration and retention of people with an illness/disability in the workforce as part of their corporate social responsibility. They need to examine ways in which people can manage their chronic illness or disability by more flexible working arrangements, shorter working weeks and distance working. Cost benefit analysis of workplace interventions is necessary to further develop the case for investment in work place prevention, promotion and retention. Partnership approaches, together with integration, coordination and prevention strategies, can contribute to success but can be difficult to implement. Time, skills and resources are needed to ensure effective responses. Government roles and responsibilities: National systems of incentives and support are needed for both employers and employees to encourage workplace integration and retention of people with a disability and chronic illness. A complex range of parties and sectors may be involved: for example, social protection agencies, rehabilitation agencies, public transport and housing sectors. It is necessary to ensure that remaining at work is a profitable and attractive alternative to exiting the workforce, for both employers and employees. Raising awareness and training are required to better inform employers, HR and training professionals, trade union officials, politicians and other stakeholders and partners. NGOs and disability stakeholder groups can assist in raising awareness; in clarifying best practice; in identifying appropriate occupational areas/sectors; and in training. *(No evidence was presented on the effectiveness of these interventions).*

TABLE 6d: SOCIAL SECURITY AND POLICY

(Menz et al. 2003) Research report	**Outcomes of US community-based rehabilitation programmes** There are > 8,000 community-based rehabilitation provider organizations in the US delivering a variety of services that lead to, promote, and help sustain employment of people with disabilities. They provide various combinations of services including evaluation and assessment, counselling, benefits and case management, vocational and work skills training, job placement, transitional and gainful employment, independent skills training, supportive services, residential and housing, services to employers, and other supported services. This paper analyses a national sample of 64 organizations and 828 selected consumers to identify core practices that achieve employment outcomes. Factor analysis identified 10 primary processes that appeared to be applied consistently, though on a highly individual basis within each programme: • Individualized and in-community supports • Vocational planning and actions to achieve employment • Training to acquire and keep job: Soft and hard job skills training • Supports for community participation • Direct supports to ensure job retention • Job training and supports • Job acquisition or job search and placement • Case management and supports coordination • Supports to remain in workforce • Intake and orientation to services 79.6% of clients were satisfied with their programme. 83.6% were employed within 30 days of completing the programme, compared to 53.9% at programme entry. *(The authors claim that 'the evidence is in' on vocational rehabilitation, but this analysis does not actually provide any scientific evidence on the effectiveness of these programmes, because of the lack of any control group on what the outcomes would have been without the programmes).*
(OECD 2003) Report	**Transforming disability into ability: policies to promote work and income security for disabled people** [Organisation for Economic Co-operation and Development] Analysis of employment policies in 20 OECD countries suggested that different policy approaches seem to have similar effects. While legislative approaches to employment promotion differ in many respects (rights-based, obligations-based, incentives-based), all approaches tend to benefit people already in employment much more than those who are out of work and looking for a job. Although no country had a particularly successful policy for disabled people, observation of different countries' policies and outcomes suggested the following general principles: • Recognise the status of disability independent of the work and income situation. • Introduce a culture of mutual obligations. • Design individual work/benefit packages. • Introduce new obligations for disabled people. • Involve employers in the process.

TABLE 6d: SOCIAL SECURITY AND POLICY

- Promote early intervention.
- Make cash benefits a flexible policy element.
- Reform programme administration.
- Design disability programmes as active programmes.

A key part of the proposals was to promote early intervention. Outflow from disability benefits is very low in virtually all countries, despite considerable cross-country differences in regulations on reviewing entitlements, the availability of partial benefits, work incentives, etc. This partly reflects that regulations on reviewing benefit entitlements are not stringently applied and that there is a low take-up of work incentives. In many countries disability benefit systems have functioned as a quasi-permanent exit route from the labour market. Early intervention can in many cases be the most effective measure against long-term benefit dependence. As soon as a person becomes disabled, a process of tailored vocational intervention should be initiated, where appropriate including, *e.g.* job search, rehabilitation and/or further training. Where possible, such measures should be launched while the person is in an early stage of a disease or a chronic health problem. Preventive measures at the workplace could even be de-linked from being temporarily out of work. *(It is unclear how these general principles would translate into practice in a social security context. practice. Social security systems generally only become aware of a disabled person when they apply for benefits, and in the case of Incapacity Benefit they will generally already be off work for at least 28 weeks. Unlike disability benefits in many countries, the outflow from IB in the first year is actually about 40%. It is only once a recipient has been on IB for 1-2 years that outflow falls to very low levels. 'Early' in the context of IB may therefore be as soon as possible after starting benefits or within 1-2 years or so of last working. Germany, Sweden and Norway were given as examples of early 'in-work' rehabilitation, but no evidence was presented of the effectiveness of these schemes).*

(Leech 2004)

Social security intervention

Preventing chronic disability from low back pain

(Irish Department of Social and Family Affairs)

A study in a social security setting that aimed to determine if early intervention, using international evidence-based guidelines in the assessment of claimants with back pain, would decrease the incidence of progression to chronic disability. Medical assessors were trained in evidence-based practice and the project was promoted at the professional level and patient information was made available. Results of the programme were compared with historical data.

- As expected 52% returned to work within 4 weeks of their own volition
- Approximately 1600 claimants selected to attend for medical assessment at 4 to 6 weeks from date of claim (much earlier than previously)
- On receipt of the invitation, 63% came off benefits and returned to work
- The remainder were duly assessed:
  - o 64% of LBP cases declared fit for work compared with ~20% previously
  - o There were fewer appeals and fewer successful appeals
  - o There was reduced duration of claim and reduced benefit costs

The report concluded that this early intervention in the acute stage should result not only in the improved health of back pain patients, but also in decreased health care costs, reduced absenteeism, increased production, and significant savings in long-term illness benefit schemes. *(But, these data were not collected during the 6-month project).*

TABLE 6d: SOCIAL SECURITY AND POLICY

(Scottish Executive 2004) Policy paper	**Healthy working lives: a plan for action** Defines a healthy working life as: 'one that continuously provides working age people with the opportunity, ability, support and encouragement to work in ways and in an environment which allows them to sustain and improve their health and wellbeing. It means that individuals are empowered and enabled to do as much as possible, for as long as possible, or as long as they want, in both their working and non-working lives.' Sets out a vision for the contribution that the workplace can make to health improvement and reducing health inequalities. The aim is to provide support and opportunities for individuals to maximise their functional capacity throughout their working lives. This begins with support for the development of basic skills for those who find themselves at some distance from the workplace, services to address physical or mental health conditions and advice on vocational, education or training issues. Whilst in work, it requires support to engender and facilitate a commitment to lifelong learning, ensure that people work in safe, supportive environments, maintain awareness of the importance of healthy lifestyles and provide access to a range of rehabilitation services should physical or mental health issues compromise workability. This requires a comprehensive policy approach to the promotion and management of occupational health and safety within Scottish workplaces. There are a large number of initiatives that contribute to the aim, but they need a shared vision and much closer collaboration to achieve the desired outcomes. Although the National Health Service has an important role to play it cannot work alone, but must work in partnership with other stakeholders. To support individuals to maximize their functional capacity, the long-term vision is of an easy to access network of support services within Scotland which brings together health services providing fast-track rehabilitation through specialties such as physiotherapy, occupational and sports therapy with the support services traditionally associated with the broader employability agenda such as advice on education, training, supported employment, career management and the benefits system. This also requires the commitment of Scottish employers. Small and medium sized enterprises need better support services. (*A key underlying theme throughout this document was the need for 'all players onside*).
(Macdonald & Docherty 2007) Narrative review	**Healthy working lives: the Scottish strategy for improving health in the workplace** Reviews history of publicly funded programmes which provide advice to Scottish workers and employers: • Scotland Health at Work Scheme (SHAW) was founded in 1996 and encourages employers to engage in workplace health promotions schemes and meet bronze, silver and gold standards. • NHS Scotland has 150,000 workers and has developed a comprehensive occupational service over the past 20 years. Some aspects of this have been used to provide contract services to industry and public-sector organisations. This has gradually been extended to provide a free advisory service to small and medium enterprises throughout Scotland since 2003, including a free telephone advisory service, workplace visits, a confidential health and safety risk assessment, a workplace health promotion needs assessment and a report and proposed action plan with follow-up advice. These and other services are now being brought together in the Scottish Centre for Healthy Working Lives, based within and funded by NHS Scotland. Client groups include employers, employees and individuals wishing to return to or start work. Much work remains to be done to create the necessary infrastructure and to bring together the various existing agencies, including those involved in rehabilitation and employability

TABLE 6d: SOCIAL SECURITY AND POLICY

(Thornton et al. 2003) Policy paper	**What works and looking ahead: a comparative study of UK and US policies and practices facilitating return to work for people with disabilities** *(Discussion paper prepared for UK/US Pathways to Work in the 21st Century Seminar and Workshop 1-2 May 2003 Washington D.C., USA).* The UK and the US are both striving to find solutions that will make an impact on the employment rates of disabled people. Incentives to leave benefits and take up benefit include: easy return to benefit, retaining benefits for trial work periods, supplementing earnings, and increasing awareness and take up of incentives and benefits planning. Individualised employment services include early intervention, increasing the employment expertise of benefits advisers, and employment network, and community based employment networks. Both US and UK had turned attention to intervention at the point of applying for benefits, but only very preliminary results were available. There was no overview of community based rehabilitation providers in UK, and limited evidence on their effectiveness in US. The authors concluded that neither the US nor the UK has yet found interventions that make a substantial impact and that the potential lessons learnt are only partial solutions.
(Waddell et al. 2002) Monograph	**Back pain, incapacity for work and social security benefits: an international literature review and analysis** *(Although the major focus of this monograph was LBP, the sections on rehabilitation and social security benefits reviewed generic evidence and were not specific to LBP).* In Sweden, Norway, the Netherlands and Victoria, Australia, employers have a statutory obligation to follow up absent workers and to develop a rehabilitation and return to work plan (though the timing varies between 3 weeks and 3 months sickness absence). There is little evidence on the effectiveness of such legislation or plans. Rehabilitation services include a wide range of personal support services to prevent sickness developing into disability, help recover working capacity and support re-adjustment to work. This may include a range of public services, but these are often very fragmented and uncoordinated. In most countries, the main rehabilitation services for workers who are injured or become sick are part of the social insurance system (e.g. Sweden, The Netherlands and Germany) or the workers or accident compensation system (e.g. US, Canada, Australia and New Zealand). Sweden, Germany, France and Canada all have arrangements in at least some circumstances to pay additional benefits during rehabilitation. Virtually all social security pilot studies of individual-level interventions (in UK, US and elsewhere) to help recipients of sickness or disability benefits back into work have major problems with uptake (often <5%), low-moderate rates of sustained return to work, minimal impact on benefit trends, and doubtful cost-effectiveness. Review of social security trends in individual countries provided extensive evidence that disability and incapacity benefit systems have a powerful impact on sickness absence rates and benefit claim rates in each country and over time. The balance of the evidence suggests that the structure of the social security system and the availability and ease or difficulty of getting sickness and disability benefits (i.e. the control mechanisms: eligibility criteria, the definition and assessment of incapacity, and the claims, adjudication and appeals procedures) have more impact than the financial level of the benefits on the number of claims and the duration of benefits paid.

TABLE 6d: SOCIAL SECURITY AND POLICY

(Wynne & McAnaney 2004) Policy paper	**Employment and disability: back to work strategies** [European Foundation for the Improvement of Work and Living conditions] How people with chronic illnesses become excluded from the workplace is complex. This report gathered information on relevant initiatives in 7 European countries. It proposes a new model for understanding the nature of the problem; develops an assessment tool for new initiatives in the area; and makes recommendations on how best to promote social inclusion for people with chronic illnesses. At a national level, each system examined revealed gaps and discontinuities. Social protection, rehabilitation and return to work systems were not originally designed to deal with chronic illness, nor to work in an integrated manner. They consist of layers of regulations added to a basic framework and rarely cater adequately for people with chronic illness. People who develop chronic illness for reasons other than work tend to fall between the systems. Occupational systems are of limited relevance, general health systems do not usually aim for return to work, disability systems are inaccessible due to eligibility restrictions, and social protection systems are often passive. Reintegration is not always seen as a relevant goal. Social exclusion then becomes a real possibility. The authors concluded that European policy recommendations and initiatives do not address illness and exclusion in a coordinated approach. On the contrary, a departmentalised approach to policy formulation and implementation, which focuses on traditional responses within each area, is a serious barrier to integrating key policy areas such as occupational health and safety, public health, active ageing, disability, equality, employment, social inclusion and social protection. Recommendations for policymakers: These recommendations are at the intersection of social inclusion, employment, health, disability, active ageing and social protection. It is unlikely that chronic illness and work disability can be adequately covered by addressing them in any one policy strand. Integrated and coordinated policy initiatives must acknowledge the contributions each area can make to an effective solution. Specific recommendations to policy-makers included: • Raise awareness of the issue. • Introduce more proactive policies. • Streamline policy towards return to work and reintegration. • Remove barriers to services/compensation which depend on employment or disability status. • Change expectation norms from welfare to work. • Introduce bonus-malus elements to return to work. • Specify stakeholders' roles and responsibilities in the return to work process. • Strengthen links between workplace, absent employees and service suppliers. • Improve data collection and analysis of chronic illness and leaving employment. *(There was no evidence-linking and no evidence provided on effectiveness or cost-effectiveness).*

TABLE 6d: SOCIAL SECURITY AND POLICY

(Wynne et al. 2006)	**Employment guidance services for people with disabilities**
Policy paper	[European Foundation for the Improvement of Work and Living conditions]
	Employment guidance and counselling services for people with disabilities provide the mechanism whereby people with disabilities may return to work. This paper provided an overview of such services in the Member States of the European Union, and identified 20 examples of good practice in Ireland, UK, Germany, Finland, Slovakia, Greece, Italy, Portugal, Poland and Estonia. There was a wide diversity of approach among the Member States regarding the design and the services. While there was much common ground on 15 elements of the services (with most countries having all or most of these service elements), there were great differences between countries Member States with regard to their accessibility and their ratings of effectiveness of many of the elements and the services overall. The most effective elements were not necessarily the most widely available. None of the provided all of the elements defined in the framework of good practice. Overall, the analysis suggests that while countries share a more or less common approach in terms of the types of employment guidance and counselling services offered, they differ considerably in the design and coordination of these services. The review did not find many initiatives specifically targeting people with disabilities who had worked previously, which would seem to indicate that this group does not have a high priority in many countries. *(No quantitative evidence on effectiveness).*

[IB = Incapacity Benefit; SME = small and medium enterprise; VR = vocational rehabilitation]

TABLE 7: REVIEWS AND REPORTS ON TIMING AND COORDINATION

Table 7a: Timing

TABLE 7a: TIMING	
Authors	**Key features** *(Reviewers' comments in italic)*
(Allen et al. 2007) Conceptual review	**Early intervention for depressive disorders in young people: the opportunity and the (lack of) evidence** *(Although focused on adolescents and young people, the reasoning and conclusions appear equally relevant to adults of working age).* Patients experiencing their first onset of depression are at risk of relapse and recurrence, so should be targets for early intervention and prevention efforts. Despite the argument for a significant research effort addressing these issues, the evidence regarding optimal intervention strategies for first episodes is lacking. Cognitive behaviour therapy is an effective approach to treatment and relapse prevention, and is likely to be an important component of any evidenced-based approach to early intervention. The role of medication requires further evaluation. Given the high prevalence of depressive disorders, and the significant burden of disease in our communities, early intervention in depressive disorders is a critical research agenda for the future.
(Burkhauser et al. 2001) National study	**How policy variables influence the timing of applications for Social Security Disability Insurance** *(Analysis of US Health and Retirement Study).* Analysed the impact of policy variables and employer accommodations on the timing of an application for DI benefits by workers with a work-limiting health condition. Most workers do not apply when they first develop a health condition. 16% of men and 13% of women applied within 1 year. The median working-age man with a work-limiting condition waited 7 years before applying, and the median working age woman waited 8 years. Men and women who were provided with accommodations by their employers were significantly less likely to apply for benefits in each of the first few years after their condition began to bother them than were those who were not accommodated.
(Campbell et al. 2007) Report	**Avoiding long-term incapacity for work: developing an early intervention in primary care** [Report commissioned by the UK Health Work and Wellbeing Executive on behalf of The Department for Work and Pensions] This report is described as a brief scoping study on how a pilot, concentrating on a primary care-led intervention in health and work, might look, and how it could be evaluated with the greatest value to policy makers in government and the NHS. It was based on a review of relevant scientific literature and the results of a stakeholder consultation held with general practitioners. The authors recommend that rehabilitation interventions should be offered as soon as possible for patients who have been off work for four weeks or more. The recommendations for mental health problems reflect previous work (Michie & Williams 2003; Seymour & Grove 2005), but do not make any recommendations on timing. The authors considered there was insufficient evidence on occupational outcomes in cardio-respiratory conditions to make any recommendations. The stakeholder panel considered that an intervention to facilitate early return to work was appropriate for the following groups of patients: • for a wider range of clinical indications in patients with musculoskeletal conditions as compared to mental health or cardio-vascular conditions; • those with mild/ moderate symptoms rather than those with severe symptoms; • those with symptoms lasting one month or longer;

TABLE 7a: TIMING	
	• those not already receiving/ awaiting specialist health care or interventions for their medical condition; • those on repeat, recurrent or extended sickness certification rather than those on their first sickness certification; • those without access to an occupational health service; • those who have been on sickness certification for 7 weeks or longer or those certified for 4-6 weeks if they do not have access to an occupational health service. The authors conclusions and recommendations included: 1. There is support, both in the research literature and from the general practitioner panel, for an early intervention to help sick-certified individuals to return to work. 2. Referrals are potentially best made by 7 weeks of certified sickness absence, but not prior to 4 weeks. 3. Any service model should facilitate timely access to relevant multi-professional input based on the individual's needs.
(DH 2004) Guidance note	**Improving chronic disease management** A key element of service delivery is a stepped care approach (though this term is not used): Level 1 'self-management' With the right support 70-80% of people can learn to be active participants in their own care, living with and managing their conditions. This can help them to prevent complications, slow down deterioration, and avoid getting further conditions. The majority of people with chronic conditions fall into this category – so even small improvements can have a huge impact. Level 2 'Disease/care management' For high risk patients, in which multidisciplinary teams provide high quality evidence based care to patients, is appropriate for the majority of people at this level. This means proactive management of care, following agreed protocols and pathways for managing specific diseases. It is underpinned by good information systems – patient registries, care planning, shared electronic health records. Level 3 'Case management' For patients with highly complex conditions or co-morbidities, whose care becomes disproportionately more complex and difficult for them, or the health and social care system, to manage. This calls for case management – with a key worker (often a nurse) actively managing and joining up care for these people. There is evidence that good chronic disease management can improve medication control, reduce health care consumption (especially hospitalisation) and costs, and improve patient and physician satisfaction. (See also Table 6c).
(Fordyce 1995) Policy paper	**Back pain in the workplace: management of disability in nonspecific conditions** [International Association for the Study of Pain] *(This report from a task force of the IASP attempted to apply emerging clinical guidelines on the clinical management of LBP to workers compensation policy with the aim of preventing unnecessary long-term disability). The fundamental proposal was that non-specific LBP causing prolonged sickness absence from work should be re-conceptualised as a problem of activity intolerance, not a medical problem. Recommended that medical benefits (in a US workers compensation system) should be provided unconditionally for the first two weeks, but thereafter should be contingent on a treatment plan that directly addressed activity intolerance by re-activation and that established contact with the employer to develop a RTW plan. Workers who had not RTW by 6 weeks should be referred for comprehensive, multidisciplinary evaluation, incorporating medical, psychological and vocational assessment, and leading to multi-disciplinary, biopsychosocial rehabilitation or retraining. Workers who still did not RTW should be reclassified as unemployed and disability benefits stopped. (See Waddell 2004 (Table 2b) for an analysis of the problems to these policy recommendations and for a history of the only attempt to implement the benefits proposals in the Workers Compensation Board of Nova Scotia – which led to legislative and legal challenges, ultimately causing their abandonment).*

TABLE 7a: TIMING

(Franche & Krause 2002) Narrative review	**Readiness for return to work following injury or illness: conceptualizing the interpersonal impact of health care, workplace, and insurance factors** Return to work after injury or illness is a behaviour influenced by physical, psychological, and social factors. A new Readiness for Return-to-Work Model is proposed focusing on the interpersonal context of the work-disabled employee. Employee interactions with the workplace, the health care, and insurance systems are considered as they impact the three defining dimensions of change—decisional balance, self-efficacy, and change processes. The Readiness for Return-to-Work Model has the potential to account for individual variation in optimal stage-specific timing of interventions based on an individual's readiness for return-to-work. The model therefore complements the Phase Model of Disability by allowing for an individual-level staging of the disability and recovery process within the broader group-level-derived framework of occupational disability phases. This link between the two models needs to be empirically tested in future research. *(Focus on mechanisms rather than effectiveness).*
(Frank et al. 1996) Narrative review	**Disability resulting from occupational low back pain. Part II: what do we know about secondary prevention? – a review of the scientific evidence on prevention after disability begins** A review of the natural history of LBP, the causes of disability and effectiveness of interventions for the secondary prevention of long-term disability. Current clinical guidelines are based on extensive scientific evidence but there is little evidence that the guidelines are implemented or effective. The authors conclude that there is significant scope for better treatment, rehabilitation and earlier accommodation at work to reduce more lengthy and costly disability. There may be an element of, at best, lost opportunity – and, at worst, mismanagement or iatrogenic (medically caused) disability in the development of some chronic cases. Acute: onset of symptoms – 3-4 weeks. At this stage there is ample evidence that the prognosis for most patients with non-specific LBP is so good, even without health care, that strong reassurance and only minimal investigation and treatment, is all that is warranted. Over-investigation and over-treatment ('medicalisation') can increase illness behaviour and disability, partly through deconditioning through excessive rest and partly through 'attention' and 'labelling' effects. Sub-acute: 3-4 weeks to about 12 weeks. Those who are still off work at this stage, because of their *(bio-psycho-social)* condition, are at such an elevated risk of much longer-term disability that much more aggressive measures are warranted and can be cost-effective. Chronic: more than 3 months. Most authorities consider an early pain syndrome has set in, with behavioural, psychosocial and perhaps also biological vicious circle feedback loops that make treatment much more difficult and successful outcomes more elusive. Research has consistently shown an unexplained variation in medical care and an unwarranted amount of inappropriate treatment. Successful implementation of evidence-based guidelines is a substantial challenge. Thee is also still *(in 1996)* a lack of evidence that implementing guidelines improves patient outcomes.
(Frank et al. 1998) Narrative review	**Preventing disability from work-related low back pain: new evidence gives new hope – if we can just get all the players onside** Management in the first 3-4 weeks should be conservative according to current clinical guidelines. Interventions at the sub-acute stage (between 3-4 and about 12 weeks) should focus on return to work and can reduce time lost from work by 30-50%. There is substantial evidence that appropriately modified work can reduce the duration of work loss by at least 30%. A combination of these approaches in a coordinated, guidelines-based and workplace-linked care system can reduce sickness absence due to LBP by 50% at no extra cost and, in some settings, with significant savings. *(See also Table 7b).* *(Although these reviews focus on duration of symptoms, they do not consider the practical problems around 'onset', perhaps because they are written in a North American workers compensation context. In fact, the discussion and conclusions apply better to duration of sickness absence from work).*

TABLE 7a: TIMING

(Freud 2007) UK Policy paper	**Reducing dependency, increasing opportunity: options for the future of welfare to work** The decision on when to provide individuals with more intensive support designed for the hard to help is complex. There is much evidence that early intervention for those furthest from the market is effective. However, early intervention multiplies the risk that support is targeted at people who would anyway have found employment ('deadweight'). It would be ideal to have a system that reduces this risk, through a thorough assessment of the likelihood, and costs, of finding particular individuals work, but the track record of such screening tools has been mixed. The most reliable proxy for identifying those who need extra help is the length of time they have been out of work. Until better screening is available, this review recommends that support should be directed primarily on the basis of duration off work. For most unemployed Jobseekers, the review concluded that more intensive support should be provided at 12 months. However, for Incapacity Benefit claimants, the review considered there may be an argument for people for more early provision of more intensive support – perhaps at the six month stage, or even at the 13 week stage. (*This argument is not elaborated*).
(Harris et al. 2001) Narrative review	**Returning to work: an examination of existing disability duration guidelines and their applicability to the Texas Workers' Compensation system** Noted that medically speaking, continuous or prolonged absences from work may be detrimental to physical, mental, and social well-being. Proactive efforts to return workers to productive employment quickly and safely help minimise future absences and the medical and financial impacts. The promotion of early RTW can be achieved by: • Encouraging better communication between employers and health care providers regarding the worker's ability to return to work • Education of employers to encourage proactive RTW programmes • Adopting RTW guidelines incorporating recommended durations of disability for specific conditions Reviewed three existing duration guidelines (Official Disability Guidelines; Medical Disability Advisor; Milliman & Roberston) plus those provided by the American College of Occupational and Environmental Medicine (ACOEM), and compared these with actual data from the Texas workers' compensation system. They noted a small percentage of claimants who continued to remain off work beyond the expected duration, and this indicates the need for targeted early intervention. The reviewers noted that RTW guidelines serve three important purposes: • Provide a comparison to the course of recovery that would exist in absence of treatment – that is, the natural recovery of untreated or unmanaged health problems • Provide recommended timeframes for safe RTW at various activity levels for health care providers, employers and insurance carriers • Provide recommended changes in physical activities to ensure aggravation, exacerbation or re-injury does not take place if the worker returns to work
(Joling et al. 2006) National study	**Duration dependence in sickness absence: how can we optimize disability management intervention strategies?** [Population study analysing data from a major longitudinal survey on work incapacity and return to work in The Netherlands.] The analysis found evidence for the presence of variable-duration dependence. Duration dependence means that the duration of time off work influences the return to work process. Duration dependence also affects the (positive or negative) effects of intervention, which means that the timing of interventions is critical. Authors conclusions: the findings imply that RTW intervention strategies should vary according to differences in workers' susceptibility to positive or negative duration-dependence effects.

TABLE 7a: TIMING

(Krause & Ragland 1994)

Narrative review

Occupational disability due to low back pain: a new interdisciplinary classification based on a phase model of disability

Understanding and preventing occupational disability due to LBP *(though the analysis applies equally to other conditions)* requires an inter-disciplinary approach. Purely biomedical classifications and approaches which assume the condition is 'fixed' are insufficient. An alternative classification was proposed in which the disabling process was organised in 8 consecutive phases based primarily on the presence and duration of work disability:

Phase 1: non-disabling episodes of low back pain

Phase 2: report of an injury or sickness (i.e. incapacity for work)

Phase 3: short-term disability (<1 week) – by the end of this phase medical certification is usually required

Phase 4: timely intervention (1-7 weeks) – medical and early intervention programmes are designed primarily for this phase

Phase 5: long-term disability (>7 – 12 weeks) – clinically 'chronic'; requires specialist or multidisciplinary rehabilitation focused on preventing

Phase 6: late rehabilitation (3-6 months) – <10% of cases; medical treatment designed for 'acute' phase no longer appropriate;

Phase 7: chronic disability (>6 – 18 months) – no longer primarily a biomedical problem; treatment directed to the medical condition alone is inappropriate; interventions should focus on the pain experience and occupational factors.

Phase 8: permanent disability (>18 months) – unemployment, job change, early retirement (though this may occur earlier)

Risk factors and interventions are specific to the phase. *(The timing of these phases appears to be related to the US workers compensation system and arbitrary).*

(Krause et al. 2001)

Selective literature review

Determinants of duration of disability and return to work after work-related injury and illness: challenges for future research

A literature review identified about 100 different determinants of RTW outcomes, including individual level, characteristics of the injury or illness, job level task and organisational characteristics. Different interventions were found to effect work disability at different phases.

Acute: back education +/- exercise, medical case management, physician–patient communication about job, physician recommendation of RTW.

Sub-acute: early activation programme, medical case management, physician– patient communication about job, physician recommendation of RTW.

Chronic: multimodal functional restoration, vocational rehabilitation programme; supported employment.

(Merry 2007)

Conceptual review

Prevention and early intervention for depression in young people – a practical possibility?

(Conceptual review based on a Cochrane review: although focused on adolescents, the reasoning and conclusions appear equally relevant to adults of working age). There is currently little evidence that primary prevention of depression is a practical possibility, and no clear evidence of effectiveness for universal programmes. There is more evidence to support targeted than universal interventions, with more evidence for short-term than long-term effects. There is evidence to support screening for depression and providing early intervention, but current treatments have limited effectiveness. There is a compelling need for further research in this area.

TABLE 7a: TIMING

(Mondloch et al. 2001) Systematic review	**Does how you do depend on how you think you'll do? - a systematic review of the evidence for a relation between patients' recovery expectations and health outcomes** Sixteen studies reviewed. They each showed that a patient's expectations influence their recovery. Six studies found that patients' beliefs and expectations have a large influence on how well they recover. Five studies found that patients' beliefs and expectations have a moderate effect Four studies showed that patients' beliefs and expectations have no effect. The different studies showed that a patient's expectations have an influence on a broad range of conditions including low-back pain, obesity, heart disease, alcoholism, benign prostate tumours and psychiatric conditions. They also showed that expectations influence recovery after surgery and psychological adjustment after abortion. The effect of patients' expectations on their recovery tended to be smaller in patients with psychiatric conditions than in other conditions. Expectations were found to influence the recovery of all patients, regardless of differences in things like the severity of their condition, their social position or their mental and physical health.
(OECD 2003) Policy paper	**Transforming disability into ability: policies to promote work and income security for disabled people** [Organisation for Economic Co-operation and Development] One of the key proposals of this report is early intervention: The most effective measure against long-term benefit dependence appears to be a strong focus on early intervention - as soon as a person becomes disabled. In theory, this may be immediately after a specific disabling event or, more commonly, at an early stage of a disease or a chronic health problem. *(In practice, this is likely to mean once it is medically recognized that the individual has some permanent impairment, or that their condition is 'chronic' and that they are unlikely to return to work in the near future. In a social security and policy context, particularly in UK, it is likely to mean once they are on benefits, by which time they may have been off work for 26 weeks).* At an early stage, a process of tailored intervention should be initiated. Health care, medical rehabilitation and vocational rehabilitation should run concurrently, where appropriate including, e.g. job search, rehabilitation and/or further training. Early 'in-work' intervention is most common in Germany and Sweden, where rehabilitation schemes are explicitly designed to kick in early. Norwegian active sick leave, to give another example, is designed to prevent long-term disability by combining sickness absence with either of two types of intervention: adjustment of tasks at the regular workplace, or vocational rehabilitation. Several countries (Denmark, France, Portugal, Sweden and Switzerland) have introduced a specific benefit that is paid during the rehabilitation period. In many countries, in contrast, the period of sickness absence is 'lost', because vocational intervention, if any, starts only when a person is potentially entitled to or paid a disability benefit. This means that, in some cases, the affected person will remain inactive for up to a year without any disability-related services. If a participation plan were started immediately, be it under the responsibility of the employer, like in the Netherlands and Sweden, or under the responsibility of the disability benefit or rehabilitation authority, the chances of re-integration would increase. *(Provides a strong rational argument and different countries' experience to support early intervention, but no actual evidence of the effectiveness of these policies). (See also Table 7b).*
(Pilgrim & Bentall 1999) Narrative review	**The medicalisation of misery: a critical realist analysis of the concept of depression** This paper explores some difficulties with the concept of depression First, it describe the variable, and sometimes incommensurable, ways in which the diagnosis of depression has been defined and discussed in professional mental health texts, and the resulting difficulty in drawing a line between depression and other psychological states. Secondly, it examines this confusion in relation to historical and cross-cultural work on emotions and distress. Thirdly, it considers two studies from social science which reveal the limitations of conventional *(medical)* approaches to depression. It concludes that medicalisation of mental problems as 'depression' is not always the best way of understanding and dealing with these problems.

TABLE 7a: TIMING

(Prezzia & Denniston 2001) Narrative review	**The use of evidence-based duration guidelines** Early disability duration guidelines were based on expert opinion and experience, but they are now increasingly evidence-based on actual experience datasets. Duration guidelines are used prospectively by claims professionals or case managers when managing the details of a case. Duration guidelines can be incorporated into claims management software and used to triage cases. The expected duration of disability can be compared to the guidelines and additional management resources applied to those cases that exceed or seem likely to exceed the guideline. For guidelines to have maximum effectiveness, they need to be accepted by all parties as defensible, fair, and evidence-based. Disability guidelines can help reinforce one of the most important determinants in return to work — good communication among all parties (workers, health professionals, employers and insurers). The use of duration guidelines has been shown to benefit insurers, employers and workers themselves *(though no evidence is presented to support this).*
(Rose 2007) Narrative review	**Beyond medicalisation** The term 'medicalisation' is used when a problem is created or annexed, in whole or in part, by the apparatus of medicine – with implications about the extension of medical authority beyond a legitimate boundary, and of the process being harmful. Medicalisation implies passivity on the part of the medicalised. Medicine is inextricably intertwined with the ways in which we experience and give meaning to our world. Medicine also makes us what we are through the role of medical expertise in influencing the ways we conduct our lives. Medicine has shaped our ethical regimes, our relations with ourselves, our judgments of the kinds of people we want to be, and the lives we want to lead. Medicalisation occurs not only at the individual level but also in public health and policy. This is not necessarily a bad thing. The term medicalisation might be better seen as the starting point for analysis of a problem, or a sign of the need for analysis, rather than the conclusion of an analysis.
(Stephens & Gross 2007) Research report	**The influence of a continuum of care model on the rehabilitation of compensation claimants with soft tissue disorders** *(Alberta Workers' Compensation Board study).* Rehabilitation services for workers who sustained soft tissue injuries at work in Alberta was designed to provide appropriate and timely health care in an effort to facilitate early, sustained return to work. The model was based on expected recovery times and involved three main components: 1) staged application of different types of clinical and rehabilitation services depending on the progress of recovery; 2) case management protocols and checkpoints integrated into case planning; and 3) contracted services with 4 types of rehabilitation service providers (physical therapy, chiropractors, multidisciplinary assessment centres, and multidisciplinary rehabilitation providers). Services options consisted of: 0-18 weeks: medical management 0-6 weeks: chiropractic treatment 1-4 weeks: physical therapy (mobilisation and activation) 4-6 weeks: physical therapy (work conditioning) 8-10 weeks*: multi-disciplinary assessment 10-18 weeks*: multi-disciplinary rehabilitation *(or earlier if appropriate) Data were from the WCB-Alberta administrative database from 2 years before implementation (1994 –1995) to 5 years after (1996 –2000). The intervention group was 70,116 workers filing soft tissue injury claims for the low back, ankle, knee, elbow, and shoulder. The comparison group was 101,620 workers filing claims for fractures or other traumatic non-soft tissue injuries. The median duration of wage-replacement benefits in the intervention group decreased from 13 to 8 days after introduction of the model (adjusted hazard ratio 1.54 95% CI 1.50-1.58 highly significant). The control group's median duration of benefits remained unchanged at 10 days The majority of claimants were satisfied with care received. Cost savings over a 2-year full implementation period was \$21.5 million (Canadian). *(This is a single study but included as a large-scale example of stepped care and organisation of rehabilitation services).*

TABLE 7a: TIMING

(Stucki et al. 2005) Narrative review	**Rationale and principles of early rehabilitation care after an acute injury or illness** Argues for the basic principle that early identification of rehabilitation needs and early rehabilitation care provision to minimize functioning loss and prevent disability. Patients hospitalized for acute illness or injuries are at risk of significant loss of functioning. The goal of early identification of rehabilitation needs and an early start to rehabilitation are to maintain functioning or to minimize loss of functioning and to optimize recovery and return to normal function. The ultimate goal is to prevent disability. This can reduce length of hospital stay, health care costs and the need for long-term support. The maintenance or early restoration of functioning is of particular importance in patients at high risk: critically ill patients, those with complications or long-term intensive care stays, people with disabilities or with pre-existing chronic conditions and the elderly. Two principles of rehabilitation for acute and early post-acute care can be distinguished. First, the provision of rehabilitation by health professionals in the acute hospital who are generally not specialized in rehabilitation. This is generally an integral part of nursing care and, where appropriate, some patients will require physiotherapy. Second, specialized rehabilitation care provided by an interdisciplinary team. There is large variation in how this specialized, typically post-acute rehabilitation care is organized, provided, and reimbursed. Most in-patients do not receive specialized rehabilitation at all during their stay in the acute hospital. But it is important to point out that health professionals working in acute hospitals and who are not specialized in rehabilitation need to be able to recognize patients' needs for rehabilitation care and to perform rehabilitation interventions themselves or to assign patients to appropriate rehabilitation care settings. (*This review focused on acute in-patient hospital care, but some of the principles are relevant to all health care*).

(Von Korff 1999)
 	
(Von Korff &
Moore 2001)
 	
(Balderson & Von Korff 2002)
 	
Narrative reviews
	Pain management in primary care: an individualized stepped-care approach
	
	Stepped care for back pain: activating approaches for primary care
	
	The stepped care approach to chronic back pain
	Cost-effective organisation of health care depends on a well-organised and effective primary health care service. In management of a recurrent or chronic condition, collaboration between patient and health care provider(s) and an element of self-management are important. Management in primary care faces three challenges: 1) limited consultation time at any one contact; 2) patients vary widely in severity and chronicity; 3) prognosis of subsequent progress is difficult. These challenges can be addressed by a stepped-care approach, which provides a framework for allocating finite resources to the greatest effect on a population basis, while individualising care. This approach has been used for a wide variety of medical and behavioural conditions. Care needs to be personalised to each patient's specific concerns, activity limitations, preferences and readiness, and the level of care is guided by the severity and duration of activity limitation.
	
	Step 1: relevant for most back pain patients – addresses fear-avoidance beliefs and encourages resumption of normal activities via education and reassurance:
	
	   Identify and address specific patient worries
	
	   Identify and support the patient's motivation for self-care
	
	Step 2: for moderately limited back pain patients – targets the substantial minority of patients who require more than simple advice to resume activities. Directly addresses common activity limitations, provides brief, structured interventions that support exercise and return to normal activities via education, reassurance and gradual return to normal activities (including work) guided by goal setting, problem solving and exercise.

TABLE 7a: TIMING

Support management of common activity limitations

- identify difficulties and goals
- support planning to overcome difficulties and to achieve goals
- support the patient's motivation for exercise

Referral to a low-cost self-care programme is a desirable option

Step 3: reserved for the small but important group of severely limited back pain patients – targets patients who require more intensive interventions. These efforts are reserved for the small but important group with work disability, for whom treatment efforts focus on work performance and return to work, including identifying and treating mental health difficulties such as depression, before they can return to normal activities and work.

Address work performance issues

- identify work difficulties
- prescribe early return to work (with modified duties if necessary)
- consider graded exercise and strengthening
- refer for active intervention if return to work is at risk

Identify and treat clinical depression

(Note that sickness absence from work more or less immediately moves the patient to Step 3). Stepped-care is not an intervention in itself. Stepped-care is the principle of starting with simple, low-intensity, low-cost interventions and 'stepping up' to more intensive, complex and costly interventions in patients who fail to respond. It is a method of sequencing progressively more intensive interventions and coordinating the efforts of patients, physicians and other health professionals to meet individual patient needs and to improve functional outcomes. It provides a framework for allocating limited health care and rehabilitation resources to those patients with greatest needs and to the greatest effect on a population basis. Implementation of this model is likely to require low-cost and self-management interventions in the primary care setting and the development of accessible (and reasonably priced) services to help patients with significant work disabilities. This approach should enable most patients to be managed in primary care (though with changes in the emphasis of management). It also targets services to patients with more severe activity limitations in a cost-effective way.

(Von Korff et al. 2002)	**Organising care for chronic illness**
Narrative review	*(This review applies the concept of stepped care to all chronic illness and explicitly to the organization of services rather than individual patient care).*
	Assumptions of stepped care
	1. Different individuals require different levels of care
	2. The optimal level of care is determined by monitoring outcomes
	3. Moving from lower to higher levels of care based on patient outcomes can increases effectiveness and lower costs
	Levels of stepped care
	1. Systematic routine assessment and preventive maintenance
	2. Self care with low intensity support
	3. Care management in primary care
	4. Intensive care management with specialist advice
	5. Specialist care
	(See also Table 6c).

TABLE 7a: TIMING

(Waddell & Burton 2004) Evidence synthesis	**Concepts of rehabilitation for the management of common health problems** *(Report commissioned by UK Department for Work and Pensions).* Most sick or injured workers RTW quite quickly, but the longer anyone is off work the harder it is to RTW and the higher the probability of going on to long-term incapacity. Sickness and disability are dynamic processes over time: obstacles to vocational rehabilitation and return to work, and their relative strength and importance, vary during different stages of sickness absence and incapacity. Interventions must therefore be designed to fit the point in time at which they are delivered. Within the first few weeks of sickness absence, most people are likely to recover and RTW with minimal health care. Formal vocational rehabilitation programmes are unnecessary at this stage, because they are unlikely to have any significant impact on what is already a good natural history, and they are unlikely to be cost-effective. They may even obstruct and delay natural recovery due to a combination of prescribed inactivity, physical and mental deconditioning, 'labelling' and 'attention' effects that may encourage illness behaviour, and delaying re-activation. The priorities at this stage are to support and encourage restoration of function, including remaining at work or early return to work, and to avoid iatrogenic disability. Rehabilitation principles should be an integral part of clinical and occupational management of common health problems from the very beginning. Evidence from LBP and to a lesser extent from other musculoskeletal conditions *(in 2004)* suggests that formal vocational rehabilitation interventions are likely to be most practical, effective, and cost-effective between about 1 and 6+ months off work (the exact limits are unclear). This is the time for secondary prevention interventions to prevent long-term incapacity. Rehabilitation should not be deferred until health care has failed and the patient has moved to long-term incapacity. Within that critical window, earlier interventions are likely to be simpler, more effective, cheaper and more cost-effective. For people with common health problems, the deleterious effects of further time out of work and delaying intervention are likely to outweigh any deadweight savings. There is limited evidence *(in 2004)* on effective rehabilitation interventions for people who have been out of work for more than 1-2 years, who are on long-term disability and incapacity benefits, and who are distanced from the labour market. By that time, workers become physically and mentally deconditioned, the obstacles to recovery and return to work become more complex and difficult to overcome, and the probability of successful occupational outcomes diminishes. Vocational rehabilitation need not necessarily be abandoned, but they are more complex, difficult and costly, and have a lower success rate. The strongest evidence from this review is for early intervention, by better clinical and workplace management from the very beginning and then if necessary by vocational rehabilitation interventions, before long-term incapacity ever develops.
(Waddell et al. 2003) Evidence synthesis	**Screening to identify people at risk of long-term incapacity for work** *(Report commissioned by UK Department for Work and Pensions).* Duration of sickness absence is one of the most powerful risk factors and predictors for long-term incapacity. *(The review presents evidence for musculoskeletal, mental health and other conditions, for IB claimants and UK Income Protection insurance claims).* The longer someone is off work, the lower their chances of returning to work. After 6 weeks sickness absence there is a 10-20% risk of long-term disability. After 6 months, there is only a 50% chance of returning to their previous job. After a year on Incapacity Benefit, the balance of probabilities is that they will remain on benefits for years or till they retire. The diminishing probability of returning to work with increased time on benefit could be explained by 'state dependence'[1] or by 'omitted heterogeneity'[2]. Probably both occur: there is some evidence of omitted heterogeneity in Department for Work and Pensions (DWP) clients; there is strong clinical evidence for state dependence in the development of chronic pain and disability.

TABLE 7a: TIMING

The passage of time is fundamental to the development of long-term incapacity, which involves biopsychosocial changes that may all influence further prognosis and constitute obstacles to coming off benefit and returning to work. At the acute stage (<3–4 weeks of sickness absence), most workers are statistically likely to recover and return to work quickly. By the sub-acute stage (about 4–12 weeks), the risks of long-term incapacity have increased substantially. Psychosocial issues are often more important than the biomedical condition or the physical demands of work: they form obstacles to recovery and the focus for rehabilitation interventions. By the chronic stage (>6 months), all individuals still off work are at substantial risk of long-term incapacity. Changing clinical and psychosocial condition over time has implications for intervention. At the acute stage, the prognosis is good with appropriate 'routine' care (although recurrence of many musculoskeletal and mental health conditions is common), and most people do not need any extra help. There is strong clinical evidence from musculoskeletal disorders that the sub-acute stage is the optimal time for more intensive intervention, and the point when specific intervention is most needed to help people return to work, and to reduce the chances of long-term incapacity. In principle, that is likely to apply equally to other conditions. Earlier return to work also decreases the chances of recurrent problems, further periods of incapacity, and unemployment in the longer term. The longer the further delay before intervention, the more difficult it is to return these individuals to work. By the chronic stage, psychosocial changes are more complex and entrenched, clients are increasingly distanced from the labour market, the obstacles to coming off benefit and returning to work are greater, and successful intervention is substantially more difficult. All of this evidence suggests that the most effective measure against long-term benefit dependency appears to be a strong focus on timely intervention. *(Though in the context of social security benefits and in practice, intervention tends to be after many months off work).*

For most individuals, it is generally accepted that return to work has health as well as social benefits, so arguably it would be better for these individuals, for employers, and for DWP to help them return to the labour market as rapidly as possible by timely work-focused interventions. There is inevitably a question of cost and cost-effectiveness. The starting point is that it would be worthwhile providing extra help to those clients who need it – but not all clients do. The costs (not only financial) of providing that help to everyone may be too great to be justified by the likely gains, which are also dependent on the success rate of the intervention. The general approach is accepted that if it is possible to provide help to some who would gain but not to all, then that would be better than not doing anything. It would therefore be most efficient and cost-effective if such interventions could be directed to those likely to go on to long-term incapacity. Unfortunately, this review of screening concluded that it is difficult to achieve greater than 70-80% sensitivity and/or specificity, and in widespread practice probably less. This produces large numbers of false positives (individuals given the intervention who would have returned to work without it) and false negatives (individuals not selected for the intervention who would have benefited from it). *(Despite its attractions in principle, this has thus far severely limited the use of screening in practice).*

(State dependence is when individuals get worse (e.g. because of increasing psychosocial disturbance and loss of contact with the labour market), and therefore the probability of each individual returning to work declines with time.

Omitted heterogeneity is when different individuals (e.g. a 25 year old and a 55 year old) each have intrinsically different rates of returning to work but for each individual that rate remains constant over time, so that as duration on benefits increases, those who are most likely to recover and easiest to help exit, leaving behind those who are less likely to exit and harder to help).

TABLE 7a: TIMING

(Wessely 2002) Comment	**Pros and cons of medicalisation** *(A letter to the editor of the BMJ).* Giving a health problem a medical diagnosis is an intervention in itself with costs and benefits. It is important to distinguish illness and disease. Most commonly, when used appropriately and constructively, giving symptoms and disability a diagnosis legitimises the condition, provides reassurance and enables the patient as the first step to recovery. However, crudely handled, it can perpetuate disability and exclusion. Labelling can have negative effects by influencing patients' (and others') beliefs and behaviour.
(Young et al. 2005a) Narrative review	**A developmental conceptualization of return to work** Although return to work (RTW) following work disability has been a focus of clinical practice and academic research for many years, there is still limited understanding of RTW and limited ability to improve outcomes. The traditional biomedical perspective viewed work status as being dependent upon the nature and severity of a clinical condition, and the ability to return to employment as directly related to the trajectory of recovery. More recent evidence shows the limitations of this medical approach, that non-medical factors are also important, and that RTW is much more complex. Recent studies also suggest that RTW is not a single event but a process. In this paper, RTW is presented as a complex, dynamic and evolving process, comprising four key phases: i.e., 'off work', 'work re-entry', 'retention', and 'advancement'. Multiple phase-specific outcomes may be used to evaluate RTW progress. By working sequentially through phase-specific actions and outcomes, one can identify roadblocks to achieving the RTW goal. Broader thinking about the complex return to work process holds promise for understanding and improving RTW, as it not only clarifies the importance of incremental milestones, but also facilitates intervention choice and evaluation.

[RTW = return to work]

Table 7b: Coordination: 'all players onside' and communication

TABLE 7b: COORDINATION	
Authors	**Key features** (*Reviewers' comments in italic*)
(Beaumont 2003a; Beaumont 2003b) Delphi study + consensus statement	**The interaction between general practitioners and occupational health professionals** A Delphi process generated a consensus statement which identified: the extremely important nature of rehabilitation for work; the crucial role of the GP; the central role of OH physicians in case management; and the barrier represented by the often poor communication between them. GPs are crucial because they see patients with long-term illness and incapacity, they coordinate and provide clinical management, and they provide advice about work and sick certification. For OH professionals (physicians, nurses and therapists), a core part of their role is assessment of functional ability against the requirements of the job and the workplace in order to provide advice to the individual and the employer. Their ideal role in vocational rehabilitation is one of case manager: assessing rehabilitation needs, liaising between GPs and other health care providers, managers, human resources and unions, and advising on the measures required to remove barriers to successful job retention or return to work. Communication between GPs is often poor or non-existent and at worst adversarial: this is a major barrier to rehabilitation and return to work, to the detriment of all concerned. Overcoming this barrier will involve changes in attitudes, cultures and systems. Improve mutual education and understanding of GPs and OH physicians, and a team approach to rehabilitation. This may be facilitated by GPs who work in occupational health and disability evaluation.
(Burton & Waddell 2002) Narrative review	**Educational and informational approaches** Reviews written educational material for patients with back pain, and provides empirical evidence about the information and advice that should be given. Traditional educational material about back pain has been based on a biomedical and bioengineering model, and has generally been ineffective. More modern approaches are based on a biopsychosocial model, are in line with current evidence-based management guidelines, and are directed more to patient beliefs and behaviour. Randomised controlled trials have shown that these **can** have a positive effect on patients' beliefs and clinical outcomes. (*A recent French trial (Coudeyre et al. 2006) has also shown a significant effect of written evidence-based information/advice on self-reported disability*).
(Franche et al. 2005a) Narrative review	**Workplace-based return-to-work interventions: optimizing the role of stakeholders in implementation and research** Engaging and involving stakeholders in return-to-work (RTW) intervention and research is challenging. Analysis of RTW stakeholder interests suggests that friction is inevitable; however, it is possible to encourage stakeholders to tolerate paradigm dissonance while engaging in collaborative problem solving to meet common goals. Authors challenge the assumption that involvement of all the stakeholders is a necessary condition for optimal RTW outcomes; rather, specific aspects of RTW interventions can be instrumental in resolving conflicts arising from differing paradigms: calibration of stakeholders' involvement, the role of supervisors and of insurance case managers, and procedural aspects of RTW interventions.

TABLE 7b: COORDINATION

(Frank et al. 1998) Narrative review	**Preventing disability from work-related low back pain: new evidence gives new hope – if we can just get all the players onside** Evidence-based clinical guidelines and evidence about workplace interventions have the potential to reduce sickness absence, particularly long-term disability, by 30-50%. However, the evidence suggests that piecemeal approaches based on only one stakeholder or addressing only one phase of disability and targeting only one of the underlying factors will not be very effective. The major challenge is how to bring all the relevant societal players together and to coordinate their roles to bring reason to bear on this multi-factorial problem. There is unlikely to be any easy answer. Each community should look for opportunities to persuade stakeholder with diverse interests that they can all gain from collaborative problem-solving to reduce work-related disability. It is only by engaging all those with a common stake in the problem and obtaining their active collaboration that this can be achieved. *(See also Table 7a).*
(Freeman 2004) Narrative review	**Union-management solutions for preventing workplace injury in older workers** *(Set in a US and workers compensation context, but many of the messages are much more generic and the language has been amended accordingly).* Union-management cooperation on Health & Safety issues has sometimes been hindered by historical political differences, adversarial contract and wage negotiations, mutual distrust and animosity. By its very nature, the labour-management relationship involves a certain degree of tension. Unions and workers representatives play a pivotal and prominent role in addressing health and safety issues. US organized labor has sought to improve the health and safety of their members, by negotiating terms and conditions while simultaneously lobbying the federal government for strong health and safety legislation. In seeking to improve health and safety conditions through collective bargaining, unions have adopted four avenues of redress: negotiating higher wages; contractually mandating safety and health policies and standards; forming health and safety committees; and influencing management thinking concerning technology, ergonomics, and workplace practices. The Americans with Disabilities Act 1990 provided a further impetus to unions and management to address disability issues. However, Health & Safety and Anti-Discrimination legislation is no substitute for unions and management placing higher priority on Health & Safety issues at work, changing from a culture of 'fitness' to one of 'accommodation', and working together to achieve what should be common and mutually beneficial goals.
(Lerner et al. 2005) Narrative review	**Work disability resulting from chronic health conditions** The three traditional sources of help for adults of working age with health problems (whether caused by work or not) which cause work disability are the health care system, employers and government agencies. However, these three sectors are all narrowly focused and none of them are sufficiently oriented to the primary and secondary prevention of work disability resulting from chronic health conditions. Despite the evidence that social factors play a major role in health and health care outcomes, most medical interventions remain oriented to treating disease. The workplace-system is actually a set of disjointed components that rarely work in tandem with each other, particularly for non-occupational illness. Government provisions and benefits are disjointed and fragmented to address different problems and situations. There is a general lack of communication and cooperation between health care, employers and government agencies. The gulf between the public health and employment arenas is particularly surprising given the increasing importance placed on work and productivity, and on health and well-being. The authors argue that further research is required to develop more effective health care, vocational rehabilitation and workplace interventions to help workers with chronic conditions to return to work. Critically, however, it is also necessary to determine how these can be successfully translated into practice and how they can be coordinated across the three sectors.

TABLE 7b: COORDINATION	
(Mueller et al. 2003) Narrative review	**What have physicians learned about returning chronically disabled back patients to work?** Proper timing for adequate interventions ('window of opportunity') is important for returning back pain patients to work before they are chronically disabled. The medical system takes some responsibility in the so-called medicalisation of the reported complaint of back pain. There needs to be a shift of focus the interaction between patient and physician from pain and spinal pathology toward restoration of function and ability to perform the duties of daily life, including work. For physician and physiotherapist, a time-contingent approach for functional restoration is more effective than a pain-contingent approach (*see also Fordyce 1995*). A multidimensional or biopsychosocial view and an honest partnership between physician and patient helps to reveal and address obstacles for return to work. A local network of general practitioners, physiotherapists, and surgeons with a similar approach and therapeutic language helps to better guide the patient. Different messages from the health care system will lead to insecurities on the patient's side and may prolong the pain problem. (*See also Table 3*).
(OECD 2003) Policy paper	**Transforming disability into ability: policies to promote work and income security for disabled people** [Organisation for Economic Co-operation and Development] One of the key recommendations of this report is to involve employers in the process. Involving employers is crucial to the successful reintegration of disabled persons. Different approaches exist, ranging from moral suasion and anti-discrimination legislation to compulsory employment quotas. The effectiveness of the measures depends on the willingness of employers to help disabled persons stay in or enter work (which can be influenced through incentives aimed at raising labour demand), but also on the possibilities of circumventing legislation or paying the fines imposed for non-compliance. Existing employer-employee relationships should be utilised as much as possible, both through positive incentives and through mandated obligations. In practice, however, many of these regulations are difficult to enforce. Employers need help to fulfill their obligations. Workplace and job adjustments generally require small financial investments. More crucial are technical assistance and guidance, including assessment of the problem and development of an intervention strategy for the participation plan. Financial incentives or disincentives for the employer should also be introduced or strengthened in work injury programmes. (*See also Table 7a*)
(Pransky et al. 2004) Narrative review	**Disability prevention and communication among workers, physicians, employers, and insurers--current models and opportunities for improvement** Review of prevailing models of disability management and prevention with respect to communication, with suggested alternative approaches. Effective disability management and return to work strategies have been the focus of an increasing number of intervention programmes and associated research studies, spanning a variety of worker populations and provider and business perspectives. Although primary and secondary disability prevention approaches have addressed theoretical bases, methods and costs, few identify communication as a key factor influencing disability outcomes. Four prevailing models of disability management and prevention (medical model, physical rehabilitation model, job-match model, and managed care model) are identified. The medical model emphasizes the physician's role to define functional limitations and job restrictions. In the physical rehabilitation model, rehabilitation professionals communicate the importance of exercise and muscle reconditioning for resuming normal work activities. The job-match model focuses on dissemination of acceptable standards for medical treatment and duration of work absence, requirements. The managed care model focuses on communicate the ability of employers to accurately communicate physical job requirements. The managed care model relies on the ability of employers to accurately communicate physical job requirements. The managed care model focuses on dissemination of acceptable standards for medical treatment and duration of work absence, and interventions by case managers when these standards are exceeded. Despite contrary evidence for many health impairments, these models share a common assumption that medical disability outcomes are highly predictable and unaffected by either individual or contextual factors. As a result, communication is often authoritative and unidirectional, with workers and employers in a passive role. Improvements in communication may be responsible for successes across a variety of new interventions. Communication-based interventions may further improve disability outcomes, reduce adversarial relationships, and prove cost-effective; however, controlled trials are needed.

TABLE 7b: COORDINATION

(Pransky et al. 2005) Overview	**Improving return to work research** There has been considerable multidisciplinary research on return to work (RTW). The importance of specific risk factors, advantages of functional restoration and biopsychosocial rehabilitation, and the impact of evidence-based practices are all supported by multiple investigations. There has been a shift from a purely medical models, to greater focus on the importance of individual, workplace, medical, economic and social factors in the genesis of disability and the RTW process. Despite these advances, there has been only modest progress in implementation the results, and little change in overall rates of work disability in developed countries. This review of the current state of the art selected six major themes as priority areas in RTW research: early risk prediction; psychosocial, behavioral and cognitive interventions; physical treatments; the challenge of implementing evidence in the workplace context; effective methods to engage multiple stakeholders; and identification of outcomes that are relevant to both RTW stakeholders and different phases of the RTW process. Understanding and preventing delayed RTW will require application of new concepts and study designs, better measures of determinants and outcomes, and more translational research. Greater stakeholder involvement and commitment, and methods to address the unique challenges of each situation are required. Different stakeholders often approach these issues with different perspectives, models and measures –which may not be meaningful to or meet the priorities of other stakeholders. Even though these are issues of public and occupational health, they are not addressed within a public health model of competing choices, best evidence, and cost-effectiveness. An ideal model of RTW should make sense from multiple stakeholder perspectives, and incorporate a range of their priorities—especially sustained employment, worker productivity, and costs, as well as key features of the RTW process. This may require new, cross-disciplinary approaches that are more acceptable to all the stakeholders, and perhaps more effective in driving meaningful change in RTW-related practices.
(Sawney & Challenor 2003) Editorial	**Poor communication between health professionals is a barrier to rehabilitation** There is increasing evidence that poor communication (e.g. between GPs and OH professionals, and between physicians and employers) is a problem and acts as a barrier to successful rehabilitation. All too frequently, the consequences of poor communication can be catastrophic for individuals and their families, leading to long-term incapacity, social exclusion and poverty. The General Medical Council requires good communication as an integral part of patient care; yet too often doctors give the wrong messages, both explicit and implied, about work. The origins of poor communication are complex, but many follow from a lack of clear goals and focus on rehabilitation and work outcomes. Mis-diagnosis and false assumptions about work-relatedness also contribute. What can be done to improve communication? The starting point is that doctors should help patients remain in or return to work, and communication with key stakeholders is fundamental to better sickness absence management and the prevention of long-term incapacity. Professional bodies, together with government, need to act urgently to improve basic medical and GP training in advice about work and occupational health issues. Occupational health physicians have an important role in initiating and promoting communication and contributing to wider professional education. But a fundamental change in attitudes and culture is also required. Better dialogue between primary health care and OH will help to change inappropriate assumptions and expectations about rehabilitation. A focus by all health professional on current best practice for rehabilitation and return to work would serve patients much better. This shift in thinking will be a major challenge for primary health care and occupational health, which will require leadership, innovation and partnership working. In conclusion, more effective communication could increase physicians' awareness and understanding of work issues and the facilities available to help return to work, and increase employers' awareness and understanding of health issues and the need and means to accommodate them.

TABLE 7b: COORDINATION

(Sirvastava & Chamberlain 2005) Survey	**Factors determining job retention and return to work for disabled employees: a questionnaire study of opinions of disabled people's organizations in the UK** (*UK survey of disability organisations*). The aim was to determine the views of disabled peoples organisations (as background to BSRM 2000). 24 organisations responded. The dominant findings concerning the National Health Service were, overwhelmingly, that it was perceived as impacting deleteriously on the work of disabled people with delays to consultation, investigation and rehabilitation and a lack of appreciation of workplace issues. Employers were seen as unresponsive to the needs of workers, with negative attitudes to disability. There was considerable agreement about the need for both the National Health Service and employers to be more responsive to the workplace needs of disabled people.
(Tompa et al. 2008) Systematic review	**A systematic review of disability management interventions with economic evaluations** Included 17 disability management interventions with economic analyses, of which eight were of high or medium quality. Most of the economic evaluations took a system, insurer, or public sector perspective, which appears reasonable given the complexity of many disability management programs (which involve the coordination of various specialties from outside a firm). There is strong evidence supporting the economic merits of system-level initiatives disability management interventions. For stratification by intervention components, there is moderate evidence for interventions that included an education component, moderate evidence for those with physiotherapy, limited evidence for those with a behavioural component, and moderate evidence for those with a work/vocational rehabilitation component. For stratification by intervention features, there is moderate evidence for interventions that included a work accommodation offer, contact between health care provider and workplace, early contact with worker by workplace, ergonomic work site visits, and interventions with a return-to-work coordinator. The authors concluded that there was credible evidence supporting the financial benefits of disability management interventions.
(Trevena et al. 2006) Systematic review	**A systematic review on communicating with patients about evidence** Included 10 systematic reviews and 30 additional RCTs. Communication tools in most formats (verbal, written, video, provider-delivered, computer-based) will increase patients' understanding but are more likely to do so if structured, tailored and/or interactive. Probabilistic information is best represented as event rates (natural frequencies) in relevant groups of people, rather than words, probabilities or summarized as effect measures such as relative risk reduction. Illustrations such as cartoons, or graphs (vertical bar charts) appear to aid understanding. Values clarification exercises may be better than standard utility techniques for eliciting preferences in individual decision making. Authors' conclusion: There is an increasing body of evidence supporting the design of effective evidence-based communication tools but variable access to such tools in practice.
(Young et al. 2005b) Narrative review	**Return-to-work outcomes following work disability: stakeholder motivations, interests and concerns** Stakeholders' interests in return to work (RTW) outcomes often go beyond the measures typically used in RTW research. It appears that detailed information is required regarding workers' RTW characteristics and how these impact on stakeholders' ability to achieve their goals. Further, it seems that information is needed throughout the process to maintain stakeholders' commitment to the RTW objective. Improving our understanding of the nature of the consensus and tensions among RTW stakeholders is an avenue for helping them collaborate in their planning and action. Embracing a comprehensive approach, which highlights the differing perspectives of the various stakeholders, appears a possible avenue for advancing the RTW field and facilitating better RTW outcomes for all. (*Looks more at mechanisms rather than presenting data on effectiveness*).